Table of Contents

P9-CDB-755

UNIT 3 — *Psychosocial Integrity*

UNIT 4 — *Physiological Integrity*

SECTION: *Basic Care and Comfort*

When reviewing the following chapters, keep in mind the relevant topics and tasks of the NCLEX outline, in particular:

Client Needs: Management of Care

CONCEPTS OF MANAGEMENT: Identify roles/responsibilities of health care team members.

ASSIGNMENT, DELEGATION AND SUPERVISION: Utilize the five rights of delegation.

CONTINUITY OF CARE: Perform procedures necessary to safely admit, transfer or discharge a client.

ESTABLISHING PRIORITIES: Prioritize the delivery of client care.

ETHICAL PRACTICE: Recognize ethical dilemmas and take appropriate action.

INFORMATION TECHNOLOGY: Utilize valid resources to enhance the care provided to a client.

LEGAL RIGHTS AND RESPONSIBILITIES: Identify legal issues affecting the client.

UNIT 1   SAFE, EFFECTIVE CARE ENVIRONMENT
SECTION: MANAGEMENT OF CARE

CHAPTER 1 *Health Care Delivery Systems*

Health care delivery systems incorporate interactions between health care providers and clients within the constraints of financing mechanisms and regulatory agencies.

Health care systems include the clients who participate, the settings in which health care takes place, the agencies that regulate health care, and mechanisms that provide financial support.

Most nurses deliver care within the context of health care systems. As these systems continue to become more business-driven and less service-oriented, the challenge to nursing today is to retain its caring values while practicing within a cost-containment structure.

COMPONENTS OF HEALTH CARE SYSTEMS

PARTICIPANTS

Consumers (clients)

Providers
- Licensed providers such as:
- Registered nurses
- Licensed practical nurses (also known as licensed vocational nurses)
- Advanced practice nurses (APN)
- Medical doctors
- Pharmacists
- Dentists
- Dietitians
- Physical, respiratory, and occupational therapists

Unlicensed providers, such as assistive personnel

SETTINGS

- Hospitals
- Homes
- Skilled-nursing, assisted-living, and extended-care facilities
- Community/health departments
- Adult day care centers
- Schools
- Hospices
- Providers' offices
- Ambulatory care clinics
- Occupational health clinics
- Stand-alone surgical centers
- Urgent care centers
- Complementary therapy centers

REGULATORY AGENCIES

- U.S. Department of Health and Human Services
- U.S. Food and Drug Administration (FDA)
- State and local public health agencies
- State licensing boards to ensure that health care providers and agencies comply with state regulations
- The Joint Commission (formerly JCAHO) to set quality standards for accreditation of health care facilities
- Professional Standards Review Organizations to monitor health care services provided
- Utilization review committees to monitor for appropriate diagnosis and treatment of hospitalized clients

HEALTH CARE FINANCING MECHANISMS

PUBLIC FEDERALLY FUNDED PROGRAMS
Medicare is for clients greater than 65 years of age or those with permanent disabilities.
- Part A: hospital insurance
- Part B: medical insurance
- Part C: Medicare advantage plan
- Part D: medications

Medicaid is for clients who have low incomes.
- It is federally and state funded.
- Individual states determine eligibility requirements.

Affordable Care Act of 2010, also known as Obamacare, is a controversial federal statute aimed at:
- Increasing access to health care for all individuals and instituting an individual mandate for health insurance
- Deceasing health care costs
- Providing opportunities for uninsured to become insured at an affordable cost

State Children's Health Insurance Program: Coverage for uninsured children up to age 19 at low cost to parents

PRIVATE PLANS

- Traditional insurance reimburses for services on a fee-for-service basis.
- Managed care organizations (MCOs): Primary care providers oversee comprehensive care for enrolled clients and focus on prevention and health promotion.
- Preferred provider organizations (PPOs): Clients choose from a list of contracted providers and hospitals. Using non-contracted providers increases the out-of-pocket costs.
- Exclusive provider organizations (EPOs): Clients choose from a list of providers and hospitals within a contracted organization with no out-of-network coverage.
- Long-term care insurance: Used as a supplement for long-term care expenses Medicare does not cover.

LEVELS OF HEALTH CARE

Preventive health care focuses on educating and equipping clients to reduce and control risk factors for disease. Examples include programs that promote immunization, stress management, occupational health programs, and seat belt use. QEBP

Primary health care emphasizes health promotion and includes prenatal and well-baby care, family planning, nutrition counseling, and disease control. This level of care is a sustained partnership between clients and providers. Examples include office or clinic visits, community health centers, and scheduled school- or work-centered screenings (vision, hearing, obesity).

Secondary health care includes the diagnosis and treatment of acute illness and injury. Examples include care in hospital settings (inpatient and emergency departments), diagnostic centers, and emergent care centers.

Tertiary health care, or acute care, involves the provision of specialized and highly technical care. Examples include intensive care, oncology centers, and burn centers.

Restorative health care involves intermediate follow-up care for restoring health and promoting self-care. Examples include home health care, rehabilitation centers, and skilled nursing facilities.

Continuing health care addresses long-term or chronic health care needs over a period of time. Examples include end-of-life care, palliative care, hospice, adult day care, assisted living, and in-home respite care.

RELATIONSHIP BETWEEN HEALTH CARE SYSTEMS AND LEVELS OF CARE

People: The level of care depends on the needs of the client. Licensed and unlicensed health care personnel work in every level of care.

Setting: The settings for secondary and tertiary care are usually within a hospital or specific facility. Settings for other levels of care vary.

Regulatory agencies help ensure the quality and quantity of health care and the protection of health care consumers.

Health care finance influences the quality and type of care by setting parameters for cost containment and reimbursement.

SAFETY AND QUALITY

In response to concerns about the safety and quality of client care in the United States, Quality and Safety Education for Nurses (QSEN) assists nursing programs in preparing nurses to provide safe, high-quality care. To draw attention to the six QSEN competencies, these icons appear throughout the review modules.

Safety: The minimization of risk factors that could cause injury or harm while promoting high-quality care and maintaining a secure environment for clients, self, and others. Qs

Patient-Centered Care: The provision of caring and compassionate, culturally sensitive care that addresses clients' physiological, psychological, sociological, spiritual, and cultural needs, preferences, and values. The client is included in the decision-making process. QPCC

Evidence Based Practice: The use of current knowledge from research and other credible sources on which to base clinical judgment and client care. QEBP

Informatics: The use of information technology as a communication and information-gathering tool that supports clinical decision-making and scientifically based nursing practice. QI

Quality Improvement: Care-related and organizational processes that involve the development and implementation of a plan to improve health care services and better meet clients' needs. QQI

Teamwork and Collaboration: The delivery of client care in partnership with multidisciplinary members of the health care team to achieve continuity of care and positive client outcomes. QTC

THE FUTURE OF HEALTH CARE

The ultimate issue in designing and delivering health care is ensuring the health and welfare of the population.

Application Exercises

1. A nurse is discussing restorative health care with a newly licensed nurse. Which of the following examples should the nurse include in the teaching? (Select all that apply.)

   A. Home health care

   B. Rehabilitation facilities

   C. Diagnostic centers

   D. Skilled nursing facilities

   E. Oncology centers

2. A nurse is explaining the various types of health care coverage clients might have to a group of nursing students. Which of the following health care financing mechanisms are federally funded? (Select all that apply.)

   A. Preferred provider organization (PPO)

   B. Medicare

   C. Long-term care insurance

   D. Exclusive provider organization (EPO)

   E. Medicaid

3. A nurse manager is developing strategies to care for the increasing number of clients who have obesity. Which of the following actions should the nurse include as a primary health care strategy?

   A. Collaborating with providers to perform obesity screenings during routine office visits

   B. Ensuring the availability of specialized beds in rehabilitation centers for clients who have obesity

   C. Providing specialized intraoperative training regarding surgical treatments for obesity

   D. Educating acute care nurses on postoperative complications related to obesity

4. A nurse is discussing the purpose of regulatory agencies during a staff meeting. Which of the following tasks should the nurse identify as the responsibility of state licensing boards?

   A. Monitoring evidence-based practice for clients who have a specific diagnosis

   B. Ensuring that health care providers comply with regulations

   C. Setting quality standards for accreditation of health care facilities

   D. Determining if medications are safe for administration to clients

5. A nurse is explaining the various levels of health care services to a group of newly licensed nurses. Which of the following examples of care or care settings should the nurse classify as tertiary care? (Select all that apply.)

   A. Intensive care unit

   B. Oncology treatment center

   C. Burn center

   D. Cardiac rehabilitation

   E. Home health care

PRACTICE Active Learning Scenario

A nurse on a medical-surgical unit is acquainting a group of nurses with the Quality and Safety Education for Nurses (QSEN) initiative. Use the ATI Active Learning Template: Basic Concept to complete this item.

RELATED CONTENT: List the six QSEN competencies, along with a brief description of each.

1. A. **CORRECT:** Restorative health care involves intermediate follow-up care for restoring health and promoting self-care. Home health care is a type of restorative health care.

    B. **CORRECT:** Restorative health care involves intermediate follow-up care for restoring health and promoting self-care. Rehabilitation facilities are a type of restorative health care.

    C. Secondary health care includes the diagnosis and treatment of acute injury or illness. Diagnostic centers are a type of secondary health care.

    D. **CORRECT:** Restorative health care involves intermediate follow-up care for restoring health and promoting self-care. Skilled nursing facilities are a type of restorative health care.

    E. Tertiary health care is specialized and highly technical care. An oncology center is a type of tertiary health care.

    Ⓝ *NCLEX® Connection: Management of Care, Health Promotion/Disease Prevention*

2. A. PPOs are privately funded.

    B. **CORRECT:** Medicare is federally funded.

    C. Long-term care insurance is privately funded.

    D. EPOs are privately funded.

    E. **CORRECT:** Medicaid is federally funded.

    Ⓝ *NCLEX® Connection: Management of Care, Information Technology*

3. A. **CORRECT:** The nurse should identify obesity screenings at office visits as an example of primary health care. Primary health care emphasizes health promotion and disease control, is often delivered during office visits, and includes screenings.

    B. The nurse should identify care that is provided in a rehabilitation center as an example of restorative health care.

    C. The nurse should identify specialized and highly technical care as an example of tertiary health care.

    D. The nurse should identify acute care of clients as an example of secondary health care.

    Ⓝ *NCLEX® Connection: Health Promotion and Maintenance, Health Promotion/Disease Prevention*

4. A. The nurse should identify that utilization review committees have the responsibility of monitoring for appropriate diagnosis and treatment according to evidence-based practice for diagnosis and treatment of hospitalized clients.

    B. **CORRECT:** The nurse should identify that state licensing boards are responsible for ensuring that health care providers and agencies comply with state regulations.

    C. The nurse should identify that the Joint Commission has the responsibility of setting quality standards for accreditation of health care facilities.

    D. The nurse should identify that the U.S. Food and Drug Administration has the responsibility of determining if medications are safe for administration to clients.

    Ⓝ *NCLEX® Connection: Management of Care, Information Technology*

5. A. **CORRECT:** Tertiary health care involves the provision of specialized and highly technical care, such as the care nurses deliver in intensive care units.

    B. **CORRECT:** Tertiary health care involves the provision of specialized and highly technical care, such as the care nurses deliver in oncology treatment centers.

    C. **CORRECT:** Tertiary health care involves the provision of specialized and highly technical care, such as the care nurses deliver in burn centers.

    D. This is an example of restorative care and also of tertiary prevention, but not of tertiary care.

    E. This is an example of restorative care.

    Ⓝ *NCLEX® Connection: Health Promotion and Maintenance, Health Promotion/Disease Prevention*

PRACTICE Answer

Using the ATI Active Learning Template: Basic Concept

RELATED CONTENT

- Safety: Minimization of risk factors that could cause injury or harm while promoting quality care and maintaining a secure environment for clients, self, and others.
- Patient-Centered Care: Provision of caring and compassionate, culturally sensitive care that addresses clients' physiological, psychological, sociological, spiritual, and cultural needs, preferences, and values.
- Evidence-Based Practice: Use of current knowledge from research and other credible sources, on which to base clinical judgment and client care.
- Informatics: Use of information technology as a communication and information-gathering tool that supports clinical decision-making and scientifically based nursing practice.
- Quality Improvement: Care-related and organizational processes that involve the development and implementation of a plan to improve health care services and better meet clients' needs.
- Teamwork and Collaboration: Delivery of client care in partnership with multidisciplinary members of the health care team to achieve continuity of care and positive client outcomes.

Ⓝ *NCLEX® Connection: Management of Care, Information Technology*

UNIT 1   SAFE, EFFECTIVE CARE ENVIRONMENT
SECTION: MANAGEMENT OF CARE

CHAPTER 2   *The Interprofessional Team*

RNs and practical nurses (PNs) are integral members of the interprofessional health care team. Each discipline represented on an interprofessional team uses a set of skills within the scope of practice for the specific profession. In some instances, the scope of practice for one discipline overlaps with the scope of practice or set of skills for another profession. For example, the nurse and the respiratory care therapist both possess the knowledge and skill to perform chest physiotherapy (using postural drainage, percussion, and vibration to promote drainage of secretions from the lungs).

The interprofessional health care team works collaboratively to provide holistic care to clients.

The nurse is most often the manager of care and must understand the roles and responsibilities of other health care team members to collaborate and make appropriate referrals.

INTERPROFESSIONAL PERSONNEL (NON-NURSING)

Spiritual support staff: Provides spiritual care (pastors, rabbis, priests).

> Example of when to refer: A client requests communion, or the family asks for prayer prior to the client undergoing a procedure.

Registered dietitian: Assesses, plans for, and educates regarding nutrition needs. Designs special diets, and supervises meal preparation.

> Example of when to refer: A client has a low albumin level and recently had an unexplained weight loss.

Laboratory technician: Obtains specimens of body fluids, and performs diagnostic tests.

> Example of when to refer: A provider needs to see a client's complete blood count (CBC) results immediately.

Occupational therapist: Assesses and plans for clients to regain activities of daily living (ADL) skills, especially motor skills of the upper extremities.

> Example of when to refer: A client has difficulties using an eating utensil with her dominant hand following a stroke.

Pharmacist: Provides and monitors medication. Supervises pharmacy technicians in states that allow this practice.

> Example of when to refer: A client is concerned about a new medication's interactions with any of his other medications.

Physical therapist: Assesses and plans for clients to increase musculoskeletal function, especially of the lower extremities, to maintain mobility.

> Example of when to refer: Following hip arthroplasty, a client requires assistance learning to ambulate and regain strength.

Provider: Assesses, diagnoses, and treats disease and injury. Providers include medical doctors (MDs), doctors of osteopathy (DOs), advanced practice nurses (APNs), and physician assistants (PAs). State regulations vary in their requirements for supervision of APNs and PAs by a physician (MDs and DOs).

> Example of when to refer: A client has a temperature of 39° C (102.2° F), is achy and shaking, and reports feeling cold.

Radiologic technologist: Positions clients and performs x-rays and other imaging procedures for providers to review for diagnosis of disorders of various body parts.

> Example of when to refer: A client reports severe pain in his hip after a fall, and the provider prescribes an x-ray of the client's hip.

Respiratory therapist: Evaluates respiratory status and provides respiratory treatments including oxygen therapy, chest physiotherapy, inhalation therapy, and mechanical ventilation.

> Example of when to refer: A client who has respiratory disease is short of breath and requests a nebulizer treatment.

Social worker: Works with clients and families by coordinating inpatient and community resources to meet psychosocial and environmental needs that are necessary for recovery and discharge.

> Example of when to refer: A client who has terminal cancer wishes to go home but is no longer able to perform many ADLs. The client's partner needs medical equipment in the home to care for the client.

Speech–language pathologist: Evaluates and makes recommendations regarding the impact of disorders or injuries on speech, language, and swallowing. Teaches techniques and exercises to improve function.

> Example of when to refer: A client is having difficulty swallowing a regular diet after trauma to the head and neck.

NURSING PERSONNEL

The nursing team works together to advocate for and meet the needs of clients within the health care delivery system.

Registered nurse (RN)

The RN is the lead team member, soliciting input from all nursing team members, setting priorities, sharing information with other disciplines, and coordinating client care. Qᴛᴄ

EDUCATIONAL PREPARATION
- Must meet the state board of nursing's requirements for licensure.
- Requires completion of a diploma program, an associate degree, or a baccalaureate degree in nursing prior to taking the licensure exam (licensed).

ROLES AND RESPONSIBILITIES
- Function legally under state nurse practice acts.
- Perform assessments; establish nursing diagnoses, goals, and interventions; and conduct ongoing client evaluations.
- Participate in developing interprofessional plans for client care.
- Share appropriate information among team members; initiate referrals for client assistance, including health education; and identify community resources.

Practical nurse (PN)

EDUCATIONAL PREPARATION
- Must meet the state board of nursing's requirements.
- Requires vocational or community college education prior to taking the licensure exam (licensed).

ROLES AND RESPONSIBILITIES
- Work under the supervision of the RN.
- Collaborate within the nursing process, coordinate the plan of care, consult with other team members, and recognize the need for referrals to assist with actual or potential problems.
- Possess technical knowledge and skills.
- Participate in the delivery of nursing care, using the nursing process as a framework.

Assistive personnel (AP)

This includes certified nursing assistants (CNAs) and certified medical assistants (CMAs), and non-nursing personnel such as dialysis technicians, monitor technicians, and phlebotomists.

EDUCATIONAL PREPARATION
- Must meet the state's formal or informal training requirements.
- Requirement by most states for training and examination to attain CNA status.

ROLES AND RESPONSIBILITIES
- Work under the direct supervision of an RN or PN.
- Position description in the employing facility outlines specific tasks.
- Tasks can include feeding clients, preparing nutritional supplements, lifting, basic care (grooming, bathing, transferring, toileting, positioning), measuring and recording vital signs, and ambulating clients.

EXPANDED NURSING ROLES

Advanced practice nurse (APN): Has a great deal of autonomy. APNs usually have a minimum of a master's degree in nursing (or related field), advanced education in pharmacology and physical assessment, and certification in a specialized area of practice. Included in this role are the following.
- **Clinical nurse specialist (CNS):** Typically specializes in a practice setting or a clinical field.
- **Nurse practitioner (NP):** Collaborates with one or more providers to deliver nonemergency primary health care in a variety of settings.
- **Certified registered nurse anesthetist (CRNA):** Administers anesthesia and provides care during procedures under the supervision of an anesthesiologist.
- **Certified nurse-midwife (CNM):** Collaborates with one or more providers to deliver care to maternal-newborn clients and their families.

Nurse educator: Teaches in schools of nursing, staff development departments in health care facilities, or client education departments.

Nurse administrator: Provides leadership to nursing departments within a health care facility.

Nurse researcher: Conducts research primarily to improve the quality of client care.

Application Exercises

1. A nurse is caring for a group of clients on a medical-surgical unit. For which of the following client care needs should the nurse initiate a referral for a social worker? (Select all that apply.)

   A. A client who has terminal cancer requests hospice care in her home.

   B. A client asks about community resources available for older adults.

   C. A client states that she wants her child baptized before surgery.

   D. A client requests an electric wheelchair for use after discharge.

   E. A client states that he does not understand how to use a nebulizer.

2. A goal for a client who has difficulty with self-feeding due to rheumatoid arthritis is to use adaptive devices. The nurse caring for the client should initiate a referral to which of the following members of the interprofessional care team?

   A. Social worker

   B. Certified nursing assistant

   C. Registered dietitian

   D. Occupational therapist

3. A client who is postoperative following knee arthroplasty is concerned about the adverse effects of the medication he is receiving for pain management. Which of the following members of the interprofessional care team can assist the client in understanding the medication's effects? (Select all that apply.)

   A. Provider

   B. Certified nursing assistant

   C. Pharmacist

   D. Registered nurse

   E. Respiratory therapist

4. A client who has had a cerebrovascular accident has persistent problems with dysphagia (difficulty swallowing). The nurse caring for the client should initiate a referral with which of the following members of the interprofessional care team?

   A. Social worker

   B. Certified nursing assistant

   C. Occupational therapist

   D. Speech-language pathologist

5. A nurse is acquainting a group of newly licensed nurses with the roles of the various members of the health care team they will encounter on a medical-surgical unit. When she gives examples of the types of tasks certified nursing assistants (CNAs) may perform, which of the following client activities should she include? (Select all that apply.)

   A. Bathing

   B. Ambulating

   C. Toileting

   D. Determining pain level

   E. Measuring vital signs

PRACTICE Active Learning Scenario

A nurse is teaching a group of newly licensed nurses about the various nursing roles they can aspire to after they achieve mastery in basic nursing skills. Use the ATI Active Learning Template: Basic Concept to complete this item.

RELATED CONTENT: Describe at least five types of advance practice nursing roles, including a brief description of their primary responsibilities.

Application Exercises Key

1. A. CORRECT: The nurse should initiate a referral for a social worker to provide information and assistance in coordinating hospice care for a client.

   B. CORRECT: The nurse should initiate a referral for a social worker to provide information and assistance in coordinating care for community resources available for clients.

   C. The nurse should initiate a referral for spiritual support staff if a client requests specific religious sacraments or prayers.

   D. CORRECT: The nurse should initiate a referral for a social worker to assist the client in obtaining medical equipment for use after discharge.

   E. The nurse should provide client teaching for concerns regarding the use of a nebulizer. If additional information is needed the nurse should initiate a referral for a respiratory therapist.

   Ⓝ *NCLEX® Connection: Management of Care, Referrals*

2. A. A social worker can coordinate community services to help the client, but not specifically with self-feeding devices.

   B. A certified nursing assistant can help the client with feeding, but does not typically procure adaptive devices for the client.

   C. A registered dietitian can help with educating the client about meeting nutritional needs, but cannot help with the client's physical limitations.

   D. CORRECT: An occupational therapist can assist clients who have physical challenges to use adaptive devices and strategies to help with self-care activities.

   Ⓝ *NCLEX® Connection: Management of Care, Referrals*

3. A. CORRECT: The provider must be knowledgeable about any medication he prescribes for the client, including its actions, effects, and interactions.

   B. It is not within the scope of a certified nursing assistant's duties to counsel a client about medications.

   C. CORRECT: A pharmacist must be knowledgeable about any medication she dispenses for the client, including its actions, effects, and interactions.

   D. CORRECT: A registered nurse must be knowledgeable about any medication she administers, including its actions, effects, and interactions.

   E. Although some analgesics can cause respiratory depression, requiring assistance from a respiratory therapist, it is not within this therapist's scope of practice to counsel the client about medications his provider prescribes.

   Ⓝ *NCLEX® Connection: Management of Care, Referrals*

4. A. A social worker can coordinate community services to help the client, but not specifically with dysphagia.

   B. A certified nursing assistant can help the client with feeding, but cannot assess and treat dysphagia.

   C. An occupational therapist can assist clients who have motor challenges to improve abilities with self-care and work, but cannot assess and treat dysphagia.

   D. CORRECT: A speech-language pathologist can initiate specific therapy for clients who have difficulty with feeding due to swallowing difficulties.

   Ⓝ *NCLEX® Connection: Management of Care, Referrals*

5. A. CORRECT: It is within the scope of a CNA's duties to provide basic care to clients, such as bathing.

   B. CORRECT: It is within the scope of a CNA's duties to provide basic care to clients, such as assisting with ambulation.

   C. CORRECT: It is within the scope of a CNA's duties to provide basic care to clients, such as assisting with toileting.

   D. Determining pain level is a task that requires the assessment skills of licensed personnel, such as nurses. It is outside the scope of a CNA's duties.

   E. CORRECT: It is within the scope of a CNA's duties to provide basic care to clients, such as measuring and recording vital signs.

   Ⓝ *NCLEX® Connection: Management of Care, Assignment, Delegation and Supervision*

PRACTICE Answer

Using the ATI Active Learning Template: Basic Concept

RELATED CONTENT

- Clinical nurse specialist (CNS): Typically specializes in a practice setting or a clinical field.
- Nurse practitioner (NP): Collaborates with one or more providers to deliver nonemergency primary health care in a variety of settings.
- Certified registered nurse anesthetist (CRNA): Administers anesthesia and provides care during procedures under the supervision of an anesthesiologist.
- Certified nurse-midwife (CNM): Collaborates with one or more providers to deliver care to maternal-newborn clients and their families.
- Nurse educator: Teaches in schools of nursing, staff development departments in health care facilities, or client education departments.
- Nurse administrator: Provides leadership to nursing departments within a health care facility.
- Nurse researcher: Conducts research primarily to improve the quality of client care.

Ⓝ *NCLEX® Connection: Management of Care, Concepts of Management*

CHAPTER 3 *Ethical Responsibilities*

Ethics is the study of conduct and character, and a code of ethics is a guide for the expectations and standards of a profession.

Ethical theories examine principles, ideas, systems, and philosophies that affect judgments about what is right and wrong, and good and bad. Common ethical theories are utilitarianism, deontology, consensus in bioethics, and ethics of care.

Ethical principles for individuals, groups of individuals, and societies are standards of what is right or wrong with regard to important social values and norms.

Values are personal beliefs about ideas that determine standards that shape behavior.

Morals are personal values and beliefs about behavior and decision-making.

ETHICAL DECISION-MAKING IN NURSING

Bioethics refers to the application of ethics to health and life. It addresses dilemmas such as stem cell research, organ transplantation, gender reassignment, and reproductive technologies (in vitro fertilization, surrogate parenting)

BASIC PRINCIPLES OF ETHICS

- **Advocacy:** support of clients' health, wellness, safety, and personal rights, including privacy.
- **Responsibility:** willingness to respect obligations and follow through on promises.
- **Accountability:** ability to answer for one's own actions.
- **Confidentiality:** protection of privacy without diminishing access to high-quality care.

ETHICAL PRINCIPLES FOR CLIENT CARE

- **Autonomy:** the right to make one's own personal decisions, even when those decisions might not be in that person's own best interest.
- **Beneficence:** action that promotes good for others, without any self-interest.
- **Fidelity:** fulfillment of promises.
- **Justice:** fairness in care delivery and use of resources.
- **Nonmaleficence:** a commitment to do no harm. Qs
- **Veracity:** a commitment to tell the truth.

ETHICAL DILEMMAS

- Ethical dilemmas are problems that involve more than one choice and stem from differences in the values and beliefs of the decision makers. These are common in health care, and nurses must apply ethical theory and decision-making to ethical problems.
- A problem is an ethical dilemma when:
  - A review of scientific data is not enough to solve it.
  - It involves a conflict between two moral imperatives.
  - The answer will have a profound effect on the situation and the client.

ETHICAL DECISION-MAKING

Ethical decision-making is a process that requires striking a balance between science and morality.

When making an ethical decision:

- Identify whether the issue is indeed an ethical dilemma.
- Gather as much relevant information as possible about the dilemma.
- Reflect on your own values as they relate to the dilemma.
- State the ethical dilemma, including all surrounding issues and the individuals it involves.
- List and analyze all possible options for resolving the dilemma, and review the implications of each option.
- Select the option that is in concert with the ethical principle that applies to this situation, the decision maker's values and beliefs, and the profession's values for client care. Justify selecting that one option in light of the relevant variables.
- Apply this decision to the dilemma, and evaluate the outcomes.

Ethics committees generally address unusual or complex ethical issues.

Examples of ethical guidelines for nurses are the American Nurses Association's *Code of Ethics for Nurses With Interpretive Statements* (2015) and the International Council of Nurses' *The ICN Code of Ethics for Nurses* (2012).

3.1 Nursing's roles in ethical decision-making

An agent for clients facing an ethical decision. Examples:

- Caring for an adolescent client who has to decide whether to undergo an abortion even though her parents believe it is wrong
- Discussing options with a parent who has to decide whether to consent to a blood transfusion for a child when his religion prohibits such treatment

A decision maker for health care delivery. Examples:

- Assigning staff nurses a higher client load than previously because administration has reduced the number of nurses per shift
- Witnessing a surgeon discussing only surgical options with a client without mentioning more conservative measures

Application Exercises

1. A nurse is caring for a client who decides not to have surgery despite significant blockages in his coronary arteries. The nurse understands that this client's choice is an example of which of the following ethical principles?
   - A. Fidelity
   - B. Autonomy
   - C. Justice
   - D. Nonmaleficence

2. A nurse offers pain medication to a client who is postoperative prior to ambulation. The nurse understands that this aspect of care delivery is an example of which of the following ethical principles?
   - A. Fidelity
   - B. Autonomy
   - C. Justice
   - D. Beneficence

3. A nurse is instructing a group of nursing students about the responsibilities organ donation and procurement involve. When the nurse explains that all clients waiting for a kidney transplant have to meet the same qualifications, the students should understand that this aspect of care delivery is an example of which of the following ethical principles?
   - A. Fidelity
   - B. Autonomy
   - C. Justice
   - D. Nonmaleficence

4. A nurse questions a medication prescription as too extreme in light of the client's advanced age and unstable status. The nurse understands that this action is an example of which of the following ethical principles?
   - A. Fidelity
   - B. Autonomy
   - C. Justice
   - D. Nonmaleficence

5. A nurse is instructing a group of nursing students about how to know and what to expect when ethical dilemmas arise. Which of the following situations should the students identify as an ethical dilemma?
   - A. A nurse on a medical-surgical unit demonstrates signs of chemical impairment.
   - B. A nurse overhears another nurse telling an older adult client that if he doesn't stay in bed, she will have to apply restraints.
   - C. A family has conflicting feelings about the initiation of enteral tube feedings for their father, who is terminally ill.
   - D. A client who is terminally ill hesitates to name her spouse on her durable power of attorney form.

PRACTICE Active Learning Scenario

A nurse is teaching a group of nursing students about the process of resolving ethical dilemmas. Use the ATI Active Learning Template: Basic Concept to complete this item.

UNDERLYING PRINCIPLES: Define the ethical decision-making process.

NURSING INTERVENTIONS: List the steps of making an ethical decision.

1. A. Fidelity is the fulfillment of promises. The nurse has not made any promises; this is the client's decision.

    B. **CORRECT:** In this situation, the client is exercising his right to make his own personal decision about surgery, regardless of others' opinions of what is "best" for him. This is an example of autonomy.

    C. Justice is fairness in care delivery and in the use of resources. Because the client has chosen not to use them, this principle does not apply.

    D. Nonmaleficence is a commitment to do no harm. In this situation, harm can occur whether or not the client has surgery. However, because he chooses not to, this principle does not apply.

    Ⓝ *NCLEX® Connection: Management of Care, Ethical Practice*

2. A. Fidelity is the fulfillment of promises. Unless the nurse has specifically promised the client a pain-free recovery, which is unlikely, this principle does not apply to this action.

    B. Autonomy is the right to make personal decisions, even when they are not necessarily in the person's best interest. In this situation, the nurse is delivering responsible client care. This principle does not apply.

    C. Justice is fairness in care delivery and in the use of resources. Pain management is available for all clients who are postoperative, so this principle does not apply.

    D. **CORRECT:** Beneficence is action that promotes good for others, without any self-interest. By administering pain medication before the client attempts a potentially painful exercise like ambulation, the nurse is taking a specific and positive action to help the client.

    Ⓝ *NCLEX® Connection: Management of Care, Ethical Practice*

3. A. Fidelity is the fulfillment of promises. Because donor organs are a scarce resource compared with the numbers of potential recipients who need them, no one can promise anyone an organ. Thus, this principle does not apply.

    B. Autonomy is the right to make personal decisions, even when they are not necessarily in the person's best interest. No personal decision is involved with the qualifications for organ recipients.

    C. **CORRECT:** Justice is fairness in care delivery and in the use of resources. By applying the same qualifications to all potential kidney transplant recipients, organ procurement organizations demonstrate this ethical principle in determining the allocation of these scarce resources.

    D. Nonmaleficence is a commitment to do no harm. In this situation, harm can occur to organ donors and to recipients. The requirements of the organ procurement organizations are standard procedures and do not address avoidance of harm or injury.

    Ⓝ *NCLEX® Connection: Management of Care, Ethical Practice*

4. A. Fidelity is the fulfillment of promises. The nurse is not addressing a specific promise when she determines the appropriateness of a prescription for the client. Thus, this principle does not apply.

    B. Autonomy is the right to make personal decisions, even when they are not necessarily in the person's best interest. No personal decision is involved when the nurse questions the client's prescription.

    C. Justice is fairness in care delivery and in the use of resources. In this situation, the nurse is delivering responsible client care and is not assessing available resources. This principle does not apply.

    D. **CORRECT:** Nonmaleficence is a commitment to do no harm. In this situation, administering the medication could harm the client. By questioning it, the nurse is demonstrating this ethical principle.

    Ⓝ *NCLEX® Connection: Management of Care, Ethical Practice*

5. A. Delivering client care while showing signs of a substance use disorder is a legal issue, not an ethical dilemma.

    B. A nurse who threatens to restrain a client has committed assault. This is a legal issue, not an ethical dilemma.

    C. **CORRECT:** Making the decision about initiating enteral tube feedings is an example of an ethical dilemma. A review of scientific data cannot resolve the issue, and it is not easy to resolve. The decision will have a profound effect on the situation and on the client.

    D. The selection of a person to make health care decisions on a client's behalf is a legal decision, not an ethical dilemma.

    Ⓝ *NCLEX® Connection: Management of Care, Ethical Practice*

PRACTICE Answer

Using the ATI Active Learning Template: Basic Concept

UNDERLYING PRINCIPLES: Ethical decision-making is a process that requires striking a balance between science and morality.

NURSING INTERVENTIONS
*   Identifying whether the issue is an ethical dilemma
*   Gathering as much relevant information as possible about the dilemma
*   Reflecting on one's own values as they relate to the dilemma
*   Stating the ethical dilemma, including all surrounding issues and individuals it involves
*   Listing and analyzing all possible options for resolving the dilemma with implications of each option
*   Selecting the option that is in concert with the ethical principle that applies to this situation, the decision maker's values and beliefs, and the profession's values for client care
*   Justifying the selection of one option in light of relevant variables

Ⓝ *NCLEX® Connection: Management of Care, Ethical Practice*

UNIT 1   SAFE, EFFECTIVE CARE ENVIRONMENT
SECTION: MANAGEMENT OF CARE

CHAPTER 4 *Legal Responsibilities*

Understanding the laws governing nursing practice helps nurses protect clients' rights and reduce the risk of nursing liability.

Nurses are accountable for practicing nursing within the confines of the law to shield themselves from liability; advocate for clients' rights; provide care that is within the nurse's scope of practice; discern the responsibilities of nursing in relationship to the responsibilities of other members of the health care team; and provide safe, proficient care consistent with standards of care.

SOURCES OF LAW

FEDERAL REGULATIONS

Federal laws affecting nursing practice
- Health Insurance Portability and Accountability Act (HIPAA)
- Americans with Disabilities Act (ADA)
- Mental Health Parity Act (MHPA)
- Patient Self-Determination Act (PSDA)

CRIMINAL AND CIVIL LAWS

- Criminal law is a subsection of public law and relates to the relationship between an individual and the government. A nurse who falsifies a record to cover up a serious mistake can be guilty of breaking a criminal law.
- Civil laws protect individual rights. One type of civil law that relates to the provision of nursing care is tort law. **(4.1)**

STATE LAWS

- Each state has enacted statutes that define the parameters of nursing practice and give the authority to regulate the practice of nursing to its state board of nursing.
- In turn, the boards of nursing have the authority to adopt rules and regulations that further regulate nursing practice. Although the practice of nursing is similar among states, it is critical that nurses know the laws and rules governing nursing in the state in which they practice.
- Boards of nursing have the authority to issue and revoke a nursing license.
- Boards also set standards for nursing programs and further delineate the scope of practice for RNs, practical nurses (PNs), and advanced practice nurses.

LICENSURE

In general, nurses must have a current license in every state in which they practice. The states (about half of them) that have adopted the nurse licensure compact are exceptions. This model allows licensed nurses who reside in a compact state to practice in other compact states under a multistate license. Within the compact, nurses must practice in accordance with the statues and rules of the state in which they provide care.

4.1 Types of torts

Unintentional torts
NEGLIGENCE: A nurse fails to implement safety measures for a client at risk for falls.

MALPRACTICE (PROFESSIONAL NEGLIGENCE): A nurse administers a large dose of medication due to a calculation error. The client has a cardiac arrest and dies.

Quasi-intentional torts
BREACH OF CONFIDENTIALITY: A nurse releases a client's medical diagnosis to a member of the press.

DEFAMATION OF CHARACTER: A nurse tells a coworker that she believes the client has been unfaithful to her partner.

Intentional torts

ASSAULT	BATTERY	FALSE IMPRISONMENT
The conduct of one person makes another person fearful and apprehensive	Intentional and wrongful physical contact with a person that involves an injury or offensive contact	A person is confined or restrained against his will
A nurse threatens to place an NG tube in a client who is refusing to eat.	A nurse restrains a client and administers an injection against her wishes.	A nurse uses restraints on a competent client to prevent his leaving the health care facility.

PROFESSIONAL NEGLIGENCE

Professional negligence is the failure of a person who has professional training to act in a reasonable and prudent manner. The terms "reasonable" and "prudent" generally describe a person who has the average judgment, intelligence, foresight, and skill that a person with similar training and experience would have.

- Negligence issues that prompt most malpractice suits include failure to:
  - Follow professional and facility-established standards of care.
  - Use equipment in a responsible and knowledgeable manner. Qs
  - Communicate effectively and thoroughly with clients.
  - Document care the nurse provided.
  - Notify the provider of a change in the client's condition.
  - Complete a prescribed procedure.
- Nursing students face liability if they harm clients as a result of their direct actions or inaction. They should not perform tasks for which they are not prepared, and they should have supervision as they learn new procedures. If a student harms a client, the student, instructor, educational institution, and facility share liability for the wrong action or inaction. **(4.2)**
- Nurses can avoid liability for negligence by:
  - Following standards of care.
  - Giving competent care.
  - Communicating with other health team members and clients. Qtc
  - Developing a caring rapport with clients.
  - Fully documenting assessments, interventions, and evaluations.
  - Being familiar with and following a facility's policies and procedures.

CLIENTS' RIGHTS

Nurses are accountable for protecting the rights of clients. Examples include informed consent, refusal of treatment, advance directives, confidentiality, and information security.
- Clients' rights are legal privileges or powers clients have when they receive health care services.
- Clients using the services of a health care institution retain their rights as individuals and citizens.
- The American Hospital Association identifies patients' rights in health care settings. See The Patient Care Partnership at www.aha.org.
- Nursing facilities that participate in Medicare programs also follow Resident Rights statutes that govern their operation.

NURSING ROLE IN CLIENTS' RIGHTS

- Nurses must ensure that clients understand their rights, and must protect their clients' rights.
- Regardless of the client's age, nursing needs, or health care setting, the basic tenets are the same. The client has the right to:
  - Understand the aspects of care to be active in the decision-making process.
  - Accept, refuse, or request modification of the plan of care.
  - Receive care from competent individuals who treat the client with respect.

4.2 The five elements necessary to prove negligence

ELEMENT OF LIABILITY	EXPLANATION	EXAMPLE: CLIENT WHO IS A FALL RISK
1. Duty to provide care as defined by a standard	Care a nurse should give or what a reasonably prudent nurse would do	The nurse should complete a fall risk assessment for all clients during admission.
2. Breach of duty by failure to meet standard	Failure to give the standard of care	The nurse does not perform a fall risk assessment during admission.
3. Foreseeability of harm	Knowledge that failing to give the proper standard of care could harm the client	The nurse should know that failure to take fall risk precautions could endanger a client at risk for falls.
4. Breach of duty has potential to cause harm (combines elements 2 and 3)	Failure to meet the standard had potential to cause harm – relationship must be provable	Without a fall risk assessment, the nurse does not know the client's risk for falls and does not take the proper precautions.
5. Harm occurs	Actual harm to the client occurs	The client falls out of bed and fractures his hip.

INFORMED CONSENT

- Informed consent is a legal process by which a client or the client's legally appointed designee has given written permission for a procedure or treatment. Consent is informed when a provider explains and the client understands:
  - The reason the client needs the treatment or procedure.
  - How the treatment or procedure will benefit the client.
  - The risks involved if the client chooses to receive the treatment or procedure.
  - Other options to treat the problem, including not treating the problem.
- The nurse's role in the informed consent process is to witness the client's signature on the informed consent form and to ensure that the provider has obtained the informed consent responsibly.

INFORMED CONSENT GUIDELINES

Clients must consent to all care they receive in a health care facility.

- For most aspects of nursing care, implied consent is adequate. Clients provide implied consent when they adhere to the instructions the nurse provides. For example, the nurse is preparing to perform a tuberculosis skin test, and the client holds out his arm for the nurse.
- For an invasive procedure or surgery, the client must provide written consent.
- State laws prescribe who is able to give informed consent. Laws vary regarding age limitations and emergencies. Nurses are responsible for knowing the laws in the state(s) in which they practice.
- A competent adult must sign the form for informed consent. The person who signs the form must be capable of understanding the information from the health care professional who will perform the service, such as a surgical procedure, and the person must be able to communicate with the health care professional. When the person giving the informed consent is unable to communicate due to a language barrier or a hearing impairment, a trained medical interpreter must intervene. Many health care facilities contract with professional interpreters who have additional skills in medical terminology to assist with providing information.

- Individuals who may grant consent for another person include the following.
  - Parent of a minor
  - Legal guardian
  - Court-specified representative
  - An individual who has durable power of attorney authority for health care
- Emancipated minors (minors who are independent from their parents, such as a married minor) may consent for themselves.
- Include a mature adolescent in the informed consent process by allowing them to sign an assent as a part of the informed consent document. **(4.3)**
- The nurse must verify that consent is informed and witness the client signing the consent form.

REFUSAL OF TREATMENT

- The PSDA stipulates that staff must inform clients they admit to a health care facility of their right to accept or refuse care. Competent adults have the right to refuse treatment, including the right to leave a facility without a discharge prescription from the provider.
- If the client refuses a treatment or procedure, the client signs a document indicating that he understands the risk involved with refusing the treatment or procedure and that he has chosen to refuse it.
- When a client decides to leave the facility against medical advice (without a discharge prescription), the nurse notifies the provider and discusses with the client the risks to expect when leaving the facility prior to discharge.
- The nurse asks the client to sign an Against Medical Advice form and documents the incident.

4.3 Responsibilities for informed consent

Provider
Obtains informed consent. To do so, the provider must give the client

- The purpose of the procedure.
- A complete description of the procedure.
- A description of the professionals who will perform and participate in the procedure.
- A description of the potential harm, pain, or discomfort that might occur.
- Options for other treatments.
- The option to refuse treatment and the consequences of doing so.

Client
Gives informed consent. To give informed consent, the client must

- Give it voluntarily (no coercion involved).
- Be competent and of legal age or be an emancipated minor. When the client is unable to provide consent, another authorized person must give consent.
- Receive enough information to make a decision based on an understanding of what to expect.

Nurse
Witnesses informed consent. This means the nurse must

- Ensure that the provider gave the client the necessary information.
- Ensure that the client understood the information and is competent to give informed consent.
- Have the client sign the informed consent document.
- Notify the provider if the client has more questions or appears not to understand any of the information. The provider is then responsible for giving clarification.
- Document questions the client has, notification of the provider, reinforcement of teaching, and use of an interpreter.

STANDARDS OF CARE (PRACTICE)

- Nurses base practice on established standards of care or legal guidelines for care, such as the following.
  - The nurse practice act of each state.
  - Published standards of nursing practice from professional organizations and specialty groups, including the American Nurses Association (ANA), the American Association of Critical Care Nurses (AACN), and the American Association of Occupational Health Nurses (AAOHN).
  - Health care facilities' policies and procedures, which establish the standard of practice for employees of that facility. They provide detailed information about how the nurse should respond to or provide care in specific situations and while performing client care procedures.
- Standards of care define and direct the level of care nurses should give, and they implicate nurses who did not follow these standards in malpractice lawsuits.
- Nurses should refuse to practice beyond the legal scope of practice or outside of their areas of competence regardless of reason (staffing shortage, lack of appropriate personnel).
- Nurses should use the formal chain of command to verbalize concerns related to assignment in light of current legal scope of practice, job description, and area of competence.

IMPAIRED COWORKERS

Impaired health care providers pose a significant risk to client safety. Qs
- A nurse who suspects a coworker of any behavior that jeopardizes client care or could indicate a substance use disorder has a duty to report the coworker to the appropriate manager.
- Many facilities' policies provide access to assistance programs that facilitate entry into a treatment program.
- Each state has laws and regulations that govern the disposition of nurses who have substance use disorders. Criminal charges could apply.

ADVANCE DIRECTIVES

The purpose of advance directives is to communicate a client's wishes regarding end-of-life care should the client become unable to do so.
- The PSDA requires asking all clients on admission to a health care facility whether they have advance directives.
- Staff should give clients who do have advance directives written information that outlines their rights related to health care decisions and how to formulate advance directives.
- A health care representative should be available to help with this process.

Types of advance directives

Living will
- A living will is a legal document that expresses the client's wishes regarding medical treatment in the event the client becomes incapacitated and is facing end-of-life issues.
- Most state laws include provisions that protect health care providers who follow a living will from liability.

Durable power of attorney for health care
A durable power of attorney for health care is a document in which clients designate a health care proxy to make health care decisions for them if they are unable to do so. The proxy may be any competent adult the client chooses.

Provider's orders
Unless a provider writes a "do not resuscitate" (DNR) or "allow natural death" (AND) prescription in the client's medical record, the nurse initiates cardiopulmonary resuscitation (CPR) when the client has no pulse or respirations. The provider consults the client and the family prior to administering a DNR or AND.

NURSING ROLE IN ADVANCE DIRECTIVES
Nursing responsibilities include the following.
- Provide written information about advance directives.
- Document the client's advance directives status.
- Ensure that the advance directives reflect the client's current decisions.
- Inform all members of the health care team of the client's advance directives. Qtc

MANDATORY REPORTING

Health care providers have a legal obligation to report their findings in accordance with state law in the following situations.

ABUSE
Nurses must report any suspicion of abuse (child or elder abuse, domestic violence) following facility policy.

COMMUNICABLE DISEASES
Nurses must report communicable disease diagnoses to the local or state health department. For a complete list of reportable diseases and a description of the reporting system, go to the Centers for Disease Control and Prevention's website, www.cdc.gov. Each state mandates which diseases to report in that state.
- Reporting allows officials to:
  - Ensure appropriate medical treatment of diseases (tuberculosis).
  - Monitor for common-source outbreaks (foodborne, hepatitis A).
  - Plan and evaluate control and prevention plans (immunizations).
  - Identify outbreaks and epidemics.
  - Determine public health priorities based on trends.

Application Exercises

1. A nurse observes an assistive personnel (AP) reprimanding a client for not using the urinal properly. The AP tells him she will put a diaper on him if he does not use the urinal more carefully next time. Which of the following torts is the AP committing?

   A. Assault

   B. Battery

   C. False imprisonment

   D. Invasion of privacy

2. A nurse is caring for a competent adult client who tells the nurse that he is thinking about leaving the hospital against medical advice. The nurse believes that this is not in the client's best interest, so she prepares to administer a PRN sedative medication the client has not requested along with his usual medication. Which of the following types of tort is the nurse about to commit?

   A. Assault

   B. False imprisonment

   C. Negligence

   D. Breach of confidentiality

3. A nurse in a surgeon's office is providing preoperative teaching for a client who is scheduled for surgery the following week. The client tells the nurse that he will prepare his advance directives before he goes to the hospital. Which of the following statements made by the client should indicate to the nurse an understanding of advance directives?

   A. "I'd rather have my brother make decisions for me, but I know it has to be my wife."

   B. "I know they won't go ahead with the surgery unless I prepare these forms."

   C. "I plan to write that I don't want them to keep me on a breathing machine."

   D. "I will get my regular doctor to approve my plan before I hand it in at the hospital."

4. A nurse is caring for a client who is about to undergo an elective surgical procedure. The nurse should take which of the following actions regarding informed consent? (Select all that apply.)

   A. Make sure the surgeon obtained the client's consent.

   B. Witness the client's signature on the consent form.

   C. Explain the risks and benefits of the procedure.

   D. Describe the consequences of choosing not to have the surgery.

   E. Tell the client about alternatives to having the surgery.

5. A nurse has noticed several occasions in the past week when another nurse on the unit seemed drowsy and unable to focus on the issue at hand. Today, she found the nurse asleep in a chair in the break room when she was not on a break. Which of the following actions should the nurse take?

   A. Alert the American Nurses Association.

   B. Fill out an incident report.

   C. Report the observations to the nurse manager on the unit.

   D. Leave the nurse alone to sleep.

PRACTICE Active Learning Scenario

A nurse is teaching a group of nursing students about avoiding liability for negligence. Use the ATI Active Learning Template: Basic Concept to complete this item.

UNDERLYING PRINCIPLES: List the five elements necessary to prove negligence.

NURSING INTERVENTIONS: List at least four ways nurses can avoid liability for negligence.

Application Exercises Key

1. A. **CORRECT:** By threatening the client, the AP is committing assault. Her threats could make the client become fearful and apprehensive.

   B. Battery is actual physical contact without the client's consent. Because the AP has only verbally threatened the client, battery has not occurred.

   C. Unless the AP restrains the client, there is no false imprisonment involved.

   D. Invasion of privacy involves disclosing information about a client to an unauthorized individual.

   (N) *NCLEX® Connection: Management of Care, Legal Rights and Responsibilities*

2. A. Assault is an action that threatens harmful contact without the client's consent. The nurse has made no threats in this situation.

   B. **CORRECT:** The nurse gave the medication as a chemical restraint to keep the client from leaving the facility against medical advice. This is false imprisonment because the client neither requested nor consented to receiving the sedative.

   C. Negligence is a breach of duty that results in harm to the client. It is unlikely that the medication the nurse administered without his consent actually harmed the client.

   D. The nurse has not disclosed any protected health information, so there is no breach of confidentiality involved in this situation.

   (N) *NCLEX® Connection: Management of Care, Legal Rights and Responsibilities*

3. A. The client may designate any competent adult to be his health care proxy. It does not have to be his spouse.

   B. The hospital staff must ask the client whether he has prepared advance directives and provide written information about them if he has not. The nurse should document whether the client has signed the advance directives. The hospital staff cannot refuse care based on the lack of advance directives.

   C. **CORRECT:** The client has the right to decide and specify which medical procedures he wants when a life-threatening situation arises.

   D. The client does not need his provider's approval to submit his advance directives. However, he should give his primary care provider a copy of the document for his records.

   (N) *NCLEX® Connection: Management of Care, Advance Directives/Self–Determination/Life Planning*

4. A. **CORRECT:** It is the nurse's responsibility to verify that the surgeon obtained the client's consent and that he understands the information the surgeon gave him.

   B. **CORRECT:** It is the nurse's responsibility to witness the client's signing of the consent form, and to verify that he is consenting voluntarily and appears to be competent to do so. The nurse also should verify that he understands the information the surgeon gave him.

   C. It is the surgeon's responsibility to explain the risks and benefits of the procedure.

   D. It is the surgeon's responsibility to describe the consequences of choosing not to have the surgery.

   E. It is the surgeon's responsibility to tell the client about any available alternatives to having the surgery.

   (N) *NCLEX® Connection: Management of Care, Informed Consent*

5. A. The nurse should not alert the American Nurses Association. The state's board of nursing regulates disciplinary action and can revoke a nurse's license for substance use.

   B. The nurse should not fill out an incident report. Incident reports are filed to document an accident or unusual occurrence.

   C. **CORRECT:** Any nurse who notices behavior that could jeopardize client care or could indicate a substance use disorder has a duty to report the situation immediately to the nurse manager.

   D. The nurse should not leave the nurse alone to sleep. Although the nurse is not responsible for solving the problem, she does have a duty to take action since she has observed the problem.

   (N) *NCLEX® Connection: Management of Care, Legal Rights and Responsibilities*

PRACTICE Answer

Using the ATI Active Learning Template: Basic Concept

UNDERLYING PRINCIPLES
- Duty to provide care as defined by a standard
- Breach of duty by failure to meet standard
- Foreseeability of harm
- Breach of duty has potential to cause harm
- Harm occurs

NURSING INTERVENTIONS
- Following standards of care
- Giving competent care
- Communicating with other health team members
- Developing a caring rapport with clients
- Fully documenting assessments, interventions, and evaluations

(N) *NCLEX® Connection: Management of Care, Legal Rights and Responsibilities*

UNIT 1   SAFE, EFFECTIVE CARE ENVIRONMENT
SECTION: MANAGEMENT OF CARE

CHAPTER 5 *Information Technology*

The chart or medical record is the legal record of care.

The medical record is a confidential, permanent, and legal document that is admissible in court. Nurses are legally and ethically responsible for ensuring confidentiality. Only health care providers who are involved directly in a client's care may access that client's medical record.

Nurses document the care they provide as documentation or charting, and it should reflect the nursing process.

There is a rapidly growing trend for maintaining medical records electronically, which creates challenges in protecting the privacy and safety of health information. Q

Information to document includes assessments, medication administration, nursing actions, treatments and responses, and client education.

DOCUMENTATION

Documentation is a standard for many accrediting agencies, including The Joint Commission (formerly JCAHO). The Joint Commission mandates the use of computerized databases to expedite the accreditation process. Health care facilities use the computerized data for budget management, quality improvement programs, research, and many other endeavors.
- Purposes for medical records include communication, legal documentation, financial billing, education, research, and auditing.
- The purpose of reporting is to provide continuity of care and enhance communication among all team members who provide care to the same clients, thus promoting client safety.
- Nurses should conduct reporting in a confidential manner.

ELEMENTS OF DOCUMENTATION

Factual: Subjective and objective data
- Nurses should document **subjective data** as direct quotes, within quotation marks, or summarize and identify the information as the client's statement. Subjective data should be supported by objective data so charting is as descriptive as possible.
- **Objective data** should be descriptive and should include what the nurse sees, hears, feels, and smells. Document without derogatory words, judgments, or opinions. Document the client's behavior accurately. Instead of writing "client is agitated," write "client pacing back and forth in his room, yelling loudly."

Accurate and concise: Document facts and information precisely (what the nurse sees, hears, feels, smells) without any interpretations of the situation. Unnecessary words and irrelevant detail are avoided. Exact measurements establish accuracy. Only abbreviations and symbols approved by The Joint Commission and the facility are acceptable.

Complete and current: Document information that is comprehensive and timely. Never pre-chart an assessment, intervention, or evaluation.

Organized: Communicate information in a logical sequence.

LEGAL GUIDELINES

- Begin each entry with the date and time.
- Record entries legibly, in nonerasable black ink, and do not leave blank spaces in the nurses' notes.
- Do not use correction fluid, erase, scratch out, or blacken out errors in the medical record. Make corrections promptly, following the facility's procedure for error correction.
- Sign all documentation as the facility requires, generally with name and title.
- Documentation should reflect assessments, interventions, and evaluations, not personal opinions or criticism about client or other health care professionals' care.

DOCUMENTATION FORMATS

Flow charts show trends in vital signs, blood glucose levels, pain level, and other frequent assessments.

Narrative documentation records information as a sequence of events in a story-like manner.

Charting by exception uses standardized forms that identify norms and allows selective documentation of deviations from those norms.

Problem-oriented medical records are organized by problem or diagnosis and consist of a database, problem list, care plan, and progress notes. Examples include SOAP, PIE, and DAR. **(5.1)** Q

Electronic health records are replacing manual formats in many settings.
- Advantages include standardization, accuracy, confidentiality, easy access for multiple users, providing ease in maintaining ongoing health record of client's condition, and rapid acquisition and transfer of clients' information.
- Challenges include learning the system, knowing how to correct errors, and maintaining security.
- Documentation rules and formats are similar to those for paper charting.

REPORTING FORMATS

Change-of-shift report Q℡

Nurses give this report at the conclusion of each shift to the nurse assuming responsibility for the clients.
- Formats include face to face, audiotaping, or presentation during walking rounds in each client's room (unless the client has a roommate or visitors are present).
- An effective report should:
  - Include significant objective information about the client's health problems.
  - Proceed in a logical sequence.
  - Include no gossip or personal opinion.
  - Relate recent changes in medications, treatments, procedures, and the discharge plan.

Telephone reports

Telephone reports are useful when contacting the provider or other members of the interprofessional team.
- It is important to:
  - Have all the data ready prior to contacting any member of the interprofessional team.
  - Use a professional demeanor.
  - Use exact, relevant, and accurate information.
  - Document the name of the person who made the call and to whom the information was given; the time, content of the message; and the instructions or information received during the report.

Telephone or verbal prescriptions

It is best to avoid these, but they are sometimes necessary during emergencies and at unusual times.
- Have a second nurse listen to a telephone prescription.
- Repeat it back, making sure to include the medication's name (spell if necessary), dosage, time, and route. Qs
- Question any prescription that seems inappropriate for the client.
- Make sure the provider signs the prescription in person within the time frame the facility specifies, typically 24 hr.

Transfer (hand-off) reports

These should include demographic information, medical diagnosis, providers, an overview of health status (physical, psychosocial), plan of care, recent progress, any alterations that might become an urgent or emergent situation, directives for any assessments or client care essential within the next few hours, most recent vital signs, medications and last doses, allergies, diet, activity, specific equipment or adaptive devices (oxygen, suction, wheelchair), advance directives and resuscitation status, discharge plan (teaching), and family involvement in care and health care proxy.

Incident reports (unusual occurrences)

Incident/variance reports are an important part of a facility's quality improvement plan.
- An incident is the occurrence of an accident or an unusual event. Examples of incidents are medication errors, falls, omission of prescription, and needlesticks.
- Document facts without judgment or opinion.
- Do not refer to an incident report in a client's medical record.
- Incident reports contribute to changes that help improve health care quality.

INFORMATION SECURITY

Mandatory adherence with the Health Insurance Portability and Accountability Act of 1996 (HIPAA) began in 2003 to help ensure the confidentiality of health information.
- A major component of HIPAA, the Privacy Rule, promotes the use of standard methods of maintaining the privacy of protected health information (PHI) among health care agencies.
- It is essential for nurses to be aware of clients' rights to privacy and confidentiality. Facilities' policies and procedures help ensure adherence with HIPAA regulations.

Privacy rule

The Privacy Rule requires that nurses protect all written and verbal communication about clients. Components of the Privacy Rule include the following.
- Only health care team members directly responsible for a client's care may access that client's record. Nurses may not share information with other clients or staff not caring for the client.
- Clients have a right to read and obtain a copy of their medical record.
- Nurses may not photocopy any part of a medical record except for authorized exchange of documents between facilities and providers.
- Staff must keep medical records in a secure area to prevent inappropriate access to the information. They may not use public display boards to list client names and diagnoses.
- Electronic records are password-protected. The public may not view them. Staff must use only their own passwords to access information.

- Nurses must not disclose clients' information to unauthorized individuals or family members who request it in person or by telephone or email.
  - Many hospitals use a code system to identify those individuals who may receive information about a client.
  - Nurses should ask any individual inquiring about a client's status for the code and disclose information only when the individual can give the code.
- Communication about a client should only take place in a private setting where unauthorized individuals cannot overhear it.
- To adhere to HIPAA regulations, each facility has specific policies and procedures to monitor staff adherence, technical protocols, computer privacy, and data safety.

Information security protocols
- Log off from the computer before leaving the workstation to ensure that others cannot view protected health information on the monitor.
- Never share a user ID or password with anyone.
- Never leave a medical record or other printed or written PHI where others can access it.
- Shred any printed or written client information for reporting or client care after use.

5.1 Problem-oriented medical records

SOAP	*PIE*	*DAR*
		focus charting
S Subjective data	**P** Problem	**D** Data
O Objective data	**I** Intervention	**A** Action
A Assessment *includes a nursing diagnosis based on the assessment*	**E** Evaluation	**R** Response
P Plan		

Social media precautions
- Know the implications of HIPAA before using social networking sites for school– or work–related communication.
- Become familiar with your facility's policies regarding the use of social networking.
- Do not use or view social networking media in clinical settings.
- Do not post information about your facility, clinical sites, clinical experiences, clients, and other health care staff on social networking sites
- Do not take pictures that show clients or their family members.

Application Exercises

1. A nurse is preparing information for change-of-shift report. Which of the following information should the nurse include in the report?
   - A. Input and output for the shift
   - B. Blood pressure from the previous day
   - C. Bone scan scheduled for today
   - D. Medication routine from the medication administration record

2. A nurse is discussing the HIPAA Privacy Rule with nurses during new employee orientation. Which of the following information should the nurse include? (Select all that apply.)
   - A. A single electronic records password is provided for nurses on the same unit.
   - B. Family members should provide a code prior to receiving client health information.
   - C. Communication of client information can occur at the nurses' station.
   - D. A client can request a copy of her medical record.
   - E. A nurse may photocopy a client's medical record for transfer to another facility.

3. A nurse is reviewing documentation with a group of newly licensed nurses. Which of the following legal guidelines should be followed when documenting in a client's record? (Select all that apply.)
   - A. Cover errors with correction fluid, and write in the correct information.
   - B. Put the date and time on all entries.
   - C. Document objective data, leaving out opinions.
   - D. Use as many abbreviations as possible.
   - E. Wait until the end of the shift to document.

4. A nurse is discussing occurrences that require completion of an incident report with a newly licensed nurse. Which of the following should the nurse include in the teaching? (Select all that apply).
   - A. Medication error
   - B. Needlesticks
   - C. Conflict with provider and nursing staff
   - D. Omission of prescription
   - E. Missed specimen collection of a prescribed laboratory test

5. A nurse is receiving a provider's prescription by telephone for morphine for a client who is reporting moderate to severe pain. Which of the following nursing actions are appropriate? (Select all that apply.)
   - A. Repeat the details of the prescription back to the provider.
   - B. Have another nurse listen to the telephone prescription.
   - C. Obtain the provider's signature on the prescription within 24 hr.
   - D. Decline the verbal prescription because it is not an emergency situation.
   - E. Tell the charge nurse that the provider has prescribed morphine by telephone.

Application Exercises Key

1. A. Unless there is a significant change in intake and output, the oncoming nurse can read that information in the chart.

   B. Unless there is a significant change in blood pressure measurements since the previous day, the oncoming nurse can read that information in the chart.

   C. **CORRECT:** The bone scan is important because the nurse might have to modify the client's care to accommodate leaving the unit.

   D. Unless there is a significant change in the medication routine, the oncoming nurse can read that information in the chart.

   ⓝ NCLEX® Connection: Management of Care, Continuity of Care

2. A. The HIPAA Privacy Rule requires the protection of clients' electronic records. The rule states that electronic records must be password protected and each staff person should use an individual password to access information.

   B. **CORRECT:** The HIPAA Privacy Rule states that information should only be disclosed to authorized individuals to whom the client has provided consent. Many hospitals use a code system to identify those individuals and should only provide information if the individual can give the code.

   C. **CORRECT:** The HIPAA Privacy Rule states that communication about a client should only take place in a private setting where unauthorized individuals cannot overhear it. A unit nurses' station is considered a private and secure location.

   D. **CORRECT:** The HIPAA Privacy Rule states that clients have a right to read and obtain a copy of their medical record.

   E. **CORRECT:** The HIPAA Privacy Rule states that nurses may only photocopy a client's medical record if it is to be used for transfer to another facility or provider.

   ⓝ NCLEX® Connection: Safety and Infection Control, Irregular Occurrence/Variance

3. A. Correction fluid implies that the nurse might have tried to hide the previous documentation or deface the medical record.

   B. **CORRECT:** The day and time confirm the recording of the correct sequence of events.

   C. **CORRECT:** Documentation must be factual, descriptive, and objective, without opinions or criticism.

   D. Too many abbreviations can make the entry difficult to understand. Nurses should minimize use of abbreviations, and use only those the facility approves.

   E. Documentation should be current. Waiting until the end of the shift can result in data omission.

   ⓝ NCLEX® Connection: Management of Care, Information Technology

4. A. **CORRECT:** The nurse should complete an incident report regarding a medication error.

   B. **CORRECT:** The nurse should complete an incident report regarding a needlestick.

   C. The nurse should report a conflict with a provider and nursing staff to the charge nurse or nurse manager.,

   D. **CORRECT:** The nurse should complete an incident report following an omission of a prescription.

   E. The nurse should report missed specimen collection of a prescribed laboratory test.

   ⓝ NCLEX® Connection: Safety and Infection Control, Reporting of Incident/Event/Irregular Occurrence/Variance

5. A. **CORRECT:** The nurse should repeat the medication's name, dosage, time or interval, route, and any other pertinent information back to the provider and receive and document confirmation.

   B. **CORRECT:** Having another nurse listen to the telephone prescription is a safety precaution that helps prevent medication errors due to miscommunication.

   C. **CORRECT:** The provider must sign the prescription within the time frame the facility specifies in its policies (generally 24 hr).

   D. Unrelieved pain can become an emergency situation without the appropriate pain management interventions.

   E. There is no need to inform the charge nurse every time a nurse receives a medication prescription, whether by telephone, verbally, or in the medical record.

   ⓝ NCLEX® Connection: Safety and Infection Control, Accident/Error/Injury Prevention

A nurse is introducing a group of newly licensed nurses to the various approaches to problem-oriented documentation. Use the ATI Active Learning Template: Basic Concept to complete this item.

UNDERLYING PRINCIPLES: List three common methods of problem-oriented charting with definitions of their acronyms.

Using the ATI Active Learning Template: Basic Concept

UNDERLYING PRINCIPLES

- SOAP
  - S: Subjective data
  - O: Objective data
  - A: Assessment (includes a nursing diagnosis based on the assessment)
  - P: Plan
- PIE
  - P: Problem
  - I: Intervention
  - E: Evaluation
- DAR (focus charting)
  - D: Data
  - A: Action
  - R: Response

ⓝ NCLEX® Connection: Management of Care, Information Technology

CHAPTER 6 # Delegation and Supervision

Delegation is the process of transferring the performance of a task to another member of the health care team while retaining accountability for the outcome. Qrc

Supervision is the process of directing, monitoring, and evaluating the performance of tasks by another team member. Nurses are responsible for supervising the performance of client care tasks they delegate to others.

Licensed personnel are nurses who have completed a course of study in nursing and successfully passed either a PN or RN examination.

Unlicensed personnel are individuals who have had training to function in an assistive role to licensed nurses in providing client care.

These unlicensed individuals might be nursing personnel, such as certified nursing assistants (CNAs) or certified medication assistants (CMAs), or they might be non-nursing personnel, such as dialysis technicians, monitor technicians, or phlebotomists.

Some facilities differentiate between licensed and unlicensed personnel by using the acronym NAP for nursing assistive personnel or AP for assistive personnel.

DELEGATION

A licensed nurse is responsible for providing clear directions when delegating a task initially and for periodic reassessment and evaluation of the outcome of the task.
- RNs may delegate to other RNs, PNs, and AP.
  - RNs must be knowledgeable about their state's nurse practice act and the regulations that guide the use of PNs and AP.
  - RNs must delegate tasks so that they can complete higher-level tasks that only RNs can perform. This allows more efficient use of all team members.
- PNs may delegate to other PNs and to AP.

DELEGATION FACTORS

- Nurses may only delegate tasks appropriate for the skill and education level of the individual who is receiving the assignment (the delegatee). Qs
- RNs may not delegate the nursing process, client education, or tasks that require nursing judgment to PNs or to APs.

TASK FACTORS: Prior to delegating client care, nurses should consider the:
- **Predictability of the outcome:** Will the completion of the task have a predictable outcome?
  - Is it a routine treatment?
  - Is it a new treatment for that client?
- **Potential for harm**
  - Is there a chance that something negative could happen to the client (bleeding, aspiration)?
  - Is the client unstable?
- **Complexity of care**
  - Does the client's care require complex tasks?
  - Does the state's practice act or the facility's policy allow the delegatee to perform the task, and does she have the necessary skills?
- **Need for problem solving and innovation**
  - Is judgment essential while performing the task?
  - Does it require nursing assessment or data-collection skills?
- **Level of interaction with the client:** Does the delegatee need psychosocial support or education during the performance of the task?

DELEGATEE FACTORS

- Education, training, and experience
- Knowledge and skill to perform the task
- Level of critical thinking the task requires
- Ability to communicate with others as it pertains to the task
- Demonstration of competence
- The facility's policies and procedures Qs
- Licensing legislation (state's nurse practice acts) (6.1)

6.1 Examples of tasks nurses may delegate to PNs and APs
(provided the facility's policy and state's practice guidelines permit)

TO PNs
- Monitoring findings (as input to the RN's ongoing assessment)
- Reinforcing client teaching from a standard care plan
- Performing tracheostomy care
- Suctioning
- Checking NG tube patency
- Administering enteral feedings
- Inserting a urinary catheter
- Administering medication (excluding IV medication in some states)

TO APs
- Activities of daily living (ADLs)
  - Bathing
  - Grooming
  - Dressing
  - Toileting
  - Ambulating
  - Feeding (without swallowing precautions)
  - Positioning
- Routine tasks
  - Bed making
  - Specimen collection
  - Intake and output
  - Vital signs (for stable clients)

DELEGATION AND SUPERVISION GUIDELINES

- Use the five rights of delegation to decide. **(6.2)**
  - Tasks to delegate (right task)
  - Under what circumstances (right circumstances, such as setting and resources)
  - To whom (right person)
  - What information to communicate (right direction and communication)
  - How to oversee and appraise (right supervision and evaluation)
- Use professional judgment and critical thinking skills when delegating.

Right task

- Identify which tasks are appropriate to delegate for each specific client.
- A right task is repetitive, requires little supervision, and is relatively noninvasive for the client.
- Delegate activities to appropriate levels of team members (RN, PN, AP) according to professional standards of practice, legal and facility guidelines, and available resources.

> **RIGHT TASK:** Delegate an AP to assist a client who has pneumonia to use a bedpan.

> **WRONG TASK:** Delegate an AP to administer a nebulizer treatment to a client who has pneumonia.

Right circumstances

- Determine the health status and complexity of care the client requires.
- Match the complexity of care demands to the skill level of the delegatee.
- Consider the workload of the delegatee.

> **RIGHT CIRCUMSTANCE:** Delegate an AP to measure the vital signs of a client who is postoperative and stable.

> **WRONG CIRCUMSTANCE:** Delegate an AP to measure the vital signs of a client who is postoperative and required naloxone to reverse respiratory depression.

6.2 The five rights of delegation

Right task
Right circumstance
Right person
Right direction and communication
Right supervision and evaluation

Right person

- Determine and verify the competence of the delegatee.
- The task must be within the delegatee's scope of practice or job description.
- The delegatee must have the necessary competence and training.
- Continually review the performance of the delegatee and determine care competence.
- Evaluate the delegatee's performance according to standards, and when necessary, take steps to remediate any failure to meet standards.

> **RIGHT PERSON:** Delegate an PN to administer enteral feedings to a client who has a head injury.

> **WRONG PERSON:** Delegate an AP to administer enteral feedings to a client who has a head injury.

Right direction and communication in writing, orally, or both

- Communicate what data to collect.
- Provide a method and timeline for reporting, including when to report concerns and assessment findings.
- Communicate specific task(s) to perform and client-specific instructions.
- Detail expected results, timelines, and expectations for follow-up communication.

> **RIGHT DIRECTION AND COMMUNICATION:** Delegate an AP to assist Mr. Martin in room 312 with a shower before 0900.

> **WRONG DIRECTION AND COMMUNICATION:** Delegate an AP to assist Mr. Martin in room 312 with morning hygiene.

Right supervision and evaluation Q℞

- Provide supervision, either directly or indirectly (assigning supervision to another licensed nurse).
- Monitor performance.
- Intervene if necessary (for unsafe clinical practice).
- Provide feedback:
  - Did the delegatee complete the tasks on time?
  - Was the delegatee's performance satisfactory?
  - Did the delegatee document and report unexpected findings?
  - Did the delegatee need help completing the tasks on time?
- Evaluate the client and determine the client's outcome status.
- Evaluate task performance and identify needs for performance-improvement activities and additional resources.

> **RIGHT SUPERVISION:** Delegate an AP to assist with ambulating a client after the RN completes the admission assessment.

> **WRONG SUPERVISION:** Delegate an AP to assist with ambulating a client prior to the RN performing an admission assessment.

1. A nurse on a medical-surgical unit has received change-of-shift report and will care for four clients. Which of the following client's needs should the nurse assign to an assistive personnel (AP)?

    A. Updating the plan of care for a client who is postoperative

    B. Reinforcing teaching with a client who is learning to walk using a quad cane

    C. Reapplying a condom catheter for a client who has urinary incontinence

    D. Applying a sterile dressing to a pressure ulcer

2. A nurse manager of a medical-surgical unit is assigning care responsibilities for the oncoming shift. A client is awaiting transfer back to the unit from the PACU following thoracic surgery. To which of the following staff members should the nurse assign this client?

    A. Charge nurse

    B. RN

    C. Practical nurse (PN)

    D. Assistive personnel (AP)

3. A nurse is delegating the ambulation of a client who had knee arthroplasty 5 days ago to an AP. Which of the following information should the nurse share with the AP? (Select all that apply.)

    A. The roommate ambulates independently.

    B. The client ambulates with his slippers on over his antiembolic stockings.

    C. The client uses a front-wheeled walker when ambulating.

    D. The client had pain medication 30 min ago.

    E. The client is allergic to codeine.

    F. The client ate 50% of his breakfast this morning.

4. An RN is making assignments for a practical nurse (PN) at the beginning of the shift. Which of the following assignments should the PN question?

    A. Assisting a client who is 24-hr postoperative to use an incentive spirometer

    B. Collecting a clean-catch urine specimen from a client who has a wound infection

    C. Providing nasopharyngeal suctioning for a client who has pneumonia

    D. Teaching a client who has asthma to use a metered-dose inhaler

5. A nurse is preparing an in-service program about delegation. Which of the following elements should she identify when presenting the five rights of delegation? (Select all that apply.)

    A. Right client

    B. Right supervision and evaluation

    C. Right direction and communication

    D. Right time

    E. Right circumstances

PRACTICE Active Learning Scenario

A nurse manager is reviewing the responsibilities of delegation with a group of nurses on a medical unit. Use the ATI Active Learning Template: Basic Concept to complete this item.

NURSING INTERVENTIONS: List at least five tasks the delegating nurse must perform when supervising and evaluating a delegatee.

Application Exercises Key

1. A. It would be inappropriate to delegate the updating of a plan of care to an AP because this is beyond the range of function for the role. It is the responsibility of the RN to establish and update the plan of care for a client.

   B. Either an RN or an PN, not an AP, may reinforce teaching.

   C. **CORRECT:** The application of a condom catheter is a noninvasive, routine procedure that the nurse may delegate to an AP.

   D. Either an RN or an PN, not an AP, may apply a sterile dressing.

   Ⓝ *NCLEX® Connection: Management of Care, Assignment, Delegation and Supervision*

2. A. Although the charge nurse can provide all the care this client requires in the immediate postoperative period, administrative responsibilities might prevent the close monitoring and assessment this client needs.

   B. **CORRECT:** A client returning from surgery requires an RN's assessment and establishment of a plan of care, especially if the client is potentially unstable.

   C. Although PNs can perform some of the tasks crucial in the immediate postoperative period, they cannot provide the comprehensive care this client needs at this time.

   D. Although APs can perform some of the tasks crucial in the immediate postoperative period, they cannot provide the comprehensive care this client needs at this time, particularly assessment.

   Ⓝ *NCLEX® Connection: Management of Care, Assignment, Delegation and Supervision*

3. A. The AP does not need to know the status of the client's roommate to complete this assignment.

   B. **CORRECT:** To complete this assignment safely, the AP should make sure the client wears stockings and slippers.

   C. **CORRECT:** To complete this assignment safely, the AP should make sure the client uses a front-wheeled walker.

   D. **CORRECT:** To complete this assignment safely, the AP should know that the client should be feeling the effects of the pain medication.

   E. The AP does not need to know the client's allergy status to complete this assignment.

   F. The AP does not need to know the client's food intake to complete this assignment.

   Ⓝ *NCLEX® Connection: Management of Care, Continuity of Care*

4. A. Assisting a client to use an incentive spirometer is within the scope of practice of the PN.

   B. Collecting a clean-catch urine specimen is within the scope of practice of the PN.

   C. Providing nasopharyngeal suctioning is within the scope of practice of the PN.

   D. **CORRECT:** The RN is responsible for primary teaching. The PN may only reinforce teaching.

   Ⓝ *NCLEX® Connection: Management of Care, Concepts of Management*

5. A. The right client is one of the rights of medication administration, not of delegation.

   B. **CORRECT:** The right supervision and evaluation is one of the five rights of delegation. They also include the right task and the right person.

   C. **CORRECT:** Right direction and communication is one of the five rights of delegation. They also include the right task and the right person.

   D. Although the delegatee needs to know whether there is a time frame or a specific time to perform the task, the right time is not one of the five rights of delegation. It is one of the rights of medication administration.

   E. **CORRECT:** The right circumstances is one of the five rights of delegation. They also include the right task and the right person.

   Ⓝ *NCLEX® Connection: Management of Care, Assignment, Delegation and Supervision*

PRACTICE Answer

Using the ATI Active Learning Template: Basic Concept

NURSING INTERVENTIONS

- Provide supervision, either directly or indirectly (assigning supervision to another licensed nurse).
- Monitor performance.
- Intervene if necessary (for unsafe clinical practice).
- Provide feedback:
  - Did the delegatee complete the tasks on time?
  - Was the delegatee's performance satisfactory?
  - Did the delegatee document and report unexpected findings?
  - Did the delegatee need help completing the tasks on time?
- Evaluate the client and determine the client's outcome status.
- Evaluate task performance and identify needs for performance-improvement activities and additional resources.

Ⓝ *NCLEX® Connection: Management of Care, Assignment, Delegation and Supervision*

CHAPTER 7 *Nursing Process*

The nursing process is a cyclical, critical thinking process that consists of five steps to follow in a purposeful, goal-directed, systematic way to achieve optimal client outcomes. It is a variation of scientific reasoning that helps nurses organize nursing care and apply the optimal available evidence to care delivery.

The nursing process is a dynamic, continuous, client-centered, problem-solving, and decision-making framework that is foundational to nursing practice.

The nursing process provides a framework throughout which nurses can apply knowledge, experience, judgment, and skills, as well as established standards of nursing practice to the formulation of a plan of nursing care. This plan is applicable to any client system, including individuals, families, groups, and communities.

The nursing process helps nurses integrate critical thinking creatively to base nursing judgments on reason.

The nursing process promotes the professionalism of nursing while differentiating the practice of nursing from the practice of medicine and that of other health care professionals.

ASSESSMENT/DATA COLLECTION

- Assessment/data collection involves the systematic collection of information about clients' present health status to identify needs and additional data to collect based on findings. Nurses can collect data during an initial assessment (baseline data), focused assessment, and ongoing assessments.
- Methods of data collection include observation, interviews with clients and families, medical history, comprehensive or focused physical examination, diagnostic and laboratory reports, and collaboration with other members of the health care team.
- To collect data effectively, nurses must ask clients appropriate questions, listen carefully to responses, and have excellent head–to–toe physical assessment skills. Nurses also must employ clinical judgment and critical thinking in accurately recognizing when to collect assessment data. They also must recognize the need to collect assessment data prior to interventions.
- Nurses collect subjective data (symptoms) during a nursing history. They include clients' feelings, perceptions, and descriptions of health status. Clients are the only ones who can describe and verify their own symptoms.
- Nurses observe and measure objective data (signs) during a physical examination. They feel, see, hear, and smell objective data through observation or physical assessment of the client. **(7.2)**
- During this assessment/data collection, the nurse validates, interprets, and clusters data.
- Documentation of the assessment data must be thorough, concise, and accurate.

7.1 Nursing process framework

The nursing process includes sequential but overlapping steps: <ul><li>Assessment/data collection*</li><li>Analysis/data collection*</li><li>Planning</li><li>Implementation</li><li>Evaluation</li></ul> *PNs combine the assessment and analysis steps into a single data collection step.*	The accuracy and thoroughness of assessment/analysis/data collection and planning have a direct impact on implementation and evaluation. Use of the nursing process results in a comprehensive, individualized, client-centered plan of nursing care that nurses can deliver in a timely and reasonable manner. ○PCC

7.2 Sources of data for collection and assessment

Primary sources
SUBJECTIVE: What the client tells the nurse
  "My shoulder is really, really sore."

OBJECTIVE: Data the nurse obtains through observation and examination:
  Client grimaces when attempting to brush her hair with her left arm.

Secondary sources
SUBJECTIVE: What others tell the nurse based on what the client has told them:
  "She told me that her shoulder is sore every morning."

OBJECTIVE: Data the nurse collects from other sources (family, friends, caregivers, health care professionals, literature review, medical records):
  Physical therapy note in chart indicates client has decreased range of motion of left shoulder.

ANALYSIS/DATA COLLECTION

- Nurses use critical thinking skills (a diagnostic reasoning process) to identify clients' health status or problem(s), interpret or monitor the collected database, reach an appropriate nursing judgment about health status and coping mechanisms, and provide direction for nursing care.
- Analysis/data collection requires nurses to look at the data and
  - Recognize patterns or trends.
  - Compare the data with expected standards or reference ranges.
  - Arrive at conclusions to guide nursing care.
- RNs make multiple analyses based on their interpretations of collected data. They decide, using reasoning and judgment, which data account for clients' health status or problems. At times, this requires further data collection and analysis. As nurses again cluster the collected data, a specific finding might serve as an alert to a specific problem that requires planning and intervention.
- As with the assessment/data collection step, complete and accurate documentation is essential. Documentation should focus on facts and should be highly descriptive.

PLANNING

- When planning client care (RN) or contributing to a client's plan of care (PN), nurses must establish priorities and optimal outcomes of care they can readily measure and evaluate. These established priorities and outcomes of client care then direct nurses in selecting interventions to include in a plan of care to promote, maintain, or restore health.
- Nurses do three types of planning. Initially, they develop a comprehensive plan of care for clients based on comprehensive assessments they complete, for example, on admission to a health care facility or to a home health organization.

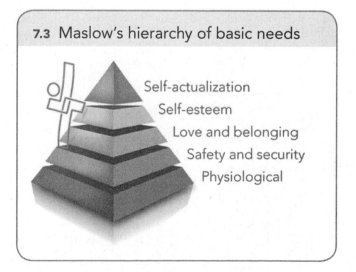

7.3 Maslow's hierarchy of basic needs

Self-actualization
Self-esteem
Love and belonging
Safety and security
Physiological

- Nurses do ongoing planning throughout the provision of care. While obtaining new information and evaluating responses to care, they modify and individualize the initial plan of care.
- Discharge planning is a process of anticipating and planning for clients' needs after discharge. To be effective, discharge planning must begin during admission.
- Throughout the planning process, nurses set priorities, determine client outcomes, and select specific nursing interventions.
- Nurses participate in priority setting when they identify a preferential order of problems. This guides the delivery of nursing care. They can use guidelines to set priorities, such as Maslow's hierarchy of basic needs. (7.3)
- Nurses work with clients to identify goals and outcomes.
  - Goals identify optimal status, whereas outcomes identify the observable criterion that will determine success or failure of the goal.
  - Often these terms are interchangeable. With any format, the goal/outcome must be client-centered, singular, observable, measurable, time-limited, mutually agreeable, and reasonable.
  - Concise, measurable goals help nurses and clients evaluate progress:
  - Nurses use short- and long-term goals to guide the client toward the planned outcome and determine the effectiveness of nursing care.
- Nurses identify actions and interventions that help achieve optimal outcomes. Scientific principles provide the rationale for nursing interventions. Q EBP
  - **Nurse-initiated/independent interventions:** Nurses use evidence and scientific rationale to take autonomous actions to benefit clients. They base these actions on identified problems and health care needs, and make sure they are within their scope of practice. Nurses perform or delegate the interventions and are accountable for them. An example is repositioning a client at least every 2 hr to prevent skin breakdown.
  - **Provider-initiated/dependent interventions:** Interventions nurses initiate as a result of a provider's prescription (written, standing, or verbal) or the facility's protocol, such as blood administration procedures.
  - **Collaborative interventions:** Interventions nurses carry out in collaboration with other health care team professionals, such as ensuring that a client receives and eats his evening snack. Q TC
- The nursing care plan (NCP) is the end product of the planning step. Nurses organize the NCP for quick identification of problems, outcomes, and interventions to implement.

IMPLEMENTATION

- In this step of the nursing process, nurses base the care they provide on assessment data, analyses, and the plan of care they developed in the previous steps of the nursing process. In this step, they must use problem-solving, clinical judgment, and critical thinking to select and implement appropriate therapeutic interventions using nursing knowledge, priorities of care, and planned goals or outcomes to promote, maintain, or restore health. Nurses also use interpersonal skills (therapeutic communication) and technical skills (psychomotor performance) when implementing nursing interventions.
- Therapeutic interventions also include measures nurses take to minimize risk, such as wearing personal protective equipment. Nurses intervene to respond to unplanned events, such as an observation of unsafe practice, a change in a status, or the emergence of a life-threatening situation.
- Nurses use evidence-based rationale for the selection and implementation of all therapeutic interventions. Additionally, caring and professional behavior should be at the center of all therapeutic nursing interventions. Q EBP
- During implementation, nurses perform nursing actions, delegate tasks, supervise other health care staff, and document the care and clients' responses.

EVALUATION

- In this step of the nursing process, nurses evaluate clients' responses to nursing interventions and form a clinical judgment about the extent to which clients have met the goals and outcomes.
- Nurses continuously evaluate the client's progress toward outcomes, and use the client data to determine whether or not to modify the plan of care.
- Nurses determine the effectiveness of the nursing care plan. They collect data based on the outcome criteria then compare what actually happened with the planned outcomes. This helps determine what further actions to take. Q PCC
- QUESTIONS TO CONSIDER
  - "Did the client meet the planned outcomes?"
  - "Were the nursing interventions appropriate and effective?"
  - "Should I modify the outcomes or interventions?"
- Client outcomes in specific, measurable terms are easier to evaluate.
- FACTORS THAT CAN LEAD TO LACK OF GOAL ACHIEVEMENT
  - An incomplete database
  - Unrealistic client outcomes
  - Nonspecific nursing interventions
  - Inadequate time for the client to achieve the outcomes

Application Exercises

1. By the second postoperative day, a client has not achieved satisfactory pain relief. Based on this evaluation, which of the following actions should the nurse take, according to the nursing process?

   A. Reassess the client to determine the reasons for inadequate pain relief.

   B. Wait to see whether the pain lessens during the next 24 hr.

   C. Change the plan of care to provide different pain relief interventions.

   D. Teach the client about the plan of care for managing his pain.

2. A newly licensed nurse is reporting to the charge nurse about the care she gave to a client. She states, "The client said his leg pain was back, so I checked his medical record, and he last received his pain medication 6 hours ago. The prescription reads every 4 hours PRN for pain, so I decided he needs it. I asked the unit nurse to observe me preparing and administering it. I checked with the client 40 minutes later, and he said his pain is going away." The charge nurse should inform the newly licensed nurse that she left out which of the following steps of the nursing process?

   A. Assessment

   B. Planning

   C. Intervention

   D. Evaluation

3. A charge nurse is reviewing the steps of the nursing process with a group of nurses. Which of the following data should the charge nurse identify as objective data? (Select all that apply.)

   A. Respiratory rate is 22/min with even, unlabored respirations.

   B. The client's partner states, "He said he hurts after walking about 10 minutes."

   C. Pain rating is 3 on a scale of 0 to 10

   D. Skin is pink, warm, and dry.

   E. The assistive personnel reports the client walked with a limp.

4. A charge nurse is talking with a newly licensed nurse and is reviewing nursing interventions that do not require a provider's prescription. Which of the following interventions should the charge nurse include? (Select all that apply.)

   A. Writing a prescription for morphine sulfate as needed for pain.

   B. Inserting a nasogastric (NG) tube to relieve gastric distention.

   C. Showing a client how to use progressive muscle relaxation.

   D. Performing a daily bath after the evening meal.

   E. Repositioning a client every 2 hr to reduce pressure ulcer risk.

5. A nurse is discussing the nursing process with a newly hired nurse. Which of the following statements by the newly hired nurse should the nurse identify as appropriate for the planning step of the nursing process?

   A. "I will determine the most important client problems that we should address."

   B. "I will review the past medical history on the client's record to get more information."

   C. "I will go carry out the new prescriptions from the provider."

   D. "I will ask the client if his nausea has resolved."

Application Exercises Key

1. A. **CORRECT:** The nurse should collect further data on the client to determine why he has not achieved satisfactory pain relief, because various factors might be interfering with his comfort. The nursing process repeats in an ongoing manner across the span of client care.

   B. The nurse should not wait longer to see how the client would respond, but should to take action to determine why the client is not reaching achieving satisfactory pain relief.

   C. The nurse should not make random changes to the plan of care without gathering evidence to guide the nurse in knowing what new interventions can be necessary.

   D. The action by the nurse does not acknowledge the client's condition or that the current plan is ineffective.

   Ⓝ *NCLEX® Connection: Reduction of Risk Potential, System Specific Assessments*

2. A. **CORRECT:** The newly licensed nurse should have used the assessment step of the nursing process by asking the client to evaluate the severity of his pain on a 0 to 10 scale. She also should have asked about the characteristics of his pain and assessed for any changes that might have contributed to worsening of the pain.

   B. The newly licensed nurse used the planning step of the nursing process when she decided that it was appropriate to administer the medication and, recognizing her level of experience in administering pain medication, prepared the dose under supervision from the unit staff.

   C. The newly licensed nurse used the implementation step of the nursing process when she administered the medication.

   D. The newly licensed nurse used the evaluation step of the nursing process when she checked the effectiveness of the pain medication in relieving the client's pain.

   Ⓝ *NCLEX® Connection: Health Promotion and Maintenance, Techniques of Physical Assessment*

3. A. **CORRECT:** Objective data includes information the nurse measures, such as vital signs.

   B. Subjective data includes a client's reported symptoms, even if told by a secondary source.

   C. Subjective data includes a client's reported symptoms.

   D. **CORRECT:** Objective data includes information the nurse observes, such as skin appearance.

   E. **CORRECT:** Objective data includes information on observations of others, such as family and staff.

   Ⓝ *NCLEX® Connection: Health Promotion and Maintenance, Techniques of Physical Assessment*

4. A. The nurse must have a prescription from the provider to administer a medication. After obtaining the prescription, the nurse has the flexibility to determine when to administer a PRN medication.

   B. The nurse must have a prescription from the provider for the insertion of an NG tube. This is a provider-initiated intervention.

   C. **CORRECT:** Showing a client how to use progressive muscle relaxation is an appropriate nurse-initiated intervention for stress relief. Unless it is a contraindication for a specific client, the nurse can use this technique with clients without a provider's prescription.

   D. **CORRECT:** Performing a bath is a routine nursing care procedure. Unless it is a contraindication for a specific client, the nurse can determine when bathing is optimal for a client without a provider's prescription.

   E. **CORRECT:** Repositioning a client every 2 hr is an appropriate nurse-initiated intervention for clients. Unless it is a contraindication for a specific client, the nurse can use this strategy without a provider's prescription.

   Ⓝ *NCLEX® Connection: Health Promotion and Maintenance, Techniques of Physical Assessment*

5. A. **CORRECT:** The nurse should prioritize client problems during the planning step of the nursing process

   B. The nurse should review the client's history during the assessment/data collection step of the nursing process

   C. The nurse should implement nurse- and provider-initiated actions during the intervention step of the nursing process.

   D. The nurse should gather information about whether the client's problems have been resolved during the evaluation step of the nursing process

   Ⓝ *NCLEX® Connection: Management of Care, Legal Rights and Responsibilities*

PRACTICE Active Learning Scenario

A nurse educator is reviewing with a group of nursing students the actions and thought processes nurses use during the steps of the nursing process. Use the ATI Active Learning Template: Basic Concept to complete this item.

NURSING INTERVENTIONS
- List at three actions to take during the analysis or data collection step.
- List four factors to consider during the evaluation step when clients have not achieved their goals.

PRACTICE Answer

Using the ATI Active Learning Template: Basic Concept

NURSING INTERVENTIONS

Analysis/data collection
- Recognize patterns or trends.
- Compare the data with expected standards or reference ranges.
- Arrive at conclusions to guide nursing care.

Factors to consider during evaluation for unmet goals
- An incomplete database
- Unrealistic client outcomes
- Nonspecific nursing interventions
- Inadequate time for the client to achieve the outcomes

Ⓝ *NCLEX® Connection: Health Promotion and Maintenance, Techniques of Physical Assessment*

CHAPTER 8 *Critical Thinking and Clinical Judgment*

Nursing practice requires the application of knowledge from biological, social, and physical sciences; knowledge of pathophysiology; and knowledge of nursing procedures and skills. Nurses also must use multiple thinking skills—including critical thinking skills such as interpretation, analysis, evaluation, inference, and explanation—to make clinical judgments about problems in nursing practice. A nursing knowledge base with foundational thinking skills, including recall and comprehension, is a prerequisite to critical thinking in nursing.

In nursing, critical thinking is an active, orderly, well thought-out reasoning process that guides a nurse in various approaches to making a nursing judgment by applying knowledge and experience, problem-solving, logic, reasoning, and decision-making. A critical thinker prioritizes, explores various courses of action, keeps ethics in mind, and determines appropriate outcomes.

To have a positive effect on a client's health status, a nurse must be able to think critically, correctly identify problems, and both devise and implement the best solutions (interventions). Critical thinking discourages quick judgments that lead to single-focused solutions.

CRITICAL THINKING

- Critical thinking requires lifelong learning and the ability to acquire relevant experiences that can be reflected on continuously to improve nursing judgment.
- The components of critical thinking include knowledge, experience, critical thinking competencies, attitudes, and intellectual and professional standards.
- Critical thinking incorporates reflection, language, and intuition, and it evolves through three distinct levels as a nurse gains knowledge and experience while maturing into a competent nursing professional.

Reflection

Purposefully thinking back or recalling a situation to discover its meaning and gain insight into the event. A nurse should reflect on the following:
- "Why did I say that or do this?"
- "Did the original plan of care achieve optimal client outcomes?"
  - If so: "Which interventions were successful?"
  - If not: "Which interventions were unsuccessful?"

Language

Precise, clear language demonstrating focused thinking and communicating unambiguous messages and expectations to clients and other health care team members. A nurse should ask the following:
- "Did I use language appropriate for the client?"
- "Did I communicate the message clearly to the provider?"

Intuition

An inner sensing that facts do not currently support something. Intuition should spark the nurse to search the data to confirm or disprove the feeling. The nurse should ask the following:
- "Did the vital signs reflect any changes that account for the client's present status?"
- "When the client's status changed in this way last month, there was a specific reason for it. Is that what is happening here?"

LEVELS OF CRITICAL THINKING

Basic critical thinking

- A nurse trusts the experts and thinks concretely based on the rules.
- Basic critical thinking results from limited nursing knowledge and experience, as well as inadequate critical thinking experience.

> Example: A client reports pain 1 hr after receiving a pain medication. Instead of reassessing the client's pain, the nurse tells the client he must wait two more hours before he can receive another dose.

Complex critical thinking

- The nurse begins to express autonomy by analyzing and examining data to determine the best alternative.
- Complex critical thinking results from an increase in nursing knowledge, experience, intuition, and more flexible attitudes.

> Example: A nurse realizes that a client is not ambulating as often as prescribed because of a fear of missing her daughter's phone call. The nurse assures the client that the staff will listen for and answer her phone when she is out of her room.

Commitment

- The nurse expects to make choices without help from others and fully assumes the responsibility for those choices.
- Commitment results from an expert level of knowledge, experience, developed intuition, and reflective, flexible attitudes.

> Example: A nurse increases the rate of an IV fluid infusion when a client's blood pressure indicates hypovolemic shock 24 hr after surgery.

COMPONENTS OF CRITICAL THINKING

Knowledge

Information that's specific to nursing and comes from:
- Basic nursing education
- Use of evidence based practice
- Continuing education courses
- Advanced degrees and certifications

Experience

Decision-making ability derived from opportunities to observe, sense, and interact with clients followed by active reflection. A nurse:
- Demonstrates an understanding of clinical situations.
- Recognizes and analyzes cues for relevance.
- Incorporates experience into intuition.

Competence

Cognitive processes a nurse uses to make nursing judgments.

General critical thinking
- Scientific method
- Problem-solving
- Decision-making
- Diagnostic reasoning and inference
- Clinical decision-making; collaboration

Specific critical thinking in nursing: The nursing process (8.1)

Attitudes

Mindsets that affect how a nurse approaches a problem. Attitudes of critical thinkers include:
- **Confidence:** Feels sure of abilities.
- **Independence:** Analyzes ideas for logical reasoning.
- **Fairness:** Is objective, nonjudgmental.
- **Responsibility:** Adheres to standards of practice.
- **Risk taking:** Takes calculated chances in finding better solutions to problems.
- **Discipline:** Develops a systematic approach to thinking.
- **Perseverance:** Continues to work at a problem until there's a resolution.
- **Creativity:** Uses imagination to find solutions to unique client problems.
- **Curiosity:** Requires more information about clients and problems.
- **Integrity:** Practices truthfully and ethically.
- **Humility:** Acknowledges weaknesses.

8.1 Critical thinking and the nursing process

Assessment/Data collection
Collect information about a client's present health status to identify needs, and to identify additional data to collect based on findings.

CRITICAL THINKING SKILLS
- Observe.
- Use correct techniques for collecting data.
- Differentiate between relevant and irrelevant data, and between important and unimportant data.
- Organize, categorize, and validate data.
- Interpret assessment data and draw a conclusion.

Analysis/Data collection
Interpret or monitor the collected database, reach an appropriate nursing judgment about a client's health status and coping mechanisms, and provide direction for nursing care.

CRITICAL THINKING SKILLS
- Identify clusters and cues.
- Detect inferences.
- Recognize an actual or potential problem or risk.
- Avoid making judgments.

Planning
Establish priorities and optimal outcomes of care to measure and evaluate. Then, select the nursing interventions to include in a client's plan of care to promote, maintain, or restore health.

CRITICAL THINKING SKILLS
- Identify goals and outcomes for client care.
- Set priorities.
- Determine appropriate strategies and interventions for inclusion on a client's plan of care or teaching plan.
- Take knowledge and apply it to more than one situation.
- Create outcome criteria.
- Theorize.
- Consider the consequences of implementation.

Implementation
Provide care based on assessment data, analyses, and the plan of care.

CRITICAL THINKING SKILLS
- Use knowledge base.
- Use appropriate skills and teaching strategies.
- Test theories.
- Delegate and supervise nursing care.
- Communicate appropriately in response to a situation.

Evaluation
Examine a client's response to nursing interventions and form a clinical judgment about meeting goals and outcomes.

CRITICAL THINKING SKILLS
- Determine accuracy of theories.
- Evaluate outcomes based on specific criteria.
- Determine understanding of teaching.

Standards

Model for comparing care to determine acceptability, excellence, and appropriateness.
- Intellectual standards ensure the thorough application of critical thinking.
- Professional standards
  - Nursing judgment based on ethical criteria
  - Evaluation that relies on evidence based practice
  - Demonstration of professional responsibility
  - Promotes maximal level of nursing care

> **PRACTICE** Active Learning Scenario
>
> A nurse is reviewing with a group of newly licensed nurses the critical thinking skills nurses used during each of the steps of the nursing process. Use the ATI Active Learning Template: Basic Concept to complete this item.
>
> **NURSING INTERVENTIONS:** List at three critical thinking skills for each of the five steps of the nursing process.

Application Exercises

1. A nurse is caring for a client who is 24 hr postoperative following an inguinal hernia repair. The client is tolerating clear liquids well, has active bowel sounds, and is expressing a desire for "real food." The nurse tells the client that she will call the surgeon and ask. The surgeon hears the nurse's report and prescribes a full liquid diet. The nurse used which of the following levels of critical thinking?
   - A. Basic
   - B. Commitment
   - C. Complex
   - D. Integrity

2. A nurse receives a prescription for an antibiotic for a client who has cellulitis. The nurse checks the client's medical record, discovers that she is allergic to the antibiotic, and calls the provider to request a prescription for a different antibiotic. Which of the following critical thinking attitudes did the nurse demonstrate?
   - A. Fairness
   - B. Responsibility
   - C. Risk taking
   - D. Creativity

3. A nurse is caring for a client who is 24 hr postoperative following abdominal surgery. The nurse suspects the client's acute pain management is inadequate. Which of the following data reinforce this suspicion? (Select all that apply.)
   - A. The client seems easily agitated.
   - B. The client is nonadherent with coughing, deep breathing, and dangling.
   - C. The client may have pain medication every 4 to 6 hr but accepts it every 6 to 7 hr.
   - D. The client reports tenderness in his right lower leg.
   - E. The client's vital signs are heart rate 124/min, respiratory rate 22/min, temperature 37° C (98.6° F), and blood pressure 156/80 mm Hg.

4. A nurse is caring for a client who has a new prescription for antihypertensive medication. Prior to administering the medication, the nurse uses an electronic database to gather information about the medication and the effects it might have on this client. Which of the following components of critical thinking is the nurse using when he reviews the medication information?
   - A. Knowledge
   - B. Experience
   - C. Intuition
   - D. Competence

5. A nurse uses a head-to-toe approach to conduct a physical assessment of a client who will undergo surgery the following week. Which of the following critical thinking attitudes did the nurse demonstrate?
   - A. Confidence
   - B. Perseverance
   - C. Integrity
   - D. Discipline

Application Exercises Key

1. A. **CORRECT:** At the basic level, thinking is concrete and based on a set of rules, such as obtaining the prescription for diet progression.

   B. At the commitment level, the nurse expects to have to make choices without help from others and fully assumes the responsibility for those choices. However, postoperative protocols generally involve obtaining a prescription for diet progression.

   C. Advanced experience and knowledge at the complex level will prompt the nurse to request diet progression to full liquids based on active bowel sounds and the client's tolerance of clear liquid, not solely on the client's request.

   D. Integrity is a critical thinking attitude that comes into play when the nurse's opinion differs from that of the client. The nurse must then review her own position and decide how to proceed to help achieve outcomes satisfactory to all parties.

   Ⓝ *NCLEX® Connection: Management of Care, Advocacy*

2. A. Fairness is using a nonjudgmental, objective approach in looking at clients and situations. This attitude does not apply here.

   B. **CORRECT:** The nurse is responsible for administering medications in a safe manner and according to standards of practice. Checking the medical record for allergies helps ensure safety.

   C. Risk taking is a calculated approach to solving a problem that is not responding to traditional methods. This attitude does not apply here.

   D. Creativity is an approach that uses imagination to find solutions to unique client problems. This problem is not unique, and it requires a straightforward solution.

   Ⓝ *NCLEX® Connection: Safety and Infection Control, Accident/Error/Injury Prevention*

3. A. Without more data, this finding alone does not suggest that the client has unrelieved pain. It might be his usual disposition, a result of hospitalization and surgery, or many other factors.

   B. **CORRECT:** Refusal to perform interventions that could increase his pain level (coughing, deep breathing) supports that the client has unrelieved pain.

   C. **CORRECT:** Acceptance of pain medication only at or beyond the maximum interval suggests that the client has pain between the time the effects of the previous dose subside and the new dose takes effect.

   D. Sudden tenderness or swelling in a lower extremity is more likely to suggest a new problem, such as deep-vein thrombosis.

   E. **CORRECT:** Elevated blood pressure and pulse rate without elevated temperature or other signs of distress support that the client has unrelieved acute pain.

   Ⓝ *NCLEX® Connection: Pharmacological and Parenteral Therapies, Pharmacological Pain Management*

4. A. **CORRECT:** By using the electronic database, the nurse takes the initiative to increase his knowledge base, which is the first component of critical thinking.

   B. The nurse has had no prior experience with administering this medication to this client.

   C. Intuition requires experience, which the nurse lacks in administering this medication to this client.

   D. Competence involves making judgments, but no one can make a judgment about how the nurse handles researching and administering this medication to this client until he performs those tasks.

   Ⓝ *NCLEX® Connection: Pharmacological and Parenteral Therapies, Medication Administration*

5. A. Confidence is feeling sure of one's own abilities. The nurse might feel confident of her physical assessment skills, but choosing a particular method or sequence requires another attitude.

   B. Perseverance is continuing to work at a problem until the nurse resolves it. This attitude does not apply here.

   C. Integrity is a practicing truthfully and ethically. This specific attitude does not apply here.

   D. **CORRECT:** Discipline is developing a systematic approach to thinking. Proceeding head to toe is a systematic approach to collecting the data a physical assessment yields.

   Ⓝ *NCLEX® Connection: Health Promotion and Maintenance, Techniques of Physical Assessment*

PRACTICE Answer

Using the ATI Active Learning Template: Basic Concept

NURSING INTERVENTIONS

- Assessment/Data collection
  - Observe.
  - Use correct techniques for collecting data.
  - Differentiate between relevant and irrelevant data and between important and unimportant data.
  - Organize, categorize, and validate data.
  - Interpret assessment data and draw a conclusion.
- Analysis/Data Collection
  - Identify clusters and cues.
  - Detect inferences.
  - Recognize an actual or potential problem or risk.
  - Avoid making judgments.

- Planning
  - Identify goals and outcomes for client care.
  - Set priorities.
  - Determine appropriate strategies and interventions for inclusion on a plan of care or teaching plan.
  - Take knowledge and apply it to more than one situation.
  - Create outcome criteria.
  - Theorize.
  - Consider the consequences of implementation.

- Implementation
  - Use knowledge base.
  - Use appropriate skills and teaching strategies.
  - Test theories.
  - Delegate and supervise nursing care.
  - Communicate appropriately in response to a situation.
- Evaluation
  - Determine accuracy of theories.
  - Evaluate outcomes based on specific criteria.
  - Determine understanding of teaching.

Ⓝ *NCLEX® Connection: Management of Care, Legal Rights and Responsibilities*

UNIT 1   SAFE, EFFECTIVE CARE ENVIRONMENT
SECTION: MANAGEMENT OF CARE

CHAPTER 9   *Admissions, Transfers, and Discharge*

Responsibilities of nurses include ensuring continuity of care and information sharing throughout the processes of admission, transfers, and discharge. The admission assessment provides baseline data to use in the development of the nursing care plan. Comparisons with future assessments help monitor client status and response to treatment.

Many clients experience anxiety, fear of the unknown, and loss of independence and self-identity at the time of admission to the hospital or health care facility. Children can experience separation anxiety if parents are not present during the hospitalization. When nurses recognize clients' concerns and provide respectful, culturally sensitive care, the clients' experiences will be more positive.

NURSING CONSIDERATIONS

- Discharge planning is an interprofessional process that starts at admission. Nurses conduct discharge planning with clients and families for optimal results. Qᴛᴄ
- Nurses establish the ability of clients to participate in the admission assessment. Clients in distress or who have mental status changes might need to have a family member provide necessary information.
- Nurses begin establishing the therapeutic relationship with clients and families during the admission process.
- Nurses promote professional communication between providers.
- Nurses use the nursing process as a guide to plan teaching and interventions for clients during discharge.
- Nurses use standard handoff communication tools, such as Introduction, Situation, Background, Assessment, Recommendation (ISBAR) to facilitate transfers and discharges.

Admission process

EQUIPMENT

Prior to arrival of the client, bring necessary equipment into the room. This should include appropriate documentation forms, equipment to measure vital signs, a pulse oximeter, and hospital attire for the client.

PROCEDURE

- Introduce yourself and identify your role.
- Explain the roles of other care delivery staff.
- If in a semiprivate room, introduce the client to his roommate.
- Provide hospital attire and assist as necessary.
- Position the client comfortably.
- Apply the identification bracelet and allergy band, if needed.
- Provide facility-specific brochures and informational material.
- Provide information about advance directives.
- Document the client's advance directives status in the medical record. Place a copy in the medical record if it is available.

ASSESS/COLLECT DATA

Baseline data: Vital signs, height, weight, allergy status

Biographical information

Client's reason for seeking health care

Present illness and symptoms

Health history
- Current illness
- Current medications (prescription and over-the-counter)
- Prior illnesses, chronic diseases
- Surgeries
- Previous hospitalizations
- Other relevant data

Family history (hypertension, cancer, heart disease, diabetes mellitus)

Psychosocial assessment
- Alcohol, tobacco, drug, and caffeine use
- History of mental illness
- History of abuse or homelessness
- Home situation/significant others

Nutrition
- Current diet, any chewing or swallowing problems
- Recent weight gain/loss
- Use of nutritional or herbal supplements
- Dentures

Spiritual health/quality-of-life concerns
- Religion
- Advance directives, living will

Review of systems

Safety assessments Qs
- History of falls
- Sensory deficits (vision, hearing)
- Use of assistive devices (walker, cane, crutches, wheelchair)

Discharge information
- Family members in the home
- Transportation for discharge
- Relevant phone numbers
- Medical equipment needs at home
- Home health care needs at home

INVENTORY PERSONAL ITEMS

Examples are clothing, jewelry, money, credit cards, assistive devices (eyeglasses, contacts, hearing aids, cane, dentures), medications, cell phones and other technology devices, and religious articles.
- Discourage keeping valuables at the bedside.
- Document communication with client related to items left within the room, and valuables locked in the facility's safe.

ORIENTATION

Orient the client and family to the room and the facility. Share information, including the following. Qs
- Call light operation
- Electric bed operation
- Telephone services/television controls
- Overhead lighting operation
- Smoking policy
- Restroom locations
- Waiting areas
- Meal times
- Usual time for providers' visits
- Dining/vending services
- Visiting policies

Transfer and discharge process

INDICATIONS FOR TRANSFER AND DISCHARGE

- The level of care changed (e.g., health status improved so a client no longer needs intensive care).
- Another setting is required to provide necessary care (e.g., transfer from medical unit to surgical suite).
- The facility does not offer the type of care a client now requires (e.g., after the acute phase of a stroke, the client requires care in a skilled facility).
- The client no longer needs inpatient care and is ready to return home.

DISCHARGE PLANNING

This should begin on admission for every patient.
- Assess whether the client will be able to return to his previous residence.
- Determine whether the client needs or has someone to assist him at home.
- Assess the residence to see if the client needs adaptations or specific equipment. Qs
- Make a referral to the social worker to arrange for community services.
- Communicate health status and needs to community service providers.
- The provider documents that the client may be discharged. However, a client who is legally competent has the right to leave the facility at any time. The nurse notifies the client's provider, has the client sign the proper forms if possible, and provides discharge teaching.
- Involve the client and family as much as possible in the discharge planning.

DISCHARGE EDUCATION

The nurse discusses the discharge instructions with the client and provides a printed copy.
- Instructions should use clear, concise language that the client will understand.
- The nurse should verify understanding of the instructions by the client.

Standards for discharge education
- Identifying safety concerns at home
- Reviewing symptoms of potential complications and when to contact emergency care or the provider
- Providing the phone number of the provider
- Providing names and phone numbers of community resources that give care at the client's residence
- Step-by-step instructions for performing continuing treatments, such as dressing changes
- Dietary restrictions and guidelines, including those that pertain to medication administration
- Amount and frequency of therapies to perform to support continued independence at home
- Directions how to take medications, potential interactions, and why adherence is important

EQUIPMENT

Items to transfer/discharge with the client

- Personal belongings at the bedside and from dresser drawers and closet (flowers, books, clothing, personal care items)
- Valuables from the safe (if leaving the facility)
- Medications (especially that belong to the client or that cannot be returned to the pharmacy for credit)
- Assistive devices
- Medical records or a transfer form

PROCEDURE

RESPONSIBILITIES OF THE NURSE

Transferring/discharging a client

- On the day and time of transfer, confirm that the receiving facility or unit is expecting the client, and that the room or bed is available.
- Communicate the time the client will transfer to the receiving facility or unit.
- Complete documentation (medical records, transfer form).
- Give a verbal transfer report in person or via telephone.
- Confirm the mode of transportation the client will use to complete the transfer or discharge (car, wheelchair, ambulance).
- Make sure the client is dressed appropriately if going outside the facility.
- Account for all the client's valuables.

Receiving a transferred client

- Have any specialized equipment ready.
- If appropriate, inform the client's roommate of the impending admission or transfer.
- Inform other health care team members of the client's arrival and needs.
- Meet with the client and family on arrival to complete the admission process and orient the client and family to the new facility or unit.
- Assess how the client tolerates the transfer.
- Review transfer documentation.
- Implement appropriate nursing interventions in a timely manner.

TRANSFER DOCUMENTATION

- Medical diagnosis and care providers
- Demographic information
- Overview of health status, plan of care, and recent progress
- Alterations that can precipitate an immediate concern
- Notification of assessments or care essential within the next few hours
- Most recent vital signs and medications, including PRN
- Allergies
- Diet and activity orders **Qs**
- Specific equipment or adaptive devices (oxygen, suction, wheelchair)
- Advance directives and emergency code status
- Family involvement in care and health care proxy, if applicable

DISCHARGE DOCUMENTATION

- Type of discharge (provider prescription or against medical advice [AMA])
- Date and time of discharge, who went with the client, and transportation (wheelchair to car, gurney to ambulance)
- Where the client went (home, long-term care facility)
- Summary of the client's condition at discharge (steady gait, ambulating independently, in no apparent distress)
- Description of any unresolved difficulties and procedures for follow up
- Disposition of valuables, medications brought from home, and prescriptions

DISCHARGE INSTRUCTIONS

Documentation of understanding of instructions by the client.

- Written instructions in the client's language
- Diet at home
- Step-by-step instructions for procedures at home
- Precautions to take when performing procedures or administering medications
- Signs and symptoms of complications to report
- Names and numbers of providers and community services to contact
- Plans for follow-up care and therapies

Application Exercises

1. A nurse is performing an admission assessment for an older adult client. After gathering the assessment data and performing the review of systems, which of the following actions is a priority for the nurse?

    A. Orient the client to his room.

    B. Conduct a client care conference.

    C. Review medical prescriptions.

    D. Develop a plan of care.

2. A nurse is admitting a client who has acute cholecystitis to a medical-surgical unit. Which of the following actions are essential steps of the admission procedure? (Select all that apply.)

    A. Explain the roles of other care delivery staff.

    B. Begin discharge planning.

    C. Inform the client that advance directives are required for hospital admission.

    D. Document the client's wishes about organ donation.

    E. Introduce the client to his roommate.

3. A nurse is caring for a client who had a stroke and is scheduled for transfer to a rehabilitation center. Which of the following tasks are the responsibility of the nurse at the transferring facility? (Select all that apply.)

    A. Ensure that the client has possession of his valuables.

    B. Confirm that the rehabilitation center has a room available at the time of transfer.

    C. Assess how the client tolerates the transfer.

    D. Give a verbal transfer report via telephone.

    E. Complete a transfer form for the receiving facility.

4. A nurse is preparing the discharge summary for a client who has had knee arthroplasty and is going home. Which of the following information about the client should the nurse include in the discharge summary? (Select all that apply.)

    A. Advance directives status

    B. Follow-up care

    C. Instructions for diet and medications

    D. Most recent vital sign data

    E. Contact information for the home health care agency

5. As part of the admission process, a nurse at a long-term care facility is gathering a nutrition history for a client who has dementia. Which of the following components of the nutrition evaluation is the priority for the nurse to determine from the client's family?

    A. Body mass index

    B. Usual times for meals and snacks

    C. Favorite foods

    D. Any difficulty swallowing

PRACTICE Active Learning Scenario

A nurse is reviewing with a group of newly licensed nurses the essential components of an admission assessment. Use the ATI Active Learning Template: Basic Concept to complete this item.

NURSING INTERVENTIONS: List at least three aspects of the health history the nurse must gather and document, as well as at least three aspects of the psychosocial evaluation the nurse must gather and document.

Application Exercises Key

1. A. **CORRECT:** The greatest risk to this client is injury from unfamiliar surroundings. Therefore, the priority action is to orient the client to the room. Before the nurse leaves the room, the client should know how to use the call light and other equipment at the bedside.

   B. The nurse should conduct a client care conference. However, another action is the priority.

   C. The nurse should review prescriptions in the medical record. However, another action is the priority.

   D. The nurse should develop a plan of care. However, another action is the priority.

   Ⓝ *NCLEX® Connection: Management of Care, Continuity of Care*

2. A. **CORRECT:** The client's hospitalization is likely to be more positive if the client understands who can perform which care activities.

   B. **CORRECT:** Unless the client is entering a long-term care facility, discharge planning should begin on admission.

   C. The Patient Self-Determination Act does not require that clients have advance directives prior to hospital admission. The act requires asking clients if they have advance directives.

   D. **CORRECT:** Upon hospital admission, required request laws direct providers to ask clients older than 18 years if they are organ or tissue donors.

   E. **CORRECT:** Any action that can reduce the stress of hospitalization is therapeutic. Introductions to other clients and staff can encourage communication and psychological comfort.

   Ⓝ *NCLEX® Connection: Management of Care, Continuity of Care*

3. A. **CORRECT:** The nurse should account for all of the client's valuable at the time of transfer.

   B. **CORRECT:** On the day of the transfer, the nurse should confirm that the receiving facility is expecting the client and that the room is available.

   C. It is the responsibility of the nurse at the receiving facility to assess the client upon arrival to determine how he tolerated the transfer.

   D. **CORRECT:** The nurse should provide the nurse at the receiving facility with a verbal transfer report in person or via telephone.

   E. **CORRECT:** The nurse should complete any documentation for the transfer, including a transfer form and the client's medical records.

   Ⓝ *NCLEX® Connection: Management of Care, Continuity of Care*

4. A. Advance directives status is important in transfer documentation, when other care providers will take over a client's care. They are not an essential component of a discharge summary for a client who is returning to his home.

   B. **CORRECT:** It is essential to include the names and contact information of providers and community resources the client will need after he returns home.

   C. **CORRECT:** The client will need written information detailing his medication and dietary therapy at home. A client who has had knee arthroscopy typically requires analgesics, possibly anticoagulants, and dietary instructions for avoiding postoperative complications such as constipation.

   D. Vital sign measurements are important in transfer documentation, when other care providers will take over a client's care. They are not an essential component of a discharge summary for a client who is returning home.

   E. **CORRECT:** It is essential to include the names and contact information of providers and community resources the client will need after returning home. For example, a client who had a knee arthroplasty might require physical therapy at home until he can travel to a physical therapy department or facility.

   Ⓝ *NCLEX® Connection: Management of Care, Continuity of Care*

5. A. It is important to calculate body mass index to help determine appropriateness of the client's weight status and related risks. However, there is a higher priority.

   B. It is important for the nurse to know and try to follow the meal schedule the client follows at home. However, there is a higher priority.

   C. It is important for the nurse to know which foods are the client's favorites in case it becomes difficult to get the client to consume adequate nutrients. However, there is a higher priority.

   D. **CORRECT:** The greatest risk to this client related to a nutrition-related evaluation is from difficulty swallowing, or dysphagia. It puts the client at risk for aspiration, which can be life-threatening.

   Ⓝ *NCLEX® Connection: Basic Care and Comfort, Nutrition and Oral Hydration*

PRACTICE Answer

Using the ATI Active Learning Template: Basic Concept

NURSING INTERVENTIONS

Health history
- Current illness
- Current medications (prescription, herbal supplements, and over the counter)
- Prior illnesses, chronic diseases
- Surgeries
- Previous hospitalizations

Psychosocial assessment
- Alcohol, tobacco, drug, and caffeine use
- History of mental illness
- History of abuse or homelessness
- Home situation/significant others

Ⓝ *NCLEX® Connection: Management of Care, Continuity of Care*

When reviewing the following chapters, keep in mind the relevant topics and tasks of the NCLEX outline, in particular:

Client Needs: Safety and Infection Control

ACCIDENT/ERROR/INJURY PREVENTION: Identify deficits that may impede client safety.

ERGONOMIC PRINCIPLES: Assess client ability to balance, transfer, and use assistive devices prior to planning care.

HOME SAFETY: Educate client on home safety issues.

REPORTING OF INCIDENT/EVENT/IRREGULAR OCCURRENCE/ VARIANCE: Acknowledge and document practice error.

SAFE USE OF EQUIPMENT: Teach client about the safe use of equipment needed for health care.

STANDARD PRECAUTIONS/TRANSMISSION-BASED PRECAUTIONS/ SURGICAL ASEPSIS: Apply principles of infection control.

CHAPTER 10 *Medical and Surgical Asepsis*

Asepsis is the absence of illness-producing micro-organisms. Hand hygiene is the primary behavior.

Medical asepsis refers to the use of precise practices to reduce the number, growth, and spread of micro-organisms ("clean technique"). It applies to administering oral medication, managing nasogastric tubes, providing personal hygiene, and performing many other common nursing tasks.

Surgical asepsis refers to the use of precise practices to eliminate all micro-organisms from an object or area and prevent contamination ("sterile technique"). It applies to parenteral medication administration, insertion of urinary catheters, surgical procedures, sterile dressing changes, and many other common nursing procedures.

Before beginning any task or procedure that requires aseptic technique, health care team members must check for latex allergies. If the client or any member of the team has a latex allergy, the team must use latex-free gloves, equipment, and supplies. Qs

PRACTICES THAT PROMOTE MEDICAL ASEPSIS

HAND HYGIENE

Always use hand hygiene. Handwashing with an antimicrobial or plain soap and water; using alcohol-based products such as gels, foams, and rinses; or performing a surgical scrub.
- The three essential components of handwashing are the following:
  ○ Soap
  ○ Running water
  ○ Friction
- All health care personnel must perform hand hygiene, either with an alcohol-based product or with soap and water, before and after every client contact, and after removing gloves. When hands are visibly soiled, after contact with body fluids, before eating, and after using the restroom, wash them with a nonantimicrobial or antimicrobial soap and water. It is also important for clients and visitors to practice hand hygiene.
- Perform hand hygiene using recommended antiseptic solutions when caring for clients who are immunocompromised or have infections with multidrug-resistant or extremely virulent micro-organisms.
- Perform hand hygiene after contact with anything in clients' rooms and after touching any contaminated items, whether or not gloves were worn, and before putting gloves on and after taking them off. Performing hand hygiene might be necessary between tasks and procedures on the same client to prevent cross-contamination of different body sites.
- Wash hands with soap and warm water. Rub hands together vigorously, and rinse under running water. Wash for at least 15 seconds to remove transient flora and up to 2 min when hands are more soiled. After washing, dry hands with a clean paper towel before turning off the faucet. If the sink does not have foot or knee pedals for turning off the water, use a clean, dry paper towel to turn off the faucet(s). Q EBP
- For hand hygiene with an alcohol-based product, dispense the manufacturer's recommended amount (usually 3 to 5 mL) in the palm of the hand. Rub hands together vigorously, remembering to cover all surfaces of both hands and fingers. Continue to rub until both hands are completely dry.

ADDITIONAL PERSONAL HYGIENE MEASURES

- Emphasize the importance of covering the mouth and nose when coughing or sneezing, using and disposing of facial tissues, and performing hand hygiene to prevent spraying and spreading droplet infections. Encourage clients and visitors to practice respiratory hygiene/cough etiquette. Ensure spatial separation of 3 ft from those with a cough, or have them wear a mask.
- Wash hair frequently and keep it short or pulled back to prevent contamination of the care area or the clients.
- Keep natural nails short and clean and free of nail gels and acrylic nails. The area around and under the nails can harbor micro-organisms.
- Remove jewelry from hands and wrists to facilitate hand disinfection.

PROTECTIVE CLOTHING

Use masks, gloves, gowns, and protective eyewear to help control the contact and spread of micro-organisms to staff and clients.

PHYSICAL ENVIRONMENT

Additional examples of practices that reduce the growth and spread of micro-organisms are changing linens daily, cleaning floors and bedside stands, and separating clean from contaminated materials.

- Do not place items on the floor (even soiled laundry). The floor is grossly contaminated.
- Do not shake linens because doing so can spread micro-organisms in the air. Keep soiled items from touching clothing.
- Clean the least soiled areas first to prevent moving more contaminants into the cleaner areas.
- Use plastic bags for moist, soiled items, following facility protocol for bag selection, to prevent further contamination of items or of individuals handling the soiled items. Put all soiled items directly into the appropriate receptacle to avoid handling soiled items more than once.
- Place all laboratory specimens in biohazard containers or bags for transport or disposal.
- Pour any liquids used for client care directly into the drain and avoid splattering to prevent spreading droplets. Empty body fluids at water level of toilet to avoid splashing.

PRACTICES THAT MAINTAIN A STERILE FIELD

Prolonged exposure to airborne micro-organisms can make sterile items nonsterile.
- Avoid coughing, sneezing, and talking directly over a sterile field.
- Advise clients to avoid sudden movements, refrain from touching supplies, drapes, or the nurse's gloves and gown, and avoid coughing, sneezing, or talking over a sterile field.

Only sterile items may be in a sterile field.
- The outer wrappings and 1-inch edges of packaging that contains sterile items are not sterile. The inner surface of the sterile drape or kit, except for that 1-inch border around the edges, is the sterile field to which other sterile items may be added. To position the field on the table surface, grasp the 1-inch border before donning sterile gloves. Discard any object that comes into contact with the 1-inch border. **Qs**
- Touch sterile materials only with sterile gloves.
- Consider any object held below the waist or above the chest contaminated.
- Sterile materials may touch other sterile surfaces or materials; however, contact with nonsterile materials at any time contaminates a sterile area, no matter how short the contact.

Microbes can move by gravity from a nonsterile item to a sterile item.
- Do not reach across or above a sterile field.
- Do not turn your back on a sterile field.
- Hold items to add to a sterile field at a minimum of 6 inches above the field.

Any sterile, non-waterproof wrapper that comes in contact with moisture becomes nonsterile by a wicking action that allows microbes to travel rapidly from a nonsterile surface to the sterile surface.
- Keep all surfaces dry.
- Discard any sterile packages that are torn, punctured, or wet.

NURSING INTERVENTIONS

EQUIPMENT

- Select a clean area above waist level in the client's environment (a bedside stand) to set up the sterile field.
- Check that all sterile packages (additional dressings, sterile bowl, sterile gloves, and solution) are dry and intact and have a future expiration date. Any chemical tape must show the appropriate color change.
- Make sure an appropriate waste receptacle is nearby.

PROCEDURE

Perform hand hygiene.

STERILE FIELD SETUP
- Open the covering of the package per the manufacturer's directions, slipping the package onto the center of the workspace with the top flap of the wrapper opening away from the body.
- Grasp the tip of the top flap of the package, and with arm positioned away from the sterile field, unfold the top flap away from body. **Qs**
- Next, open the side flaps, using the right hand for the right flap and the left hand for the left flap.
- Grasp the last flap and turn it down toward the body.

ADDITIONAL STERILE PACKAGES

- Open next to the sterile field by holding the bottom edge with one hand and pulling back on the top flap with the other hand. Place the packages that will be used last furthest from the sterile field; open these first.
- Add them directly to the sterile field. Lift the package from the dry surface, holding it 15 cm (6 in) above the sterile field, pulling the two surfaces apart, and dropping it onto the sterile field.

POUR STERILE SOLUTIONS

- Removing the bottle cap.
- Placing the bottle cap face up on a clean (nonsterile) surface.
- Holding the bottle with the label in the palm of the hand so that the solution does not run down the label.
- First pouring a small amount (1 to 2 mL) of the solution into an available receptacle.
- Pouring the solution (without splashing) onto the dressing or site without touching the bottle to the site.

STERILE GLOVES

- Once the sterile field is set up, don sterile gloves.
- Sterile gloving includes opening the wrapper and handling only the outside of the wrapper. Don gloves by using the following steps.
- With the cuff side pointing toward the body, use the nondominant hand and pick up the dominant-hand glove by grasping the folded bottom edge of the cuff and lifting it up and away from the wrapper.
- While picking up the edge of the cuff, pull the dominant glove onto the hand.
- With the sterile dominant-gloved hand, place the fingers of the dominant hand inside the cuff of the nondominant glove, lifting it off the wrapper and putting the nondominant hand into it.
- When both hands are gloved, adjust the fingers.
- During that time, only a sterile gloved hand may touch the other sterile gloved hand.
- At the close of the sterile procedure or if the gloves tear, remove the gloves. Take them off by grasping the outer part of one glove at the cuff area, avoiding touching the wrist and pulling the glove down over the fingers and into the hand that is still gloved. Then, place the ungloved hand inside the soiled glove and pull the glove off so that it is inside out and only the clean inside part is exposed. Discard into an appropriate receptacle.

Application Exercises

1. When entering a client's room to change a surgical dressing, a nurse notes that the client is coughing and sneezing. Which of the following actions should the nurse take when preparing the sterile field?

    A. Keep the sterile field at least 6 ft away from the client's bedside.

    B. Instruct the client to refrain from coughing and sneezing during the dressing change.

    C. Place a mask on the client to limit the spread of micro-organisms into the surgical wound.

    D. Keep a box of facial tissues nearby for the client to use during the dressing change.

2. A nurse has removed a sterile pack from its outside cover and placed it on a clean work surface in preparation for an invasive procedure. Which of the following flaps should the nurse unfold first?

    A. The flap closest to the body

    B. The right side flap

    C. The left side flap

    D. The flap farthest from the body

3. A nurse is wearing sterile gloves in preparation for performing a sterile procedure. Which of the following objects can the nurse touch without breaching sterile technique? (Select all that apply.)

    A. A bottle containing a sterile solution

    B. The edge of the sterile drape at the base of the field

    C. The inner wrapping of an item on the sterile field

    D. An irrigation syringe on the sterile field

    E. One gloved hand with the other gloved hand

4. A nurse is reviewing hand hygiene techniques with a group of assistive personnel (AP). Which of the following instructions should the nurse include when discussing handwashing? (Select all that apply.)

    A. Apply 3 to 5 mL of liquid soap to dry hands.

    B. Wash the hands with soap and water for at least 15 seconds.

    C. Rinse the hands with hot water.

    D. Use a clean paper towel to turn off hand faucets.

    E. Allow the hands to air dry after washing.

5. A nurse has prepared a sterile field for assisting a provider with a chest tube insertion. Which of the following events should the nurse recognize as contaminating the sterile field? (Select all that apply.)

    A. The provider drops a sterile instrument onto the near side of the sterile field.

    B. The nurse moistens a cotton ball with sterile normal saline and places it on the sterile field.

    C. The procedure is delayed 1 hr because the provider receives an emergency call.

    D. The nurse turns to speak to someone who enters through the door behind the nurse.

    E. The client's hand brushes against the outer edge of the sterile field.

Application Exercises Key

1. A. It would be difficult for the nurse to maintain a sterile field away from the bedside. But more important, this might not have any effect on the transmission of some micro-organisms.

   B. The client might be unable to refrain from coughing and sneezing during the dressing change.

   C. **CORRECT:** Placing a mask on the client prevents contamination of the surgical wound during the dressing change.

   D. Keeping tissues close by for the client to use still allows contamination of the surgical wound.

   Ⓝ *NCLEX® Connection: Safety and Infection Control, Standard Precautions/Transmission-Based Precautions/Surgical Asepsis*

2. A. The flap closest to the nurse's body is the innermost flap and the last one to unfold.

   B. The nurse should unfold the side flap that is closest to the top of the package before the one underneath it; however, there is another flap the nurse should unfold first.

   C. The nurse should unfold the side flap that is closest to the top of the package before the one underneath it; however, there is another flap the nurse should unfold first.

   D. **CORRECT:** The priority goal in setting up a sterile field is to maintain sterility and thus reduce the risk to the client's safety. Unless the nurse pulls the top flap (the one farthest from her body) away from her body first, she risks touching part of the inner surface of the wrap and thus contaminating it.

   Ⓝ *NCLEX® Connection: Safety and Infection Control, Standard Precautions/Transmission-Based Precautions/Surgical Asepsis*

3. A. A bottle of sterile solution is sterile on the inside and nonsterile on the outside. The nurse must prepare the sterile container of solution on the field before putting on sterile gloves.

   B. The 1-inch border at the outer edge of the sterile field is not sterile. The nurse may not touch it with sterile gloves.

   C. **CORRECT:** The inner wrappings of any objects the nurse dropped onto the sterile field are sterile. The nurse may touch them with sterile gloves.

   D. **CORRECT:** Any objects the nurse dropped onto the sterile field during the setup are sterile. The nurse may touch the syringe with sterile gloves.

   E. **CORRECT:** One sterile gloved hand may touch the other sterile gloved hand because both are sterile.

   Ⓝ *NCLEX® Connection: Safety and Infection Control, Standard Precautions/Transmission-Based Precautions/Surgical Asepsis*

4. A. The APs should apply alcohol rubs to dry hands, and wet the hands first before applying soap for handwashing.

   B. **CORRECT:** This is the amount of time it takes to remove transient flora from the hands. For soiled hands, the recommendation is 2 minutes.

   C. The APs should use warm water to minimize the removal of protective skin oils.

   D. **CORRECT:** If the sink does not have foot or knee pedals, the APs should turn off the water with a clean paper towel and not with their hands.

   E. The APs should dry their hands with a clean paper towel. This helps prevent chapped skin.

   Ⓝ *NCLEX® Connection: Safety and Infection Control, Standard Precautions/Transmission-Based Precautions/Surgical Asepsis*

5. A. As long as the provider has not reached over the sterile field, such as by placing the instrument on a near portion of the field, the field remains sterile.

   B. **CORRECT:** Fluid permeation of the sterile drape or barrier contaminates the field.

   C. **CORRECT:** Prolonged exposure to air contaminates a sterile field.

   D. **CORRECT:** Turning away from a sterile field contaminates the field because the nurse cannot see if a piece of clothing or hair made contact with the field.

   E. The 1-inch border at the outer edge of the sterile field is not sterile. Unless the client reached farther into the field, the field remains sterile.

   Ⓝ *NCLEX® Connection: Safety and Infection Control, Standard Precautions/Transmission-Based Precautions/Surgical Asepsis*

PRACTICE Active Learning Scenario

A nurse is reviewing with a newly licensed nurse the procedure for putting on sterile gloves. Use the ATI Active Learning Template: Nursing Skill to complete this item.

DESCRIPTION OF SKILL: List the steps involved in putting on a pair of sterile gloves.

PRACTICE Answer

Using the ATI Active Learning Template: Nursing Skill

DESCRIPTION OF SKILL

- With the cuff side pointing toward the body, use the nondominant hand to pick up the dominant-hand glove by grasping the folded bottom edge of the cuff and lifting it up and away from the wrapper.
- While picking up the edge of the cuff, pull the dominant glove onto the hand.
- With the sterile dominant-gloved hand, place the fingers of the dominant hand inside the cuff of the nondominant glove, lifting it off the wrapper and putting the nondominant hand into it.
- Adjust the fingers.

Ⓝ *NCLEX® Connection: Safety and Infection Control, Standard Precautions/Transmission-Based Precautions/Surgical Asepsis*

CHAPTER 11 *Infection Control*

An infection occurs when the presence of a pathogen leads to a chain of events. All components of the chain must be present and intact for the infection to occur. A nurse uses infection control practices (medical asepsis, surgical asepsis, standard precautions) to break the chain and thus stop the spread of infection.

TYPES OF PATHOGEN

Pathogens are the micro-organisms or microbes that cause infections.
- **Bacteria** (*Staphylococcus aureus*, *Escherichia coli*, *Mycobacterium tuberculosis*)
- **Viruses**: Organisms that use the host's genetic machinery to reproduce (HIV, hepatitis, herpes zoster, herpes simplex)
- **Fungi**: Molds and yeasts (*Candida albicans*, Aspergillus)
- **Prions**: Protein particles (new variant Creutzfeldt-Jakob disease)
- **Parasites**: Protozoa (malaria, toxoplasmosis) and helminths (worms [flatworms, roundworms], flukes [Schistosoma])

Virulence is the ability of a pathogen to invade and injure a host.

Herpes zoster is a common viral infection that erupts years after exposure to chickenpox and invades a specific nerve tract.

IMMUNE DEFENSES

Nonspecific innate

Native immunity restricts entry or immediately responds to a foreign organism (antigen) through the activation of phagocytic cells, complement, and inflammation. This occurs with all micro-organisms, regardless of previous exposure.

Passive: Antibodies are produced by an external source.
- Temporary immunity that does not have memory of past exposures
- Intact skin, the body's first line of defense
- Mucous membranes, secretions, enzymes, phagocytic cells, and protective proteins
- Inflammatory response with phagocytic cells, the complement system, and interferons localize the invasion and prevent its spread

Specific adaptive immunity

Specific adaptive immunity allows the body to make antibodies in response to a foreign organism (antigen). This reaction directs against an identifiable micro-organism.

Active: Antibodies are produced in response to an antigen.
- Requires time to react to antigens
- Provides permanent immunity
- Involves B– and T–lymphocytes
- Produces specific antibodies against specific antigens (immunoglobulins [IgA, IgD, IgE, IgG, IgM])

INFECTION PROCESS

Chain of infection (11.1)

Causative agent (bacteria, virus, fungus, prion, parasite)

Reservoir (human, animal, food, organic matter on inanimate surfaces, water, soil, insects)

Portal of exit from (means for leaving) the host
- Respiratory tract (droplet, airborne): *Mycobacterium tuberculosis* and *Streptococcus pneumoniae*
- Gastrointestinal tract: Shigella, *Salmonella enteritidis*, *Salmonella typhi*, hepatitis A
- Genitourinary tract: *Escherichia coli*, hepatitis A, herpes simplex virus (type 1), HIV
- Skin/mucous membranes: Herpes simplex virus and varicella
- Blood/body fluids: HIV and hepatitis B and C
- Transplacental

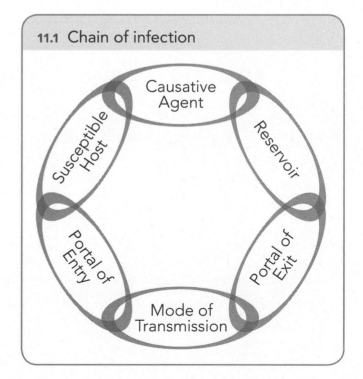

11.1 Chain of infection

Mode of transmission

- Contact
  - Direct physical contact: Person to person
  - Indirect contact with an inanimate object: Object to person
  - Fecal–oral transmission: Handling food after using a restroom and failing to wash hands
- Droplet: Sneezing, coughing, and talking
- Airborne: Sneezing and coughing
- Vector borne: Animals or insects as intermediaries (ticks transmit Lyme disease; mosquitoes transmit West Nile and malaria)

Portal of entry to the host: Might be the same as the portal of exit

Susceptible host: Compromised defense mechanisms (immunocompromised, breaks in skin) leave the host more susceptible to infections.

Stages of an infection

Incubation: interval between the pathogen entering the body and the presentation of the first symptom.

Prodromal stage: interval from onset of general symptoms to more distinct symptoms. During this time, the pathogen is multiplying.

Illness stage: interval when symptoms specific to the infection occur.

Convalescence: interval when acute symptoms disappear. Total recovery could take days to months.

11.2 Health-care associated infections

Health-care associated infections (HAIs) are infections that a client acquires while receiving care in a health care setting. Formerly called nosocomial infections, these can come from an exogenous source (from outside the client) or an endogenous source (inside the client when part of the client's flora is altered).

- Often occur in the intensive care unit.
- The best way to prevent HAIs is through frequent and effective hand hygiene.
- A common site of HAIs is the urinary tract and these are often caused by *Escherichia coli, Staphylococcus aureus,* and enterococci. Other sites of HAIs are surgical wounds, the respiratory tract, and the bloodstream.
- An iatrogenic infection is a type of HAI resulting from a diagnostic or therapeutic procedure.
- HAIs are not always preventable and are not always iatrogenic.
- Use current evidence-based practice guidelines to prevent HAIs due to multidrug-resistant organisms.

ASSESSMENT/DATA COLLECTION

RISK FACTORS

A nurse should assess each client for the risks of infection specific to the client, the disease or injury, and the environment. The most common risks include:

- Inadequate hand hygiene (client and caregivers).
- Individuals who have compromised health or defenses against infection, which include:
  - Those who are immunocompromised.
  - Those who have had surgery.
  - Those with indwelling devices.
  - A break in the skin (the body's best protection against infection).
  - Those with poor oxygenation.
  - Those with impaired circulation.
  - Those who have chronic or acute disease, such as diabetes mellitus, adrenal insufficiency, renal failure, hepatic failure, or chronic lung disease.
- Caregivers using medical or surgical asepsis that does not follow the established standards. **(11.2)**
- Clients who have poor personal hygiene or poor nutrition, smoke, or consume excessive amounts of alcohol, and those experiencing stress.
- Clients who live in a very crowded environment.
- **OLDER ADULT CLIENTS:** Older adults have a slowed response to antibiotic therapy, slowed immune response, loss of subcutaneous tissue and thinning of the skin, decreased vascularity and slowed wound healing, decreased cough and gag reflexes, chronic illnesses, decreased gastric acid production, decreased mobility, bowel and bladder incontinence, dementia, and greater incidence of invasive devices such as a urinary catheter or feeding tube. Ⓖ
- Individuals who make poor lifestyle choices that put them at risk, which include:
  - Clients who use IV drugs and share needles.
  - Clients who engage in unprotected sex.
- Clients who have recently been exposed to:
  - Poor sanitation.
  - Mosquito–borne or parasitic diseases.
  - Diseases endemic to the area visited, but not in the client's home country.

EXPECTED FINDINGS

- Findings identifiable in the nursing assessment of generalized or systemic infection include the following.
  - Fever
  - Presence of chills, which occur when temperature is rising, and diaphoresis, which occurs when temperature is decreasing
  - Increased pulse and respiratory rate (in response to the high fever)
  - Malaise
  - Fatigue
  - Anorexia, nausea, and vomiting
  - Abdominal cramping and diarrhea
  - Enlarged lymph nodes (repositories for "waste")

- OLDER ADULT CLIENTS
  - Older adults have a reduced inflammatory and immune response and thus might have an advanced infection before it is identified. Atypical findings such as agitation, confusion, or incontinence can be the only manifestations. Ⓒ
  - Other findings can vary depending on the site of the infection (dyspnea, cough, purulent sputum, and crackles in lung fields, dysuria, urinary frequency, hematuria and pyuria, rash, skin lesions, purulent wound drainage, erythema and odynophagia, dysphagia, hyperemia, enlarged tonsils, change in level of consciousness, nuchal rigidity, photophobia, headache)
- Inflammation is the body's local response to injury or infection. The inflammatory response has three stages.
  - Findings during the first stage of the inflammatory response (local infection) include the following.
    - Redness (from dilation of arterioles bringing blood to the area)
    - Warmth of the area on palpation
    - Edema
    - Pain or tenderness
    - Loss of use of the affected part
  - In the second stage, the micro-organisms are killed. Fluid containing dead tissue cells and WBCs accumulates and exudate appears at the site of the infection. The exudate leaves the body by draining into the lymph system. The types of exudate are:
    - Serous (clear).
    - Sanguineous (contains red blood cells).
    - Purulent (contains leukocytes and bacteria).
  - In the third stage, damaged tissue is replaced by scar tissue. Gradually, the new cells take on characteristics that are similar in structure and function to the old cells.

LABORATORY TESTS

- Leukocytosis (WBCs greater than 10,000/µL)
- Increases in the specific types of WBCs on differential (left shift = an increase in neutrophils)
- Elevated erythrocyte sedimentation rate (ESR) over 20 mm/hr; an increase indicates an active inflammatory process or infection
- Presence of micro-organisms on culture of the specific fluid/area

DIAGNOSTIC PROCEDURES

- Gallium scan: Nuclear scan that uses a radioactive substance to identify hot spots of WBCs
- Radioactive gallium citrate: Injected by IV and accumulates in area of inflammation
- X-rays, CT scan, magnetic resonance imaging (MRI), and biopsies to determine the presence of infection, abscesses, and lesions

PATIENT-CENTERED CARE

NURSING CARE

- Use frequent and effective hand hygiene before and after care.
- Educate the client about the required and recommended immunizations and where to obtain them. The target groups include children, older adults, those with chronic disease, and those who are immunocompromised and their families and contacts.
- Educate the client and ask for a return demonstration of good oral hygiene. Good oral hygiene decreases the protein (which attracts micro-organisms) in the oral cavity, which thereby decreases the growth of micro-organisms that can migrate through breaks in the oral mucosa.
- Encourage the client to consume an adequate amount of fluids. Adequate fluid intake prevents the stasis of urine by flushing the urinary tract and decreasing the growth of micro-organisms. Adequate hydration also keeps the skin from breaking down. Intact skin prevents micro-organisms from entering the body.
- For immobile clients, ensure that pulmonary hygiene (turning, coughing, deep breathing, incentive spirometry) is done every 2 hr, or as prescribed. Good pulmonary hygiene decreases the growth of micro-organisms and the development of pneumonia by preventing stasis of pulmonary excretions, stimulating ciliary movement and clearance, and expanding the lungs.
- Use of aseptic technique and proper personal protective equipment (such as gloves, masks, gowns, and goggles) in the provision of care to all clients prevents unnecessary exposure to micro-organisms.
- Teach and use respiratory hygiene/cough etiquette. It applies to anyone entering a health care setting (clients, visitors, staff) with signs or symptoms of illness, whether diagnosed or undiagnosed. This includes cough, congestion, rhinorrhea, or an increase in the production of respiratory secretions. The components of respiratory hygiene and cough etiquette include:
  - Covering the mouth and nose when coughing and sneezing.
  - Using facial tissues to contain respiratory secretions and disposing of them promptly into a hands-free receptacle.
  - Wearing a surgical mask when coughing to minimize contamination of the surrounding environment.
  - Turning the head when coughing and staying a minimum of 3 ft away from others, especially in common waiting areas.
  - Performing hand hygiene after contact with respiratory secretions and contaminated objects/materials.

ISOLATION GUIDELINES

- Isolation guidelines are a group of actions that include hand hygiene and the use of barrier precautions, which intend to reduce the transmission of infectious organisms.
- The precautions apply to every client, regardless of the diagnosis, and implementation of them must occur whenever there's anticipation of coming into contact with a potentially infectious material.
- Change personal protective equipment after contact with each client and between procedures with the same client if in contact with large amounts of blood and body fluids.
- Clients in isolation are at a higher risk for depression and loneliness. Assist the client and their family to understand the reason for isolation and provide sensory stimulation.

Standard precautions (tier one)

This tier of standard precautions applies to all body fluids (except sweat), nonintact skin, and mucous membranes. A nurse should implement standard precautions for all clients.

- Hand hygiene using an alcohol-based waterless product is recommended after contact with the client when the hands are not visibly soiled or contaminated with blood or body fluids and after the removal of gloves.
- Alcohol-based waterless antiseptic is preferred unless the hands are visibly dirty, because the alcohol-based product is more effective in removing micro-organisms.
- Use a nonantimicrobial soap if contamination with spores is suspected.
- Hand hygiene using nonantimicrobial soap or an antimicrobial soap and water is recommended when visibly soiled or contaminated with blood or body fluids.
- Remove gloves and complete hand hygiene between each client.
- Masks, eye protection, and face shields are required when care might cause splashing or spraying of body fluids.
- Clean gloves are worn when touching anything that has the potential to contaminate the hands of the nurse. This includes body secretions, excretions, blood and body fluids, nonintact skin, mucous membranes, and contaminated items.
- Hand hygiene is required after removal of the gown. Use a sturdy moisture-resistant bag for soiled items and tie the bag securely in a knot at the top.
- Properly clean all equipment for client care; dispose of one-time use items according to facility policy.
- Bag and handle contaminated laundry to prevent leaking or contamination of clothing or skin.
- Enable safety devices on all equipment and supplies after use; dispose of all sharps in a puncture-resistant container.
- A client does not need a private room unless he is unable to maintain appropriate hygienic practices.

Transmission precautions (tier two)

Airborne precautions

Use airborne precautions to protect against droplet infections smaller than 5 mcg (measles, varicella, pulmonary or laryngeal tuberculosis).

Airborne precautions require:
- A private room.
- Masks and respiratory protection devices for caregivers and visitors.

> Use an N95 or high-efficiency particulate air (HEPA) respirator if the client is known or suspected to have tuberculosis.

- Negative pressure airflow exchange in the room of at least six to 12 exchanges per hour, depending on the age of the structure.
- If splashing or spraying is a possibility, wear full face (eyes, nose, mouth) protection.

Droplet precautions

Droplet precautions protect against droplets larger than 5 mcg and travel 3 to 6 ft from the client (streptococcal pharyngitis or pneumonia, Haemophilus influenzae type B, scarlet fever, rubella, pertussis, mumps, mycoplasma pneumonia, meningococcal pneumonia and sepsis, pneumonic plague).

Droplet precautions require:
- A private room or a room with other clients who have the same infectious disease. Ensure that clients have their own equipment.
- Masks for providers and visitors.

Contact precautions

Contact precautions protect visitors and caregivers when they are within 3 ft of the client against direct client and environmental contact infections (respiratory syncytial virus, shigella, enteric diseases caused by micro-organisms, wound infections, herpes simplex, impetigo, scabies, multidrug-resistant organisms).

Contact precautions require:
- A private room or a room with other clients who have the same infection.
- Gloves and gowns worn by the caregivers and visitors.
- Disposal of infectious dressing material into a single, nonporous bag without touching the outside of the bag.

Protective precautions

Protective environment to protect clients who are immunocompromised, such as those who have had an allogeneic hematopoietic stem cell transplant.

A protective environment requires:
- Private room.
- Positive airflow 12 or more air exchanges/hr.
- HEPA filtration for incoming air.
- Mask for the client when out of room.

MEDICATIONS

Antipyretics

Antipyretics (acetaminophen and aspirin) are used for fever and discomfort as prescribed.

NURSING CONSIDERATIONS

- Monitor fever to determine effectiveness of medication.
- Document the client's temperature fluctuations on the medical record for trending.

Antimicrobial therapy

Antimicrobial therapy kills or inhibits the growth of micro-organisms (bacteria, fungi, viruses, protozoans). Antimicrobial medications either kill pathogens or prevent their growth. Give anthelmintics for worm infestations. (11.3)

NURSING CONSIDERATIONS

- Administer antimicrobial therapy as prescribed.
- Monitor for medication effectiveness (reduced fever, increase in the level of comfort, decreasing WBC count).
- Maintain a medication schedule to ensure consistent therapeutic blood levels of the antibiotic.

INTERPROFESSIONAL CARE

Transporting a client

If movement of the client to another area of the facility is unavoidable, the nurse takes precautions to ensure that the environment is not contaminated. For example, a surgical mask is placed on the client who has an airborne or droplet infection, and a draining wound is well covered.

Guidelines for cleaning contaminated equipment

- Always wear gloves and protective eyewear.
- Rinse first in running cold water. Hot water coagulates proteins, making them adhere.
- Wash the article in warm water with soap.
- Use a brush or abrasive to clean corners or hard-to-reach areas.
- Rinse well in warm water.
- Dry the article. It is considered clean at this point.
- Clean the equipment used in cleaning and the sink (still dirty unless a disinfectant is used).
- If indicated, follow facility policy for recommended disinfection or sterilization.
- Remove gloves and perform hand hygiene.

Reporting communicable diseases

A complete list of reportable diseases and the reporting system are available through the Centers for Disease Control and Prevention's website (www.cdc.gov). There are more than 60 communicable diseases that must be reported to the public health departments to allow for officials to:

- Ensure appropriate medical treatment of diseases (tuberculosis).
- Monitor for common-source outbreaks (foodborne—hepatitis A).
- Plan and evaluate control and prevention plans (immunizations for preventable diseases).
- Identify outbreaks and epidemics.
- Determine public health priorities based on trends.

CLIENT EDUCATION

Teach the client about:
- Any infection control measures at home.
- Self-administration of medication therapy.
- Complications to report immediately.

11.3 Multidrug-resistant infection

Antimicrobials are becoming less effective for some strains of pathogens due to the pathogen's ability to adapt and become resistant to previously sensitive antibiotics. This significantly limits the number of antibiotics that are effective against the pathogen.

Use of antibiotics, especially broad-spectrum antibiotics, has significantly decreased to prevent new strains from evolving. Taking the measures below can ensure that an antimicrobial is necessary and therapy is effective.

Methicillin-resistant *Staphylococcus aureus* (MRSA) is a strain of *Staphylococcus aureus* that is resistant to many antibiotics. Vancomycin and linezolid are used to treat MRSA.

Vancomycin-resistant *Staphylococcus aureus* (VRSA) is a strain of *Staphylococcus aureus* that is resistant to vancomycin, but so far is sensitive to other antibiotics specific to a client's strain.

NURSING ACTIONS
- Obtain specimens for culture and sensitivity prior to initiation of antimicrobial therapy.
- Monitor antimicrobial levels and ensure that therapeutic levels are maintained.

CLIENT EDUCATION
- Complete the full course of antimicrobial therapy.
- Avoid overuse of antimicrobials.

Herpes zoster (shingles)

Herpes zoster is a viral infection. It initially produces chickenpox, after which the virus lies dormant in the dorsal root ganglia of the sensory nerves. It is then reactivated as shingles later in life.

- Shingles is usually preceded by a prodromal period of several days, during which pain, tingling, or burning might occur along the involved dermatome.
- Shingles can be very painful and debilitating.

ASSESSMENT/DATA COLLECTION

RISK FACTORS

- Concurrent illness
- Stress
- Compromise to the immune system
- Fatigue
- Poor nutritional status
- OLDER ADULT CLIENTS are more susceptible to herpes zoster infection. The immune function of older adults might also be compromised, so assess them carefully for local or systemic signs of infection. Ⓖ

EXPECTED FINDINGS

- Paresthesia
- Pain that is unilateral and extends horizontally along a dermatome

PHYSICAL ASSESSMENT FINDINGS

- Vesicular, unilateral rash (the rash and lesions occur on the skin area innervated by the infected nerve)
- Rash that is erythematous, vesicular, pustular, or crusting (depending on the stage)
- Rash that usually resolves in 14 to 21 days
- Low-grade fever

LABORATORY TESTS

- Cultures provide a definitive diagnosis. But, the virus grows so slowly that cultures are often of minimal diagnostic use.
- Occasionally, an immunofluorescence assay can be done.

PATIENT-CENTERED CARE

NURSING CARE

- Assess/Monitor
  - Pain
  - Condition of the lesions
  - Presence of fever
  - Neurologic complications
  - Signs of infection
- Use an air mattress or bed cradle for pain prevention and control of affected areas.
- Isolate the client until the vesicles have crusted over.
- Maintain strict wound care precautions.
- Avoid exposing the client to infants, pregnant women who have not had chickenpox, and clients who are immunocompromised, although anyone who has not had chickenpox and has not been vaccinated is at risk.
- Use lotions to help relieve itching and discomfort.
- Administer medications as prescribed.

MEDICATIONS

Analgesics (NSAIDs, narcotics) enhance client comfort.

Antiviral agents, such as acyclovir, can shorten the clinical course.

COMPLICATIONS

Postherpetic neuralgia

- Characterized by pain that persists for longer than 1 month following resolution of the vesicular rash
- Tricyclic antidepressants might be prescribed
- Postherpetic neuralgia is common in adults older than 60 years of age. Ⓖ

PREVENTION

- Zoster vaccine reduces the risk of developing shingles
- Do not give to clients who are immunocompromised.

Application Exercises

1. A nurse is caring for a client diagnosed with severe acute respiratory syndrome (SARS). The nurse is aware that health care professionals are required to report communicable and infectious diseases. Which of the following illustrate the rationale for reporting? (Select all that apply.)

    A. Planning and evaluating control and prevention strategies

    B. Determining public health priorities

    C. Ensuring proper medical treatment

    D. Identifying endemic disease

    E. Monitoring for common-source outbreaks

2. A nurse is caring for a client who presents with linear clusters of fluid-containing vesicles with some crustings. The nurse should identify the client has manifestations of which of the following conditions?

    A. Allergic reaction

    B. Ringworm

    C. Systemic lupus erythematosus

    D. Herpes zoster

3. A nurse is caring for a client who reports a severe sore throat, pain when swallowing, and swollen lymph nodes. The client is experiencing which of the following stages of infection?

    A. Prodromal

    B. Incubation

    C. Convalescence

    D. Illness

4. A nurse educator is reviewing with a newly hired nurse the difference in manifestations of a localized versus a systemic infection. The nurse indicates understanding when she states that which of the following are manifestations of a systemic infection? (Select all that apply.)

    A. Fever

    B. Malaise

    C. Edema

    D. Pain or tenderness

    E. Increase in pulse and respiratory rate

5. A nurse is contributing to the plan of care for a client who is being admitted to the facility with a suspected diagnosis of pertussis. Which of the following interventions should the nurse include in the plan of care? (Select all that apply.)

    A. Place the client in a room that has negative air pressure of at least six exchanges per hour.

    B. Wear a mask when providing care within 3 ft of the client.

    C. Place a surgical mask on the client if transportation to another department is unavoidable.

    D. Use sterile gloves when handling soiled linens.

    E. Wear a gown when performing care that might result in contamination from secretions.

PRACTICE Active Learning Scenario

A nurse educator is teaching a module on the chain of infection during nursing orientation to a group of newly licensed nurses. Use the ATI Active Learning Template: Basic Concept to complete this item.

RELATED CONTENT: List the six links in the chain of infection that must be present for an infection to occur.

1. A. **CORRECT:** Reporting of communicable and infectious diseases assists with planning and evaluating control and prevention strategies.

    B. **CORRECT:** Reporting of communicable and infectious diseases assists with determining public health policies.

    C. **CORRECT:** Reporting of communicable and infectious diseases assists with ensuring proper medical treatment is available.

    D. Endemic disease is already prevalent within a population, so reporting is not necessary.

    E. **CORRECT:** Reporting of communicable and infectious diseases assists with monitoring for common-source outbreaks.

    Ⓝ *NCLEX® Connection: Physiological Adaptation, Illness Management*

2. A. A pink body rash is a manifestation of an allergic reaction.

    B. Red circles with white centers is a manifestation of ringworm.

    C. A red edematous rash bilaterally on the cheeks is a manifestation of systemic lupus erythematosus.

    D. **CORRECT:** Vesicles that follow along a unilateral dermatome is a manifestation of herpes zoster.

    Ⓝ *NCLEX® Connection: Physiological Adaptation, Pathophysiology*

3. A. The prodromal stage consists of nonspecific manifestations of the infection.

    B. The incubation period consists of the time when the pathogen first enters the body prior to the appearance of any manifestations of infection.

    C. During convalescence, manifestations of the infection fade.

    D. **CORRECT:** The illness stage is when the client experiences manifestations specific to the infection.

    Ⓝ *NCLEX® Connection: Physiological Adaptation, Pathophysiology*

4. A. **CORRECT:** A fever indicates that the infection is affecting the whole body, and therefore systemic.

    B. **CORRECT:** Malaise indicates that the infection is affecting the whole body, and therefore systemic.

    C. Edema is a localized manifestation indicating a localized, not systemic, infection.

    D. Pain and tenderness is a localized manifestation indicating a localized, not systemic, infection.

    E. **CORRECT:** An increase in pulse and respiratory rate indicates that the infection is affecting the whole body, and therefore systemic.

    Ⓝ *NCLEX® Connection: Physiological Adaptation, Pathophysiology*

5. A. A nurse should place a client in a private room and initiate droplet precautions if he has pertussis. Negative-pressure airflow is required for a client who is on airborne precautions.

    B. **CORRECT:** The nurse should wear a mask when within 3 ft of the client.

    C. **CORRECT:** The nurse should place a surgical mask on the client during transport to another area of the facility.

    D. The nurse should wear a gown and non-sterile gloves when performing care that might result in contamination from body fluids.

    E. **CORRECT:** A gown should be worn if the nurse's clothing or skin might be contaminated with body secretions or excretions.

    Ⓝ *NCLEX® Connection: Safety and Infection Control, Standard Precautions/Transmission–Based Precautions/Surgical Asepsis*

PRACTICE Answer

Using the ATI Active Learning Template: Basic Concept

RELATED CONTENT: The infection process (chain of infection)
- Causative agent
- Reservoir
- Portal of exit (means of leaving) from the host
- Mode of transmission
- Portal of entry to the host
- Susceptible host

Ⓝ *NCLEX® Connection: Safety and Infection Control, Standard Precautions/Transmission–Based Precautions/Surgical Asepsis*

CHAPTER 12   *Client Safety*

Safety is freedom from injury. Providing for safety and preventing injury are major nursing responsibilities.

Many factors affect the client's ability to protect himself. Those factors include the client's age, with the young and old at greater risk; mobility; cognitive and sensory awareness; emotional state; ability to communicate; and lifestyle and safety awareness.

It is the provider's responsibility to assess, report, and document clients' allergies and to provide care that avoids exposure to allergens.

NURSING ACTIONS

- Use risk assessment tools to evaluate clients and their environment for safety.
- Encourage clients to speak up and take an active role in their health care and in preventing errors.
- Create a culture of checks and balances to avoid errors when working in stressful circumstances.
- Communicate risk factors and plans of care to clients, family, and other staff.
- Use protocols for responding to dangerous situations.
- Adopt quality care priorities from the National Quality Forum, including "Never Events."
- Use current evidence to promote a culture of safety, while using the National Patient Safety Goals as a guide.
- Know the facility's disaster plan, understand the chain of command and roles, and use common terminology when communicating with the team.
- Identify and document incidents and responses according to the facility's policy. These reports help identify trends, patterns, and the root cause of adverse events. Qs
- Know the location of safety data sheets and hazardous chemicals in the environment.
- Use equipment only after adequate instruction and safety inspection.

FALLS

- Older adult clients can be at an increased risk for falls due to decreased strength, impaired mobility and balance, improper use of mobility aids, unsafe clothing, environmental hazards, endurance limitations, and decreased sensory perception. Ⓖ
- Other clients at increased risk include those with decreased visual acuity, generalized weakness, urinary frequency, gait and balance problems (cerebral palsy, injury, multiple sclerosis), and cognitive dysfunction. Adverse effects of medications (orthostatic hypotension, drowsiness) can also increase the risk for falls.
- Clients are at greater risk for falls when they have more than one risk factor.
- Prevention of client falls is a major nursing priority. Nurses must evaluate all clients in health care facilities for risk factors for falls and implement preventative measures accordingly.
- Programs to prevent falls are essential for settings that provide services to older adult clients.
- Health care facilities must actively prevent falls, especially because Medicare and Medicaid no longer reimburse for treating injuries resulting from falls.

PREVENTING FALLS

- Complete a fall-risk assessment for each client at admission and at regular intervals. Individualize the plan for each client according to the results of the fall-risk assessment. For example, instruct a client who has orthostatic hypotension to avoid getting up too quickly, to sit on the side of the bed for a few seconds prior to standing, and to stand at the side of the bed for a few seconds prior to walking.
- Be sure the client knows how to use the call light (by giving a return demonstration) that it is in reach, and to encourage its use.
- Respond to call lights in a timely manner.
- Use fall-risk alerts, such as color-coded wristbands.
- Provide regular toileting and orientation of clients who have cognitive impairment.
- Provide adequate lighting.
- Orient clients to the setting to make sure they know how to use all assistive devices (grab bars) and can locate necessary items.
- Place clients at risk for falls near the nurses' station.
- Provide hourly rounding.
- Make sure' bedside tables, overbed tables, and frequent-use items (telephone, water, facial tissues) are within reach.
- Keep the bed in the low position and lock the brakes.
- For clients who are sedated, unconscious, or otherwise compromised, keep the side rails up.
- Avoid the use of full side rails for clients who get out of bed or attempt to get out of bed without assistance.
- Provide nonskid footwear and nonskid bath mats for use in tubs and showers.
- Use gait belts and additional safety equipment when moving clients.
- Keep the floor clean, dry, and free from clutter with a clear path to the bathroom (no scatter rugs, cords, or furniture).
- Keep assistive devices nearby after validation of safe use (eyeglasses, walkers, transfer devices).

- Educate the client and family about safety risks and the plan of care. Clients and family who are aware of risks are more likely to call for assistance.
- Lock the wheels on beds, wheelchairs, and carts to prevent them from rolling during transfers or stops.
- Use electronic safety monitoring devices, such as chair or bed sensors, for clients at risk for getting up without assistance to alert staff of independent ambulation.
- Report and document all incidents. This provides valuable information that can help prevent similar incidents.

SEIZURES

A seizure is a sudden surge of electrical activity in the brain. It can occur at any time due to epilepsy, fever, or a variety of medical problems. Partial seizures (also called focal seizures) are due to electrical surges in one part of the brain, and generalized seizures involve the entire brain. Status epilepticus (a prolonged seizure) is a medical emergency.

SEIZURE PRECAUTIONS

Seizure precautions (measures to protect clients from injury during a seizure) are imperative for clients who have a history of seizures that involve the entire body and/or result in unconsciousness. Qs

- Make sure rescue equipment is at the bedside, including oxygen, an oral airway, suction equipment, and padding for the side rails. Clients at high risk for generalized seizures should have a saline lock in place for immediate IV access.
- Ensure rapid intervention to maintain airway patency.
- Inspect the client's environment for items that could cause injury during a seizure, and remove items that are not necessary for current treatment.
- Assist clients at risk for seizures with ambulation and transferring to reduce the risk of injury.
- Advise all caregivers and family not to put anything in the client's mouth (except an airway for status epilepticus) during a seizure.
- Advise all caregivers and family not to restrain the client during a seizure but to lower him to the floor or bed, protect his head, remove nearby furniture, provide privacy, put him on his side with his head flexed slightly forward if possible, and loosen his clothing.

DURING A SEIZURE

- Stay with the client, and call for help.
- Maintain airway patency and suction PRN. Qs
- Administer medications.
- Note the duration of the seizure and the sequence and type of movements.
- After a seizure, determine mental status and measure oxygenation saturation and vital signs. Explain what happened, and provide comfort, understanding, and a quiet environment for recovery.
- Document the seizure with any precipitating behavior and a description of the event (movements, injuries, duration of seizures, aura, postictal state), and report it to the provider.

SECLUSION AND RESTRAINT

- Nurses must know and follow federal, state, and facility policies for the use of restraints.
- Some clients require seclusion rooms and/or restraints.
- In general, use seclusion or restraints for the shortest duration necessary and only if less restrictive measures are not sufficient. They are for the physical protection of the client or the protection of other clients or staff.
- Clients may voluntarily request temporary seclusion if the environment is disturbing or seems too stimulating.
- Restraints can be either physical (devices that restrict movement: vest, belt, mitt, limb) or chemical, such as sedatives and neuroleptic or psychotropic medications to calm the client.
- Restraints can cause complications, including pneumonia, incontinence, and pressure ulcers.
- It is inappropriate to use seclusion or restraints for:
  ○ Convenience of the staff
  ○ Punishment for the client
  ○ Clients who are extremely physically or mentally unstable
  ○ Clients who cannot tolerate the decreased stimulation of a seclusion room
- Restraints should:
  ○ Never interfere with treatment
  ○ Restrict movement as little as is necessary
  ○ Fit properly and be as discreet as possible
  ○ Be easy to remove or change
- When all other less restrictive means have failed to prevent a client from harming himself or others (orientation to the environment, supervision of a family member or sitter, diversional activities, electronic devices), the following must occur before using seclusion or restraints.
  ○ The provider must prescribe seclusion or restraints in writing, after a face-to-face assessment of the client.

In an emergency situation when there is immediate risk to the client or others, nurses may place restraints on a client. The nurse must obtain a prescription from the provider as soon as possible according to the facility's policy (usually within 1 hr).

  ○ The prescription must include the reason for the restraints, the type of restraints, the location of the restraints, how long to use the restraints, and the type of behavior that warrants using the restraints.
  ○ The prescription allows only 4 hr of restraints for an adult, 2 hr for clients ages 9 to 17, and 1 hr for clients younger than 9 years of age. Providers may renew these prescriptions with a maximum of 24 consecutive hours.
  ○ Providers cannot write PRN prescriptions for restraints.

NURSING RESPONSIBILITIES FOR CLIENTS IN RESTRAINTS

- Explain the need for the restraints to the client and family, emphasizing that the restraints keep the client safe and are temporary.
- Ask the client or guardian to sign a consent form.
- Review the manufacturer's instructions for correct application.
    - Assess skin integrity, and provide skin care according to the facility's protocol, usually every 2 hr.
    - Offer food and fluid.
    - Provide a means for hygiene and elimination.
    - Monitor vital signs.
    - Offer range-of-motion exercises of extremities.
- Pad bony prominences to prevent skin breakdown.
- Use a quick-release knot (loose knot that is easy to remove) to tie the restraints to the bed frame where they will not tighten when raising or lowering the bed.
- Make sure the restraints are loose enough for range of motion and that there is enough room to fit two fingers between the restraints and the client.
- Remove or replace restraints frequently to ensure good circulation to the area and allow for full range of motion to the limbs.
- Conduct an ongoing evaluation of the client.
- Regularly determine the need to continue using the restraints. Qs
- Never leave the client alone without the restraints.

DOCUMENT

- Precipitating events and behavior of the client prior to seclusion or restraints
- Alternative actions to avoid seclusion or restraints
- Time of application and removal of the restraints
- Type of restraints and location
- The client's behavior while in restraints
- Type and frequency of care (range of motion, neurosensory checks, removal, integumentary checks)
- Condition of the body part in restraints
- The client's response at removal of the restraints
- Medication administration

FIRE SAFETY

Fires in health care facilities are usually due to problems with electrical or anesthetic equipment, or from smoking.

All staff must:
- Know the location of exits, alarms, fire extinguishers, and oxygen shut-off valves.
- Make sure equipment does not block fire doors.
- Know the evacuation plan for the unit and the facility.

Fire response follows the RACE sequence

R: Rescue and protect clients in close proximity to the fire by moving them to a safer location. Clients who are ambulatory may walk independently to a safe location.

A: Alarm: Activate the facility's alarm system and then report the fire's details and location.

C: Contain/Confine the fire by closing doors and windows and turning off any sources of oxygen and any electrical devices. Ventilate clients who are on life support with a bag-valve mask.

E: Extinguish the fire if possible using the appropriate fire extinguisher.

FIRE EXTINGUISHERS

To use a fire extinguisher, use the PASS sequence.

P: Pull the pin.

A: Aim at the base of the fire.

S: Squeeze the handle.

S: Sweep the extinguisher from side to side, covering the area of the fire.

Classes of fire extinguishers

Class A is for combustibles such as paper, wood, upholstery, rags, and other types of trash fires.

Class B is for flammable liquids and gas fires.

Class C is for electrical fires.

Application Exercises

1. A nurse is caring for a client who fell at a nursing home. The client is oriented to person, place, and time and can follow directions. Which of the following actions should the nurse take to decrease the risk of another fall? (Select all that apply.)

    A. Place a belt restraint on the client when he is sitting on the bedside commode.

    B. Keep the bed in its lowest position with all side rails up.

    C. Make sure that the client's call light is within reach.

    D. Provide the client with nonskid footwear.

    E. Complete a fall-risk assessment.

2. A nurse manager is reviewing with nurses on the unit the care of a client who has had a seizure. Which of the following statements by a nurse requires further instruction?

    A. "I will place the client on his side."

    B. "I will go to the nurses' station for assistance."

    C. "I will administer his medications."

    D. "I will prepare to insert an airway."

3. A nurse observes smoke coming from under the door of the staff's lounge. Which of the following actions is the nurse's priority?

    A. Extinguish the fire.

    B. Activate the fire alarm.

    C. Move clients who are nearby.

    D. Close all open doors on the unit.

4. A nurse is caring for a client who has a history of falls. Which of the following actions is the nurse's priority?

    A. Complete a fall-risk assessment.

    B. Educate the client and family about fall risks.

    C. Eliminate safety hazards from the client's environment.

    D. Make sure the client uses assistive aids in his possession.

5. A charge nurse is assigning rooms for the clients to be admitted to the unit. To prevent falls, which of the following clients should the nurse assign to the room closest to the nurses' station?

    A. A middle adult who is postoperative following a laparoscopic cholecystectomy

    B. A middle adult who requires telemetry for a possible myocardial infarction

    C. A young adult who is postoperative following an open reduction internal fixation of the ankle

    D. An older adult who is postoperative following a below-the-knee amputation

PRACTICE Active Learning Scenario

A nurse educator is addressing the safe use of seclusion and restraints with a group of newly licensed nurses. What information should the nurse include? Use the ATI Active Learning Template: Basic Concept to complete this item.

NURSING INTERVENTIONS: Describe at least six nursing responsibilities when caring for a client in either seclusion or restraints.

Application Exercises Key

1. A. By restraining the client, the nurse risks liability for false imprisonment.

    B. Full side rails for this client puts the client at risk for a fall because he might attempt to climb over the rails to get out of bed.

    C. **CORRECT:** Making sure that the call light is within reach enables the client to contact the nursing staff to ask for assistance and prevents the client from falling out of bed while reaching for the call light.

    D. **CORRECT:** Nonskid footwear keeps the client from slipping.

    E. **CORRECT:** A fall-risk assessment serves as the basis for a plan of care the nurse can then individualize for the client.

    Ⓝ *NCLEX® Connection: Safety and Infection Control, Accident/Error/Injury Prevention*

2. A. During a seizure, the nurse should place the client in a side-lying position to allow for drainage of secretions and to prevent his tongue from occluding the airway.

    B. **CORRECT:** During a seizure, the nurse should stay with the client and use the call light to summon assistance.

    C. The nurse should administer any medications the provider prescribes.

    D. The nurse should place nothing in the client's mouth except an oral airway, if he needs it. A tongue blade can cause injury and airway obstruction.

    Ⓝ *NCLEX® Connection: Physiological Adaptation, Alterations in Body Systems*

3. A. Although extinguishing the fire is part of the protocol for responding to a fire, it is not the priority action.

    B. Although activating the fire alarm is part of the protocol for responding to a fire, it is not the priority action.

    C. **CORRECT:** The greatest risk to this client is injury from the fire. Therefore, the priority intervention is to rescue the clients. The nurse should protect and move clients in close proximity to the fire.

    D. Although containing the fire by closing doors and windows is part of the protocol for responding to a fire, it is not the priority action.

    Ⓝ *NCLEX® Connection: Safety and Infection Control, Accident/Error/Injury Prevention*

4. A. **CORRECT:** The first action the nurse should take using the nursing process is to assess or collect data from the client. Therefore, the priority action is to determine the client's fall risk. This will guide the nurse in implementing appropriate safety measures.

    B. It is important for family members to be aware of the client's risk for falls. Providing instruction to the client and family is an appropriate nursing action, but this is not the priority action.

    C. It is important to eliminate safety hazards from the client's environment, but this is not the priority action.

    D. It is important for the client to use aids such as eyeglasses, hearing aids, canes, and walkers. However, this is not the priority action.

    Ⓝ *NCLEX® Connection: Safety and Infection Control, Accident/Error/Injury Prevention*

5. A. Although this client just had surgery, the client's age and type of surgery puts him at low risk for falls.

    B. Although this client requires telemetry, the client does not have as many risk factors as another client the nurse will admit.

    C. Although this client just had surgery, the client's age and type of surgery puts him at low risk for falls.

    D. **CORRECT:** The nurse should assign this client to a room near the nurses' station due to risk factors that include client's age plus the immobility and balance issues that result from this type of surgery. The client will also receive analgesics, which increase the risk for drowsiness, dizziness, and confusion.

    Ⓝ *NCLEX® Connection: Reduction of Risk Potential, System Specific Assessments*

PRACTICE Answer

Using the ATI Active Learning Template: Basic Concept

NURSING INTERVENTIONS

- Explain the need for the restraints to the client and family, emphasizing that the restraints keep the client safe and are temporary.
- Ask the client or guardian to sign a consent form.
- Review the manufacturer's instructions for correct application.
- Assess skin integrity, and provide skin care according to the facility's protocol, usually every 2 hr.

- Offer food and fluid.
- Provide a means for hygiene and elimination.
- Monitor vital signs.
- Offer range-of-motion exercises of extremities.
- Pad bony prominences to prevent skin breakdown.
- Use a quick-release knot to tie the restraints to the bed frame (loose knots that are easy to remove) where they will not tighten when raising or lowering the bed.

- Make sure the restraints are loose enough for range of motion and that there is enough room to fit two fingers between the restraints and the client.
- Remove or replace restraints frequently to ensure good circulation to the area and allow for full range of motion to the limbs.
- Conduct an ongoing evaluation of the client.

Ⓝ *NCLEX® Connection: Safety and Infection Control, Use of Restraints/Safety Devices*

CHAPTER 13 *Home Safety*

In addition to taking measures to prevent injury of clients in a health care setting, nurses play a pivotal role in promoting safety in the client's home and community. Nurses often collaborate with the client, family, and members of the interprofessional team (social workers, occupational therapists, and physical therapists) to promote the safety of the client. Q℞

To initiate a plan of care, the nurse must identify risk factors using a risk assessment tool and complete a nursing history, physical examination, and home hazard appraisal.

In the plan of care for safety preparedness, the nurse should include emergency nursing principles, such as basic first aid and CPR.

RISK FACTORS FOR CLIENT INJURY

- Age and developmental status
- Mobility and balance
- Knowledge about safety hazards
- Sensory and cognitive awareness
- Communication skills
- Home and work environment
- Community in which the client lives
- Lifestyle choices

SAFETY RISKS BASED ON AGE AND DEVELOPMENTAL STATUS

- The age and developmental status of the client create specific safety risks. Q℗cc
- Infants and toddlers are at risk for injury due to a tendency to put objects in their mouth and from hazards encountered while exploring their environment.
- Preschool- and school-age children often face injury from limited or underdeveloped motor coordination.
- Adolescents' risks for injury can stem from increased desire to make independent decisions, and relying on peers for guidance rather than family.
- Some of the accident prevention measures for specific age groups are found below.

INFANTS AND TODDLERS

Aspiration
- Keep all small objects out of reach.
- Check toys and objects for loose or small parts and sharp edges.
- Do not feed the infant hard candy, peanuts, popcorn, or whole or sliced pieces of hot dog.
- Do not place the infant in the supine position while feeding or prop the infant's bottle.
- A pacifier (if used) should be constructed of one piece and never placed on string or ribbon around the neck.

Suffocation
- Teach "back to sleep" mnemonic and always place infants on back to rest.
- Keep plastic bags out of reach.
- Make sure crib mattress fits snugly and that crib slats are no more than $2^3/_8$ inches apart.
- Never leave an infant or toddler alone in the bathtub.
- Do not place anything in crib with infant.
- Remove crib toys, such as mobiles, from over the bed as soon as the infant begins to push up.
- Keep latex balloons away from infants and toddlers.
- Fence swimming pools and use a locked gate.
- Begin swimming lessons when the child's developmental status allows for protective responses, such as closing her mouth under water.
- Teach caregivers CPR and Heimlich maneuver.
- Keep toilet lids down and bathroom doors closed.

Poisoning
- Keep houseplants and cleaning agents out of reach.
- Inspect and remove sources of lead, such as paint chips, and provide parents with information about prevention of lead poisoning.
- Place poisons, paint, and gasoline in locked cabinet.
- Keep medications in child-proof containers and locked up.
- Dispose of medications that are no longer used or are out of date.

Falls

- Keep crib and playpen rails up.
- Never leave the infant unattended on a changing table or other high surface.
- Use gates on stairs, and ensure windows have screens.
- Restrain according to manufacturer's recommendations and supervise when in high chair, swing, stroller, etc. Discontinue use when the infant or toddler outgrows size or activity limits.
- Place in a low bed when toddler starts to climb.

Motor vehicle injury

- Place infants and toddlers in a rear-facing car seat until 2 years of age or until they exceed the height and weight limit of the car seat. They can then sit in a forward-facing car seat.
- Use a car seat with a five-point harness for infants and children.
- All car seats should be federally approved and be placed in the back seat.

Burns

- Test the temperature of formula and bath water.
- Place pots on back burner and turn handle away from front of stove.
- Supervise the use of faucets.
- Keep matches and lighters out of reach.
- Cover electrical outlets.

PRESCHOOLERS AND SCHOOL-AGE CHILDREN

Drowning

- Be sure child has learned to swim and knows rules of water safety.
- Place locked fences around home and neighborhood pools.
- Provide supervision near pools or water.

Motor vehicle injury

- Use booster seats for children who are less than 4 feet 9 inches tall and weigh less than 40 lb (usually 4 to 8 years old). The child should be able to sit with his back against the car seat, and his legs should dangle over the seat.
- If car has a passenger air bag, place children under 12 years in the back seat.
- Use seat belts properly after booster seats are no longer necessary.
- Use protective equipment when participating in sports, riding a bike, or riding as a passenger on a bike.
- Supervise and teach safe use of equipment.
- Teach the child to play in safe areas and never to run after a ball or toy that goes into a road.
- Teach child safety rules of the road.

Begin sex education for school-age child.

Firearms

- Keep firearms unloaded, locked up, and out of reach.
- Teach to never touch a gun or stay at a friend's house where a gun is accessible.
- Store bullets in a different location from guns.

Play injury

- Teach to not run with candy or objects in mouth.
- Remove doors from refrigerators or other potentially confining structures.
- Ensure that bikes are the appropriate size for child.
- Teach playground safety.
- Teach to play in safe areas, and avoid heavy machinery, railroad tracks, excavation areas, quarries, trunks, and vacant buildings.
- Teach to never swim alone and to wear a life jacket in boats.
- Wear protective helmets and knee and elbow pads, when needed.
- Teach to avoid strangers and keep parents informed of strangers.

Burns

- Reduce setting on water heater to no higher than 120° F.
- Teach dangers of playing with matches, fireworks, and firearms.
- Teach school-age child how to properly use microwave and other cooking instruments.

Poison

- Teach child about the hazards of alcohol, cigarettes, and prescription, non-prescription, and illegal drugs.
- Keep potentially dangerous substances out of reach.

ADOLESCENTS

Educate on the hazards of smoking, alcohol, legal and illegal drugs, and unprotected sex.

Motor vehicle and injury

- Ensure the teen has completed a driver's education course.
- Set rules on the number of people allowed to ride in cars, seat belt use, and to call for a ride home if a driver is impaired.
- Educate on the hazards of driving while distracted (eating or drinking, making phone calls or texting).
- Reinforce teaching on proper use of protective equipment when participating in sports.
- Be alert to signs of depression, anxiety or other behavioral changes
- Teach about the hazards of firearms and safety precautions with firearms.
- Teach water safety.
- Teach to check water depth before diving.

Burns

- Teach to use sunblock and protective clothing.
- Teach the dangers of sunbathing and tanning beds.

YOUNG AND MIDDLE-AGE ADULTS

Motor vehicle crashes are the most common cause of death and injury to adults. Occupational injuries contribute to the injury and death rate of adults. High consumption of alcohol and suicide are also major concerns for adults.

CLIENT EDUCATION
- Remind clients to drive defensively and to not drive after drinking alcohol.
- Reinforce teaching about the long-term effects related to high alcohol consumption.
- Ensure home safety with smoke and carbon monoxide detectors, fire alarms, well-lit and uncluttered staircases.
- Be attuned to behaviors that suggest the presence of depression or thoughts of suicide. Referring clients as appropriate and encourage counseling.
- Teach diving and water safety.
- Encourage clients to become proactive about safety in the workplace and in the home.
- Discuss dangers of social networking and the Internet.
- Ensure that clients understand the hazards of excessive sun exposure and the need to protect the skin with the use of sun-blocking agents and protective clothing.

OLDER ADULTS

- The rate at which age-related changes occur varies greatly among older adults. Ⓖ
- Many older adults are able to maintain a lifestyle that promotes independence and the ability to protect themselves from safety hazards.
- Prevention is important because elderly clients can have longer recovery times from injuries and the risk of complications.
- A decrease in tactile sensitivity can place the client at risk for burns and other types of tissue injury.
- When the client demonstrates factors that increases the risk for injury (regardless of age), a home hazard evaluation should be conducted by a nurse, physical therapist, and/or occupational therapist. The client is made aware of the environmental factors that can pose a risk to safety and suggestion modifications to be made.

RISK FACTORS FOR FALLS IN OLDER ADULTS
- Physical, cognitive, and sensory changes
- Changes in the musculoskeletal and neurological systems
- Impaired vision and/or hearing
- Frequent trips to the bathroom at night because of nocturia and incontinence

MODIFICATIONS TO IMPROVE HOME SAFETY
- Remove items that could cause the client to trip, such as throw rugs and loose carpets.
- Place electrical cords and extension cords against a wall behind furniture.
- Monitor gait and balance, and provide aids as needed.
- Make sure that steps and sidewalks are in good repair.
- Place grab bars near the toilet and in the tub or shower, and install a stool riser.
- Use a nonskid mat in the tub or shower.
- Place a shower chair in the shower and provide a bedside commode if needed.
- Ensure that lighting is adequate inside and outside the home.

FIRE SAFETY IN THE HOME

Home fires continue to be a major cause of death and injury for people of all ages. Nurses should educate clients about the importance of a home safety plan.

ELEMENTS OF A HOME SAFETY PLAN

- Keep emergency numbers near the phone for prompt use in the event of an emergency of any type.
- Ensure that the number and placement of fire extinguishers and smoke alarms are adequate, that they are functional, and that family members understand how to operate them. Set a time to routinely change batteries in smoke alarms (e.g., in the fall when the clocks are set to standard time and spring when set to Daylight Saving Time).
- Have a family exit plan for fires that is reviewed and practiced regularly. Be sure to include closing windows and doors if able and to exit a smoke-filled area by covering the mouth and nose with a damp cloth, and getting down as close to the floor as possible.
- Review with clients of all ages that in the event that the client's clothing or skin is on fire, the mnemonic "stop, drop, and roll" should be used to extinguish the fire.
- Review oxygen safety measures. Because oxygen can cause materials to combust more easily and burn more rapidly, the client and family must be provided with information on use of the oxygen delivery equipment and the dangers of combustion. Include the following information in the teaching plan:
  ○ Use and store oxygen equipment according to the manufacturer's recommendations.
  ○ Place a "No Smoking" sign in a conspicuous place near the front door of the home. A sign can also be placed on the door to the client's bedroom.
  ○ Inform the client and family of the danger of smoking in the presence of oxygen. Family members and visitors who smoke should do so outside the home.
  ○ Ensure that electrical equipment is in good repair and well grounded.
  ○ Replace bedding that can generate static electricity (wool, nylon, synthetics) with items made from cotton.
  ○ Keep flammable materials, such as heating oil and nail polish remover, away from the client when oxygen is in use.
  ○ Follow general measures for fire safety in the home, such as having a fire extinguisher readily available and an established exit route if a fire occurs.

ADDITIONAL RISKS IN THE HOME AND COMMUNITY

Additional risks in the home and community include passive smoking, carbon monoxide poisoning, and food poisoning. Bioterrorism also has become a concern, making disaster plans a mandatory part of community safety. Nurses should teach clients about the dangers of these additional risks. Qs

Passive smoking

* Passive smoking is the unintentional inhalation of tobacco smoke.
* Exposure to nicotine and other toxins places people at risk for numerous diseases including cancer, heart disease, and lung infections.
* Low-birth-weight infants, prematurity, stillbirths, and sudden infant death syndrome (SIDS) have been associated with maternal smoking.
* Smoking in the presence of children is associated with the development of bronchitis, pneumonia, and middle ear infections.
* For children who have asthma, exposure to passive smoke can result in an increase in the frequency and the severity of asthma attacks.

CLIENT EDUCATION

Inform the client who smokes and his family about:
* The hazards of smoking
* Available resources to stop smoking (smoking cessation programs, medication support, self-help groups)
* The effect that visiting individuals who smoke or riding in the automobile of a smoker has on a nonsmoker

Carbon monoxide

Carbon monoxide is a very dangerous gas because it binds with hemoglobin and ultimately reduces the oxygen supplied to the tissues in the body.
* Carbon monoxide cannot be seen, smelled, or tasted.
* Symptoms of carbon monoxide poisoning include nausea, vomiting, headache, weakness, and unconsciousness.
* Death can occur with prolonged exposure.
* Measures to prevent carbon monoxide poisoning include ensuring proper ventilation when using fuel-burning devices (lawn mowers, wood-burning and gas fireplaces, charcoal grills).
* Gas-burning furnaces, water heaters, and appliances should be inspected annually.
* Flues and chimneys should be unobstructed.
* Carbon monoxide detectors should be installed and inspected regularly.

Food poisoning

Food poisoning is a major cause of illness in the United States. Most food poisoning is caused by bacteria such as *Escherichia coli*, *Listeria monocytogenes*, and *Salmonella*.
* Healthy individuals usually recover from the illness in a few days.
* Very young, very old, immunocompromised, and pregnant individuals are at risk for complications.
* Clients who are especially at risk are instructed to follow a low-microbial diet.
* Most food poisoning occurs because of unsanitary food practice.
* Performing proper hand hygiene, ensuring that meat and fish are cooked to the correct temperature, handling raw and fresh food separately to avoid cross contamination, and refrigerating perishable items are measures that can prevent food poisoning.
* Check expiration dates, and clean fresh fruits and vegetables.

Bioterrorism

Bioterrorism is the dissemination of harmful toxins, bacteria, viruses, and pathogens for the purpose of causing illness or death.
* Anthrax, variola, *Clostridium botulism*, and *Yersinia pestis* are examples of agents used by terrorists.
* Nurses and other health professionals must be prepared to respond to an attack by being proficient in early detection, recognizing the causative agent, identifying the affected community, and providing early treatment to affected persons.

PRIMARY SURVEY

A primary survey is a rapid assessment of life-threatening conditions. It should take no longer than 60 seconds to perform. QEBP
- The primary survey should be completed systematically so conditions are not missed.
- Standard precautions (gloves, gowns, eye protection, face masks, and shoe covers) must be worn to prevent contamination with bodily fluids.

ABCDE PRINCIPLE

The ABCDE principle guides the primary survey and emergency care.

Airway/Cervical Spine: This is the most important step in performing the primary survey. If a patent airway is not established, subsequent steps of the primary survey are futile. Protect the cervical spine if head or neck trauma is suspected.

Breathing: After achieving a patent airway, assess for the presence and effectiveness of breathing.

Circulation: After ensuring adequate ventilation, assess circulation.

Disability: Perform a quick assessment to determine the client's level of consciousness.

Exposure: Perform a quick physical assessment to determine the client's exposure to adverse elements such as heat or cold.

See the chapter on *Emergency Nursing Principles and Management* in the *Adult Medical Surgical Nursing Review Module* for further detail on the primary survey.

BASIC FIRST AID

Complete the primary survey before performing first aid.

Bleeding

- Identify any sources of external bleeding and apply direct pressure to the wound site.
- DO NOT remove impaling objects. Instead, stabilize the object.
- Internal bleeding can require intravascular volume replacement with fluids and/or blood products, or surgical intervention.

Fractures and splinting

- Assess the site for swelling, deformity, and skin integrity.
- Assess temperature, distal pulses, and mobility.
- Apply a splint to immobilize the fracture. Cover open areas with a sterile cloth if available.
- Reassess neurovascular status below the injury site after splinting.

Sprains

- Use the acronym RICE to manage sprains:
- Refrain from weight-bearing.
- Apply ice to decrease inflammation.
- Apply a compression dressing to minimize swelling.
- Elevate the affected limb.

Heat stroke

- The nurse should identify heat stroke (body temperature greater than 40° C [104° F]) quickly and treat it aggressively.
- Manifestations of heat stroke include hot, dry skin; hypotension; tachypnea; tachycardia; anxiety; confusion; unusual behavior; seizures; and coma. The client does not sweat.
- Intervene to provide rapid cooling.
  - Remove the client's clothing.
  - Place ice packs over the major arteries (axillae, chest, groin, neck).
  - Immerse the client in a cold-water bath.
  - Wet the client's body, then fan with rapid movement of air.
  - Do not allow client to shiver. If client shivers, cover her with a sheet.

Frostnip and frostbite

- Occurs when the body is exposed to freezing temperatures.
- Common sites include the earlobes, tip of the nose, fingers, and toes.
- Frostnip does not lead to tissue injury and can be treated by warming.
- Frostbite presents as white, waxy areas on exposed skin. Tissue injury occurs.
- Frostbite can be full- or partial-thickness.
- Warm the affected area in a 37° to 42° C (98.6° to 108° F) water bath.
- Provide pain medication.
- Administer a tetanus vaccination.

Burns

- Burns can result from electrical current, chemicals, radiation, or flames.
- Home hazards include pot handles that protrude over the stove, hot bath water, and electrical appliances.
- Remove the agent (electrical current, radiation source, chemical).
- Smother any flames that are present. Perform a primary survey.
- Cover the client and maintain NPO status.
- Elevate the client's extremities if not contraindicated (presence of a fracture).
- Perform a head-to-toe assessment and estimate the surface area and thickness of burns.
- Administer fluids and a tetanus toxoid.

Altitude-related illnesses

Clients can become hypoxic in high altitudes. Altitude sickness can progress to cerebral and pulmonary edema and requires immediate treatment.

EXPECTED FINDINGS
- Throbbing headache
- Nausea
- Vomiting
- Dyspnea
- Anorexia

NURSING INTERVENTIONS
- Administer oxygen.
- Descend to a lower altitude.
- Provide pharmacological therapy, such as steroids and diuretics, if indicated.
- Promote rest

CPR

CPR is a combination of basic interventions designed to sustain oxygen and circulation to vital organs until more advanced interventions can be initiated to correct the root cause of the cardiac arrest.
- Efficient CPR improves the client's chance of survival.
- Trained individuals can deliver basic interventions, but advanced interventions require training that is more sophisticated, which requires certification and use of emergency equipment.
- CPR is directed at artificially providing a client with circulation (chest compressions) and oxygenation (ventilations) in the absence of cardiac output.
- CPR is a component of basic life support (BLS).
- The goal of BLS is to provide oxygen to the vital organs until appropriate advanced resuscitation measures can be initiated or until resuscitative efforts are ordered to be stopped.
- BLS involves the CABs (Chest Compression, Airway, and Breathing) of CPR. Q EBP
  - Assess victim for a response and look for breathing. Do not take time to perform a "look, listen, and feel" assessment of breathing. If there is no breathing or no normal breathing (only gasping), call for help.
  - If alone, activate emergency response system and get an automated external defibrillator (AED), if available, and return to the client. If a second person is available, send her to activate the emergency response system and get an AED.
  - Check pulse. Begin CPR compressions alternated with breaths if a pulse is not detected.
- For further detail on CPR, visit the American Heart Association website, www.heart.org.

CLIENT EDUCATION
- Encourage family members to take basic first aid and CPR courses. Refer clients and family members to a community agency where basic first aid and CPR are taught.
- Teach clients and family members keep emergency numbers (poison control, fire/rescue, providers, and nearest hospitals and urgent care facilities) in the home.

1. A nurse is providing discharge instructions to a client who has a prescription for oxygen use at home. Which of the following information should the nurse include about home oxygen safety? (Select all that apply.)

    A. Family members who smoke must be at least 10 ft from the client when oxygen is in use.

    B. Nail polish should not be used near a client who is receiving oxygen.

    C. A "No Smoking" sign should be placed on the front door.

    D. Cotton bedding and clothing should be replaced with items made from wool.

    E. A fire extinguisher should be readily available in the home.

2. A nurse educator is presenting a module on basic first aid for newly licensed home health nurses. The nurse educator evaluates the teaching as effective when the newly licensed nurse states the client who has heat stroke will have which of the following?

    A. Hypotension

    B. Bradycardia

    C. Clammy skin

    D. Bradypnea

3. A nurse educator is conducting a parenting class for new parents of infants. Which of the following statements made by a participant indicates understanding of the instructions?

    A. "I will set my water heater at 130° F."

    B. "Once my baby can sit up, he should be safe in the bathtub."

    C. "I will place my baby on his stomach to sleep."

    D. "Once my infant starts to push up, I will remove the mobile from over the crib."

4. A home health nurse is discussing the dangers of carbon monoxide poisoning with a client. Which of the following information should the nurse include in her counseling?

    A. Carbon monoxide has a distinct odor.

    B. Water heaters should be inspected every 5 years.

    C. The lungs are damaged from carbon monoxide inhalation.

    D. Carbon monoxide binds with hemoglobin in the body.

5. A home health nurse is discussing the dangers of food poisoning with a client. Which of the following information should the nurse including in her counseling? (Select all that apply.)

    A. Most food poisoning is caused by a virus.

    B. Immunocompromised individuals are at risk for complications from food poisoning

    C. Clients who are at high risk should eat or drink only pasteurized dairy products.

    D. Healthy individuals usually recover from the illness in a few weeks.

    E. Handling raw and fresh food separately can prevent food poisoning.

PRACTICE Active Learning Scenario

A nurse educator is teaching a module on the basic principles of creating a home safety plan during nursing orientation to a group of newly appointed home health nurses. Use the ATI Active Learning Template: Basic Concept to complete this item.

NURSING INTERVENTIONS: List four key elements that a home safety plan should include.

Application Exercises Key

1. A. The nurse should remind family members who smoke to do so outside.

   B. **CORRECT:** The nurse should remind the client not to use nail polish or other flammable materials in the home.

   C. **CORRECT:** The nurse should have the client place a "No Smoking" sign near the front door, and possibly on the client's bedroom door.

   D. The nurse should tell the client to choose cotton materials for clothing and bedding. Woolen and synthetic materials create static electricity and could cause a fire.

   E. **CORRECT:** The nurse should remind all individuals to have a fire extinguisher at home. This is especially important for a client who is receiving oxygen.

   (N) *NCLEX® Connection: Safety and Infection Control, Safe Use of Equipment*

2. A. **CORRECT:** Hypotension is a manifestation of heat stroke.

   B. Tachycardia is a manifestation of heat stroke.

   C. Hot, dry skin is a manifestation of heat stroke.

   D. Dyspnea is a manifestation of heat stroke.

   (N) *NCLEX® Connection: Physiological Adaptation, Pathophysiology*

3. A. The nurse should instruct the parent to set the home water heater temperature to 120° F or less.

   B. Although the baby can hold his head above the water by sitting up, this does not make the child safe in the bathtub. The nurse should warn the parent to never leave an infant or toddler alone in the bathtub.

   C. The nurse should remind the parent to place the infant on his back to sleep, and to remove suffocation hazards from the crib.

   D. **CORRECT:** The parent should plan to remove crib toys, such as mobiles, from over the bed as soon as the infant begins to push up so the infant is unable to touch them.

   (N) *NCLEX® Connection: Safety and Infection Control, Home Safety*

4. A. The nurse should include that carbon monoxide cannot be seen, smelled, or tasted.

   B. The nurse should tell the client to inspect gas-burning furnaces, water heaters, and appliances annually.

   C. The nurse should inform the client that carbon monoxide impairs the body's ability to use oxygen, but the lungs are not damaged.

   D. **CORRECT:** The nurse should warn the client that carbon monoxide is very dangerous because it binds with hemoglobin and ultimately reduces the oxygen supplied to the tissues in the body.

   (N) *NCLEX® Connection: Safety and Infection Control, Home Safety*

5. A. The nurse should include that most food poisoning is caused by bacteria such as *Escherichia coli*, *Listeria monocytogenes*, and *Salmonella*.

   B. **CORRECT:** The nurse should warn the client that very young, very old, immunocompromised, and pregnant individuals are at risk for complications from food poisoning.

   C. **CORRECT:** The nurse should include that clients who are at high risk should follow a low-microbial diet, which includes eating or drinking only pasteurized milk, yogurt, cheese, and other dairy products.

   D. The nurse should inform the client that healthy individuals usually recover from the illness in a few days.

   E. **CORRECT:** The nurse should include interventions to prevent food poisoning, such as performing proper hand hygiene, cooking meat and fish to the correct temperature, handling raw and fresh food separately to avoid cross-contamination, and refrigerating perishable items.

   (N) *NCLEX® Connection: Physiological Adaptation, Pathophysiology*

PRACTICE Answer

Using the ATI Active Learning Template: Basic Concept

NURSING INTERVENTIONS

A home safety plan should include the following.

- Keep emergency numbers near the phone for prompt use in the event of an emergency of any type.
- Ensure that the number and placement of fire extinguishers and smoke alarms are adequate, that they are operable, and that family members know how to operate them. Set a time to routinely change the batteries in the smoke alarms (for example, in the fall when the clocks are set to standard time and spring when set to Daylight Saving Time).
- Have a family exit plan for fires that the family reviews and practices regularly. Be sure to include closing windows and doors if able and to exit a smoke filled area by covering the mouth and nose with a damp cloth and getting down as close to the floor as possible.
- Review with clients of all ages that in the event that the client's clothing or skin is on fire, the client should use the mnemonic "stop, drop, and roll" to extinguish the fire.
- Review oxygen safety measures. Because oxygen can cause materials to combust more easily and burn more rapidly, the client and family must be provided with information on use of the oxygen delivery equipment and the dangers of combustion.

(N) *NCLEX® Connection: Safety and Infection Control, Home Safety*

UNIT 1   SAFE, EFFECTIVE CARE ENVIRONMENT
SECTION: SAFETY AND INFECTION CONTROL

CHAPTER 14 *Ergonomic Principles*

Ergonomics is a science that focuses on the factors or qualities in an object's design or use that contribute to comfort, safety, efficiency, and ease of use.

Using good body mechanics when positioning and moving clients promotes safety for the client and the staff.

Before attempting to position or move a client, perform a mobility assessment. Begin with the easiest movements (range of motion) and progress as long as the client tolerates it (balance, gait, exercise).

ERGONOMIC PRINCIPLES AND BODY MECHANICS

- Body mechanics is the use of muscles to maintain balance, posture, and body alignment when performing a physical task. Nurses use body mechanics when providing care to clients by lifting, bending, and assisting clients with the activities of daily living.
- Body alignment keeps the center of gravity stable, which promotes comfort and reduces strain on the muscles.
- Good body mechanics reduces the risk of injury. Whenever possible, use mechanical lift devices to lift and transfer clients. Many facilities have "no manual lift" and "no solo lift" policies.

CENTER OF GRAVITY

- The center of gravity is the center of a mass.
- Weight is a quantity of matter on which the force of gravity acts.
- To lift an object, it is essential to overcome the weight of the object and to know the center of gravity of the object.
- When the human body is in the upright position, the center of gravity is the pelvis.
- When an individual moves, the center of gravity shifts.
- The closer the line of gravity is to the center of the base of support, the more stable the individual is.
- To lower the center of gravity, bend the hips and knees.
- Spread your feet apart to lower your center of gravity and broaden your base of support. This results in greater stability and balance.

LIFTING

- Use the major muscle groups to prevent back strain, and tighten the abdominal muscles to increase support to the back muscles.
- Distribute your weight between the large muscles of the arms and legs to decrease the strain on any one muscle group and to avoid strain on smaller muscles.
- When lifting an object from the floor, flex your hips, knees, and back. Bring the object to thigh level, bending your knees and keeping your back straight. Stand up while holding the object as close as possible to your body, bringing the load to the center of gravity to increase stability and decrease back strain.
- Use assistive devices whenever possible and seek assistance whenever you need it.

PUSHING OR PULLING

When pushing or pulling a load:
- Widen your base of support.
- When opportunity allows, pull objects toward the center of gravity rather than pushing them away.
- If pushing, move your front foot forward and, if pulling, move your rear leg back to promote stability.
- Face the direction of movement when moving a client.
- Use your own body as a counterweight when pushing or pulling to make the movement easier.
- Sliding, rolling, and pushing require less energy than lifting and offer less risk for injury.
- Avoid twisting your thoracic spine and bending your back while your hips and knees are straight.

GUIDELINES FOR PREVENTING INJURY

- Know your facility's policies for lifting and safe client handling. **Qs**
- Have one or more staff members assist with positioning clients. Moving them up in bed is a significant cause of back pain and injury.
- Plan ahead for activities that require lifting, transfer, and ambulation of a client, and ask others to be available to assist.
- Prepare the environment by removing obstacles prior to the procedure.
- Explain the process to the client and assistants to clarify their roles.
- Be aware that the safest way to lift a client is with assistive equipment.
- Rest between heavy activities to decrease muscle fatigue.
- Maintain good posture and exercise regularly to increase the strength of your arms, legs, back, and abdominal muscles, so these activities will require less energy.
- Keep your head and neck in a straight line with your pelvis to avoid neck flexion and hunched shoulders, which can cause impingement of nerves in your neck.
- Use smooth movements when lifting and moving clients to prevent injury from sudden or jerky muscle movements.

- When standing for long periods of time, flex your hips and knees by using a footrest. When sitting for long periods of time, keep your knees slightly higher than your hips.
- Avoid repetitive movements of the hands, wrists, and shoulders. Take a break every 15 to 20 min to flex and stretch joints and muscles.
- Avoid twisting your spine or bending at the waist (flexion) to minimize the risk for injury.

POSITIONING CLIENTS

- Position clients, especially those who are unable to move themselves, so that they maintain good body alignment. Frequent position changes prevent discomfort, contractures, pressure on tissues, and nerve and circulatory damage, and they stimulate postural reflexes and muscle tone. Qᴘᴄᴄ
- Use pillows, bath blankets, hand rolls, boots, splints, trochanter rolls, ankle support devices, and other aids to maintain proper body alignment.

TRANSFERS AND USE OF ASSISTIVE DEVICES

- Evaluate each situation and use an algorithm to determine the safest method to transfer or move the client. Answer these questions: Can the client bear weight? Can she assist? Is she cooperative?
- Determine the client's ability to help with transfers (balance, muscle strength, endurance, use of a trapeze bar).
- Evaluate the need for additional staff or assistive devices (transfer belt, hydraulic lift, sliding board).
- Assess and monitor the use of mobility aids (canes, walkers, crutches).
- Include assistance or mobility aids in the plan of care for safe transfers and ambulation.

BED AND CLIENT POSITIONS

Semi-Fowler's

- The client lies supine with the head of the bed elevated 15° to 45° (typically 30°).
- This position prevents regurgitation of enteral feedings and aspiration by clients who have difficulty swallowing.
- It also promotes lung expansion for clients who have dyspnea or are receiving mechanical ventilation.

Fowler's

- The client lies supine with the head of the bed elevated 45° to 60°.
- This position is useful during procedures such as nasogastric tube insertion and suctioning. It allows for better chest expansion and ventilation and better dependent drainage after abdominal surgeries.

High-Fowler's

- The client lies supine with the head of the bed elevated 60° to 90°.
- This position promotes lung expansion by lowering the diaphragm and thus helps relieve severe dyspnea.
- It also helps prevent aspiration during meals.

Supine or dorsal recumbent

- The client lies on his back with his head and shoulders elevated on a pillow and his forearms on pillows or at his side. A foot support prevents foot drop and maintains proper alignment.

Prone

- The client lies flat on his abdomen and chest with his head to one side and his back in correct alignment.
- This position promotes drainage from the mouth after throat or oral surgery, but inhibits chest expansion. It is for short-term use only.
- This position helps prevent hip flexion contractures following a lower extremity amputation.

Lateral or side-lying

- The client lies on his side with most of his weight on the dependent hip and shoulder and his arms in flexion in front of his body. He should have a pillow under his head and neck, his upper arms, and his legs and thighs to maintain body alignment.
- This is a good sleeping position, but the client needs turning regularly to prevent the development of pressure ulcers on the dependent areas. A 30° lateral position is essential for clients at risk for pressure ulcers.

Sims' or semi-prone

- The client is on his side halfway between lateral and prone positions, with his weight on his anterior ileum, humerus, and clavicle. His lower arm is behind him while his upper arm is in front. Both legs are in flexion but the upper leg is flexed at a greater angle than the lower leg at the hip as well as at the knee.
- This is a comfortable sleeping position for many clients, and it promotes oral drainage.

Orthopneic

- The client sits in the bed or at the bedside with a pillow on the overbed table, which is across the client's lap. He rests his arms on the overbed table.
- This position allows for chest expansion and is especially beneficial for clients who have COPD.

Trendelenburg

- The entire bed is tilted with the head of the bed lower than the foot of the bed.
- This position facilitates postural drainage and venous return.

Reverse Trendelenburg

- The entire bed is tilted with the foot of the bed lower than the head of the bed.
- This position promotes gastric emptying and prevents esophageal reflux.

Modified Trendelenburg

- The client remains flat with his legs above the level of his heart.
- This position helps prevent and treat hypovolemia and facilitates venous return.

PRACTICE Active Learning Scenario

A nurse is presenting the basic principles of proper lifting to a group of assistive personnel. Use the ATI Active Learning Template: Basic Concept to complete this item.

UNDERLYING PRINCIPLES: List four key elements of proper lifting techniques.

Application Exercises

1. A nurse is caring for a client who is receiving enteral tube feedings due to dysphagia. Which of the following bed positions should the nurse use for safe care of this client?

   A. Supine

   B. Semi-Fowler's

   C. Semi-prone

   D. Trendelenburg

2. A nurse is caring for a client who is sitting in a chair and asks to return to bed. Which of the following actions is the nurse's priority at this time?

   A. Obtain a walker for the client to use to transfer back to bed.

   B. Call for additional staff to assist with the transfer.

   C. Use a transfer belt and assist the client back into bed.

   D. Determine the client's ability to help with the transfer.

3. A nurse is completing discharge instructions for a client who has COPD. The nurse should identify that the client understands the orthopneic position when she states that she will do which of the following when she has difficulty breathing at night?

   A. Lie on her back with her head and shoulders on a pillow.

   B. Lie flat on her stomach with her head to one side.

   C. Sit on the side of her bed and rest her arms over pillows on top of her bedside table.

   D. Lie on her side with her weight on her hip and shoulder with her arm flexed in front of her.

4. A nurse manager is reviewing guidelines for preventing injury with staff nurses. Which of the following instructions should the nurse manager include? (Select all that apply.)

   A. Request assistance when repositioning a client.

   B. Avoid twisting your spine or bending at the waist.

   C. Keep your knees slightly lower than your hips when sitting for long periods of time.

   D. Use smooth movements when lifting and moving clients.

   E. Take a break from repetitive movements every 2 to 3 hr to flex and stretch your joints and muscles.

5. A nurse educator is reviewing proper body mechanics during employee orientation. Which of the following statements should the nurse identify as an indication that an attendee understands the teaching? (Select all that apply.)

   A. "My line of gravity should fall outside my base of support."

   B. "The lower my center of gravity, the more stability I have."

   C. "To broaden my base of support, I should spread my feet apart."

   D. "When I lift an object, I should hold it as close to my body as possible."

   E. "When pulling an object, I should move my front foot forward."

1. A. In the supine position, the client lies on his back with his head and shoulders elevated on a pillow. This angle will not prevent regurgitation.

   B. **CORRECT:** In the semi-Fowler's position, the client lies supine with the head of the bed elevated 15° to 45° (typically 30°). This position helps prevent regurgitation and aspiration by clients who have difficulty swallowing. This is the safest position for clients receiving enteral tube feedings.

   C. In the semi-prone or Sims' position, the client is on his side halfway between lateral and prone positions. This position is not safe because it promotes regurgitation.

   D. In the Trendelenburg position, the entire bed is tilted with the head of the bed lower than the foot of the bed. This position is not safe because it promotes regurgitation.

   Ⓝ *NCLEX® Connection: Reduction of Risk Potential, Potential for Complications of Diagnostic Tests/Treatments/Procedures*

2. A. Although this might be a necessary assistive device for this client, obtaining a walker is not the priority action the nurse should take.

   B. Although this might be necessary for a safe transfer, calling for assistance is the not the priority action the nurse should take.

   C. Although this might be a necessary assistive device for the transfer of this client, using a transfer belt is not the priority action the nurse should take.

   D. **CORRECT:** The first action the nurse should take using the nursing process is to assess or collect data from the client. The nurse should determine the client's ability to help with transfers and then proceed with a safe transfer.

   Ⓝ *NCLEX® Connection: Safety and Infection Control, Ergonomic Principles*

3. A. The client is describing the supine position, not the orthopneic position.

   B. The client is describing the prone position, not the orthopneic position.

   C. **CORRECT:** The client is describing the orthopneic position. This position allows for chest expansion and is especially beneficial for clients who have COPD.

   D. The client is describing the lateral or side-lying position, not the orthopneic position.

   Ⓝ *NCLEX® Connection: Safety and Infection Control, Ergonomic Principles*

4. A. **CORRECT:** To reduce the risk of injury, at least two staff members should reposition clients.

   B. **CORRECT:** Twisting the spine or bending at the waist (flexion) increases the risk for injury.

   C. When sitting for long periods of time, it is essential to keep the knees slightly higher, not lower, than the hips to decrease strain on the lower back.

   D. **CORRECT:** Using smooth movements instead of sudden or jerky muscle movements helps prevent injury

   E. It is important to take a break every 15 to 20 min, not every 2 to 3 hr, from repetitive movements to flex and stretch joints and muscles.

   Ⓝ *NCLEX® Connection: Safety and Infection Control, Ergonomic Principles*

5. A. To reduce the risk of falling, the line of gravity should fall within the base of support, not outside it.

   B. **CORRECT:** Being closer to the ground lowers the center of gravity, which leads to greater stability and balance.

   C. **CORRECT:** Spreading the feet apart increases and widens the base of support.

   D. **CORRECT:** Holding an object as close to the body as possible helps avoid displacement of the center of gravity and thus prevent injury and instability.

   E. To promote stability, the nurse should move the rear leg back when pulling on an object.

   Ⓝ *NCLEX® Connection: Safety and Infection Control, Ergonomic Principles*

PRACTICE Answer

Using the ATI Active Learning Template: Basic Concept

UNDERLYING PRINCIPLES

- Use the major muscle groups to prevent back strain, and tighten the abdominal muscles to increase support to the back muscles.
- Distribute your weight between the large muscles of the arms and legs to decrease the strain on any one muscle group and to avoid strain on smaller muscles.
- When lifting an object from the floor, flex your hips, knees, and back. Bring the object to thigh level, bending your knees and keeping your back straight. Stand up while holding the object as close as possible to your body, bringing the load to the center of gravity to increase stability and decrease back strain.
- Use assistive devices whenever possible, and seek assistance whenever you need it.

Ⓝ *NCLEX® Connection: Safety and Infection Control, Ergonomic Principles*

CHAPTER 15 *Security and Disaster Plans*

A disaster is a mass casualty or intra-facility event that at least temporarily overwhelms or interrupts the normal flow of services of a hospital. Disasters that health care facilities face include internal and external emergencies.

Internal emergencies include loss of electric power or potable water, and severe damage or casualties within the facility related to fire, weather (tornado, hurricane), explosion, or a terrorist act. Internal emergency readiness includes safety and hazardous materials protocols, and infection control policies and practices.

External emergencies include hurricanes, floods, volcano eruptions, earthquakes, disease epidemics, industrial accidents, chemical plant explosions, major transportation accidents, building collapse, and terrorist acts (including biological and chemical warfare). External emergency readiness includes a plan for participation in community-wide emergencies and disasters.

THE JOINT COMMISSION AND EMERGENCY PREPAREDNESS

The Joint Commission established emergency preparedness management standards for various types of health care facilities. These standards mandate that an institutional emergency preparedness plan is developed by all health care institutions and that these plans include institution-specific procedures for the following. Qs

- Notifying and assigning personnel.
- Notifying external authorities of emergencies.
- Managing space and supplies and providing security.
- Isolating and decontaminating radioactive or chemical agents (measures to contain contamination, decontamination at the scene of exposure).
- Evacuating and setting up an alternative care site when the environment cannot support adequate client care and treatment. Critical processes when an alternative care site is necessary include the following.
  - Client information/care packaging (medications, supplies, admissions, medical records, and tracking)
  - Interfacility communication
  - Transportation of clients, staff, and equipment
  - Cross-privileging of medical staff
- Performing triage of incoming clients.
- Managing clients during emergencies, including scheduling, modification or discontinuation of services, control of client information, and client discharge and transportation.
- Interacting with family members and the media and responding to public reaction.
- Identifying backup resources (electricity, water, fire protection, fuel sources, medical gas and vacuum) for utilities and communication.
- Orienting and educating personnel participating in implementation of the emergency preparedness plan.
- Providing crisis support for health care workers (access to vaccines, infection control recommendations, mental health counseling).
- Providing performance monitoring and evaluation related to emergency preparedness.
- Conducting two emergency preparedness drills each year.
  - Drills should include an influx of clients beyond those being treated by the facility. Qpi
  - Drills should include either an internal or an external disaster (a situation beyond the normal capacity of the facility).
- Participating in one community-wide practice drill per year.

NURSING ROLE IN DISASTER PLANNING AND EMERGENCY RESPONSE PLANS

Emergency response plans

Each health care institution must have an emergency preparedness plan developed by a planning committee. This committee reviews information regarding the potential for various types of natural and man-made emergencies depending on the characteristics of the community. Resources necessary to meet the potential emergency are determined and a plan developed that takes into consideration all of the above factors.

- Nurses, as well as a cross-section of other members of the health care team, are involved in the development of a disaster plan for such emergencies. Criteria under which the disaster plan is activated must be clear. Roles for each employee are outlined and administrative control determined. A designated area for the area command center is identified as well as a person to serve as the incident control manager.
- Communication, using common terminology, is important within any emergency management plan. Qᴛᴄ
- Nurses are expected to set up an emergency action plan for personal family needs.

TRIAGE

Principles of triage are followed in health care facilities involved in a mass casualty event. These differ from the principles of triage that are typically followed during provision of day-to-day services in an emergency or urgent care setting. During mass casualty events, casualties are separated in relation to their potential for survival, and treatment is allocated accordingly.

Categories of triage during mass casualty events

Emergent Category (Class I): Highest priority is given to clients who have life-threatening injuries but also have a high possibility of survival once they are stabilized.

Urgent Category (Class II): Second-highest priority is given to clients who have major injuries that are not yet life-threatening and can usually wait 45 to 60 min for treatment.

Nonurgent Category (Class III): The next highest priority is given to clients who have minor injuries that are not life-threatening and do not need immediate attention.

Expectant Category (Class IV): The lowest priority is given to clients who are not expected to live and are allowed to die naturally. Comfort measures can be provided, but restorative care is not.

DISCHARGE/RELOCATION OF CLIENTS

During an emergency such as a fire or a mass casualty event, decisions are made regarding discharging clients or relocating them so their beds can be given to clients who have higher-priority needs.

Criteria for identifying when clients can be safely discharged
- Ambulatory clients requiring minimal care are discharged or relocated first.
- Clients requiring assistance are next and arrangements are made for continuation of their care.
- Clients who are unstable and/or require nursing care are not discharged or relocated unless they are in imminent danger.

FIRE

- If evacuation of the unit is necessary, horizontal evacuation is done first. Lateral evacuation is done if client safety cannot be maintained.
- If a nurse discovers a fire that threatens the safety of a client, the nurse uses the RACE (Rescue, Alarm, Contain, and Extinguish) mnemonic to guide the order of actions. **(15.1)**

SEVERE THUNDERSTORM/TORNADO

- Draw shades and close drapes to protect against shattering glass.
- Lower beds to the lowest position and move away from the windows.
- Place blankets over all clients who are confined to beds.
- Close all doors.
- Relocate as many ambulatory clients as possible into the hallways (away from windows) or other secure location designated by the facility.
- Do not use elevators.
- Monitor for severe weather warnings using television, radio, or Internet.

15.1 Race mnemonic	
R RESCUE	Rescue the client and other individuals from the area.
A ALARM	Sound the fire alarm, which activates the EMS response system. Systems that could increase fire spread are automatically shut down with activation of the alarm.
C CONTAIN	After clearing the room or area, close the door leading to the area in which the fire is located as well as the fire doors. Fire doors are kept closed as much as possible when moving from area to area within the facility to avoid the spread of smoke and fire.
E EXTINGUISH	Make an attempt to extinguish small fires using a single fire extinguisher, smothering them with a blanket, or dousing with water (except with an electrical or grease fire). Complete evacuation of the area occurs if the nurse cannot put the fire out with these methods. Attempts at extinguishing the fire are only made when the employee is properly trained in the safe use of a fire extinguisher and when only one extinguisher is needed.

BIOLOGICAL PATHOGENS

Be alert to indications of a possible bioterrorism attack, as early detection and management is key. Often the manifestations are similar to other illnesses.

- Be alert for the appearance of a disease that does not normally occur at a specific time or place, has atypical manifestations, or occurs in a specific community or people group.
- In most instances, infection from biological agents is not spread from one client to another. Management of the incident includes recognition of the occurrence, directing personnel in the proper use of personal protective equipment, and, in some situations, decontamination and isolation.
- Use appropriate isolation measures as indicated.
- Transport or move clients only if needed for treatment and care.
- Take measures to protect self and others.
- Recognize indications of infection/poisoning and appropriate treatment. **(15.2)** ○EBP

CHEMICAL INCIDENTS

Chemical incidents can occur as result of an accident or due to a purposeful action such as terrorism.

- Take measures to protect self and to avoid contact.
- Assess and intervene to maintain the client's airway, breathing, and circulation. Administer first aid as needed.
- Remove the offending chemical by undressing the client, removing all identifiable particulate matter. Provide immediate and prolonged irrigations of contaminated areas. Irrigate skin with running water, with the exception of dry chemicals such as lye or white phosphorus. In the case of exposure to a dry chemical, brush the agent off of the client's clothing and skin.
- Gather a specific history of the injury, if possible (name and concentration of the chemical, duration of exposure).
- In the event of chemical attack, have knowledge of which facilities are open to exposed clients and which are only open to unexposed clients.
- Follow the facility's emergency response plans (personal protection measures, the handling and disposal of wastes, use of space and equipment, reporting procedures).

15.2 Biological pathogen manifestations, prevention, and treatment

Inhalational anthrax
MANIFESTATIONS
- Fever
- Cough
- Shortness of breath
- Muscle aches
- Mild chest pain
- Meningitis
- Shock

PREVENTION
- Anthrax vaccine for high-risk
- Ciprofloxacin & Doxycycline IV/PO

TREATMENT: includes one or two additional antibiotics such as vancomycin, penicillin and anthrax antitoxin

Cutaneous anthrax
MANIFESTATIONS
- Starts as a lesion that can be itchy
- Develops into a vesicular lesion that later becomes necrotic with the formation of black eschar
- Fever, chills

PREVENTION: Anthrax vaccine for high-risk

TREATMENT: Ciprofloxacin, Doxycycline

Botulism
MANIFESTATIONS
- Difficulty swallowing
- Double vision
- Slurred speech
- Descending progressive weakness
- Nausea, vomiting, abdominal cramps
- Difficulty breathing

PREVENTION/TREATMENT
- Airway management
- Antitoxin
- Elimination of toxin

Viral hemorrhagic fevers (e.g., Ebola, yellow fever)
MANIFESTATIONS
- Fatigue
- Kidney failure
- Elevated temperature
- Nausea, vomiting, diarrhea
- Internal and external bleeding
- Shock

PREVENTION
- Vaccination available for yellow fever, Argentine hemorrhagic fever
- Barrier protection from infected person, isolation precautions specific to disease

TREATMENT
- No cure, supportive care only
- Minimize invasive procedures

Plague
MANIFESTATIONS
- These forms can occur separately or in combination:
- Pneumonic plague: fever, headache, weakness, pneumonia with shortness of breath, chest pain, cough, and bloody or watery sputum.
- Bubonic plague: swollen, tender lymph glands, fever, headache, chills, and weakness.
- Septicemic plague: fever, chills, prostration, abdominal pain, shock, disseminated intravascular coagulation (DIC), gangrene of nose and digits.

PREVENTION: Contact precautions till decontaminated or bubos no longer drain (bubonic, septicemic); droplet precautions till 72 hr after antibiotics (pneumonic)

TREATMENT: Streptomycin/gentamicin or tetracycline/doxycycline.

Smallpox
MANIFESTATIONS
- High fever
- Fatigue
- Severe headache
- Rash
- Chills
- Vomiting
- Delirium

PREVENTION
- Vaccine; can vaccinate within 3 days of exposure
- Contact and airborne precautions

TREATMENT
- Supportive care(prevent dehydration, provide skin care, medications for pain and fever)
- Antibiotics for secondary infections

Tularemia
MANIFESTATIONS
- Sudden fever
- Chills
- Headache
- Diarrhea
- Muscle aches
- Joint pain
- Dry cough
- Progressive weakness
- If airborne, life-threatening pneumonia and systemic infection

PREVENTION: vaccine under review by the Food and Drug Administration

TREATMENT: streptomycin or gentamicin are the medications of choice; in mass causality, use doxycycline or ciprofloxacin

HAZARDOUS MATERIAL INCIDENTS

- Take measures to protect self and to avoid contact.
- Approach the scene with caution.
- Identify the hazardous material with available resources (emergency response guidebook, poison control centers). Know the location of the safety data sheets manual.
- Try to contain the material in one place prior to the arrival of the hazardous materials team.
- If individuals are contaminated, decontaminate them as much as possible at the scene or as close as possible to the scene.
  - Don gloves, gown, mask, and shoe covers to protect self from contamination.
  - With few exceptions, water is the universal antidote. For biological hazardous materials, wash skin with copious amounts of water and antibacterial soap.
  - Carefully and slowly remove contaminated clothing so that deposited material does not become airborne
  - Place all contaminated material into large plastic bags and seal them.

RADIOLOGICAL INCIDENTS

- The amount of exposure is related to the duration of the exposure, distance from source, and amount of shielding.
- The facility where victims are treated activates interventions to prevent contamination of treatment areas (floors and furniture are covered, air vents and ducts are covered, radiation-contaminated waste is disposed of according to procedural guidelines).
- Wear water-resistant gowns, double glove, and fully cover their bodies with caps, shoe covers, masks, and goggles.
- Wear radiation or dosimetry badges to monitor the amount of their radiation exposure.
- Survey clients initially with a radiation meter to determine the amount of contamination.
- Decontamination with soap, water, and disposable towels occurs prior to entering the facility. Water runoff is contaminated and contained.
- After decontamination, resurvey clients for residual contamination. Continue irrigation of the skin until the client is clean of all contamination.

BOMB THREAT

When a phone call is received:
- Extend the conversation as long as possible.
- Listen for distinguishing background noises (music, voices, traffic, airplanes).
- Note distinguishing voice characteristics of the caller.
- Ask where and when the bomb is set to explode.
- Note whether the caller is familiar with the physical arrangement of the facility.
- If a bomb-like device is located, do not touch it. Clear the area, and isolate the device as much as possible by closing doors, for example.
- Notify the appropriate authorities and personnel (police, administrator, director of nursing).
- Cooperate with police and others. Assist to conduct a search as needed, provide copies of floor plans, have master keys available, and watch for and isolate suspicious objects such as packages and boxes.
- Keep elevators available for authorities.
- Remain calm and alert and try not to alarm clients.

SECURITY PLAN

All health care facilities have security plans in place that include preventive, protective, and response measures designed for identified security needs.
- Security issues faced by health care facilities include admission of potentially dangerous individuals, vandalism, infant abduction, and information theft.
- The International Association for Healthcare Security & Safety provides recommendations for the development of security plans.

NURSING ROLE IN SECURITY PLAN

Nurses should be aware that security measures include:
- An identification system that identifies employees, volunteers, physicians, students, and regularly scheduled contract services staff as authorized personnel of the health care facility.
- Electronic security systems in high-risk areas (maternal newborn to prevent infant abductions, the emergency department to prevent unauthorized entrance).
  - Key code access into and out of high-risk areas
  - Wristbands that electronically link parents and their infants
  - Alarms integrated with closed-circuit television cameras

Nurses should prepare to take immediate action when breaches in security occur. Time is of the essence in preventing or stopping a breach in security. **Qs**

Application Exercises

1. A nurse is caring for multiple clients during a mass casualty event. Which of the following clients is the priority?

   A. A client who received crush injuries to the chest and abdomen and is expected to die

   B. A client who has a 4-inch laceration to the head

   C. A client who has partial-thickness and full-thickness burns to his face, neck, and chest

   D. A client who has a fractured fibula and tibia

2. A nurse educator is discussing the facility protocol in the event of a tornado with the staff. Which of the following should the nurse include in the instructions? (Select all that apply.)

   A. Open doors to client rooms.

   B. Place blankets over clients who are confined to beds.

   C. Move beds away from the windows.

   D. Draw shades and close drapes.

   E. Instruct ambulatory clients in the hallways to return to their rooms.

3. An occupational health nurse is caring for an employee who was exposed to an unknown dry chemical, resulting in a chemical burn. Which of the following interventions should the nurse include in the plan of care?

   A. Irrigate the affected area with running water.

   B. Wash the affected area with antibacterial soap.

   C. Brush the chemical off the skin and clothing.

   D. Leave the clothing in place until emergency personnel arrive.

4. A security officer is reviewing actions to take in the event of a bomb threat by phone to a group of nurses. Which of the following statements by a nurse indicates understanding of proper procedure?

   A. "I will get the caller off the phone as soon as possible so I can alert the staff."

   B. "I will begin evacuating clients using the elevators."

   C. "I will not ask any questions and just let the caller talk."

   D. "I will listen for background noises."

5. A nurse on a medical-surgical unit is informed that a mass casualty event occurred in the community and that it is necessary to discharge stable clients to make beds available for injury victims. Which of the following clients should the nurse recommend for discharge? (Select all that apply.)

   A. A client who is dehydrated and receiving IV fluid and electrolytes

   B. A client who has a nasogastric tube to treat a small bowel obstruction

   C. A client who is scheduled for elective surgery

   D. A client who has chronic hypertension and blood pressure 135/85 mm Hg

   E. A client who has acute appendicitis and is scheduled for an appendectomy

---

PRACTICE Active Learning Scenario

A nurse educator is teaching a module on biological pathogens during orientation to a group of newly hired nurses. What information should the nurse educator include? Use the ATI Active Learning Template: Basic Concept to complete this item.

RELATED CONTENT: List four manifestations and the recommended treatment for anthrax, botulism, pneumonic plague, and tularemia.

Application Exercises Key

1. A. The nurse should give the lowest priority to a client who is not expected to live. The nurse should provide comfort measures for this client (Expectant Category: Class IV).

   B. The nurse should give third priority to the client who has minor injury that is not life-threatening, such as a laceration to the head (Nonurgent Category: Class III).

   C. **CORRECT:** The nurse should give first priority to the client who has the greatest chance of survival with prompt intervention. If not treated immediately, a client who has burns to his face, neck, and chest is at risk for airway obstruction, but is otherwise expected to live. Therefore, this client is the highest priority (Emergent Category: Class I).

   D. The nurse should give second priority to the client who has major fractures (Urgent Category: Class II).

   Ⓝ *NCLEX® Connection: Management of Care, Establishing Priorities*

2. A. The nurse should close all client doors to minimize the threat of flying glass and debris.

   B. **CORRECT:** The nurse should place blankets over clients to protect them from shattering glass or flying debris.

   C. **CORRECT:** The nurse should move all beds away from windows to protect clients from shattering glass or flying debris.

   D. **CORRECT:** The nurse should draw shades and close drapes to protect clients against shattering glass.

   E. The nurse should instruct ambulatory clients to go to the hallways, away from windows, or other secure location designated by the facility.

   Ⓝ *NCLEX® Connection: Safety and Infection Control, Accident/Error/Injury Prevention*

3. A. The nurse should not apply water to a dry chemical exposure because it could activate the chemical and cause further harm.

   B. The nurse should wash the skin with antibacterial soap in the event of a biological exposure.

   C. **CORRECT:** The nurse should use a brush to remove the chemical off the skin and clothing.

   D. The nurse should plan to remove the client's clothing following appropriate decontamination.

   Ⓝ *NCLEX® Connection: Safety and Infection Control, Handing Hazardous and Infectious Materials*

4. A. In the event of a bomb threat, the nurse should keep the caller on the line in order to trace the call and to collect as much information as possible.

   B. The nurse should avoid using the elevators so that they are free for the authorities to use, and should not evacuate clients unless directed to by facility protocol.

   C. The nurse should ask the caller about the location of the bomb and the time it is set to explode in order to gather as much information as possible.

   D. **CORRECT:** In order to identify the location of the caller, the nurse should listen for background noises such as church bells, train whistles, or other distinguishing noises.

   Ⓝ *NCLEX® Connection: Safety and Infection Control, Handing Hazardous and Infectious Materials*

5. A. The nurse should recognize that a client who is receiving IV fluid and electrolytes requires ongoing nursing care and is therefore unstable for discharge.

   B. The nurse should recognize that a client who has a nasogastric tube requires ongoing nursing care and is therefore unstable for discharge.

   C. **CORRECT:** The nurse should identify a client who is scheduled elective surgery is stable and is therefore appropriate to recommend for discharge.

   D. **CORRECT:** A blood pressure 135/85 mm Hg is within the reference range for prehypertension. The nurse should identify this client as stable and appropriate to recommend for discharge.

   E. The nurse should recognize that a client who has an acute illness and is scheduled for surgery requires ongoing nursing care and is therefore unstable for discharge.

   Ⓝ *NCLEX® Connection: Management of Care, Establishing Priorities*

PRACTICE Active Learning Scenario

Using the ATI Active Learning Template: Basic Concept

RELATED CONTENT

Anthrax
- Manifestations
  - Fever
  - Cough
  - Shortness of breath
  - Muscle aches
  - Meningitis
  - Shock
- Nursing interventions
  - Ciprofloxacin
  - One or two additional antibiotics, such as vancomycin or penicillin

Botulism
- Manifestations
  - Difficulty swallowing
  - Double vision
  - Slurred speech
  - Descending progressive weakness
  - Nausea, vomiting, abdominal cramps
  - Difficulty breathing
- Nursing interventions
  - Airway management
  - Antitoxin
  - Elimination of toxin

Pneumonic plague
- Manifestations
  - Fever
  - Headache
  - Weakness
  - Rapidly developing pneumonia
  - Shortness of breath
  - Chest pain
  - Cough
  - Bloody or watery sputum.
- Nursing interventions
  - Early treatment is essential.
  - Streptomycin, gentamicin, the tetracyclines

Tularemia
- Manifestations
  - Sudden fever
  - Chills
  - Headache
  - Diarrhea
  - Muscle aches
  - Joint pain
  - Dry cough
  - Progressive weakness
  - If airborne, life-threatening pneumonia and systemic infection
- Nursing interventions
  - Streptomycin IV or gentamicin IV or IM are the drugs of choice.
  - In mass casualty, use doxycycline or ciprofloxacin.

Ⓝ *NCLEX® Connection: Safety and Infection Control, Handing Hazardous and Infectious Materials*

NCLEX® Connections

When reviewing the following chapters, keep in mind the relevant topics and tasks of the NCLEX outline, in particular:

Client Needs: Safety and Infection Control

ACCIDENT/ERROR/INJURY PREVENTION: Identify factors that influence accident/injury prevention.

HOME SAFETY: Educate the client on home safety issues.

Client Needs: Health Promotion and Maintenance

AGING PROCESS: Provide care and education for the adult client ages 65 through 85 years and over.

DEVELOPMENTAL STAGES AND TRANSITIONS: Identify expected physical, cognitive, and psychosocial stages of development.

HEALTH PROMOTION/DISEASE PREVENTION
Assess client's readiness to learn, learning preferences and barriers to learning.

Educate the client on actions to promote/maintain health and prevent disease.

Client Needs: Basic Care and Comfort

MOBILITY/IMMOBILITY: Assess the client for mobility, gait, strength, and motor skills.

CHAPTER 16 # Health Promotion and Disease Prevention

Nurses use traditional nursing measures and complementary therapies, such as guided imagery, massage, relaxation, and music, to help promote health and prevent disease.

Levels of prevention address health-related activities that are primary, secondary, and tertiary. Levels of prevention are not the same as levels of care. Qⓞⓘ

RISK ASSESSMENT

RISK FACTORS

Genetics: Heredity creates a predisposition for various disorders (heart disease, cancers, mental illnesses).

Gender: Some diseases are more common in one gender than in the other. For example, women have a higher incidence of autoimmune disorders, while men have a higher suicide rate.

Physiologic factors: Various physiologic states place clients at an increased risk for health problems (body mass index [BMI] above 25, pregnancy).

Environmental factors: Toxic substances and chemicals can affect health where clients live and work (water quality, pesticide exposure, air pollution).

Lifestyle-risk behaviors: Clients have control over how they choose to live, and making positive choices can reduce risk factors. Risk behaviors to screen for include stress, substance use disorders, tobacco use, diet deficiencies, lack of exercise, and sun exposure.

Age: Screening guidelines from the American Diabetes Association, American Heart Association, and American Cancer Society promote early detection and intervention. Ages vary with individual practices (for example, a woman who is sexually active before the age of 20 should start screenings when sexual activity begins).

TESTS

Frequency of some major examinations and screenings are baseline for clients who are asymptomatic and do not have risk factors:

Routine physical examination: Generally every 1 to 3 years for women and every 5 years for men from age 20 to 40, more often after age 40.

Dental assessment: Every 6 months.

Tuberculosis screen: Tuberculosis (TB) skin test every year. TB tests are generally not needed for people with a low risk of infection with TB bacteria. Higher risks include weak immune system and drug use. Health care workers should be screened annually.

Blood pressure: At least every 2 years; annually if previously elevated.

Body mass index: At each routine health care visit.

Blood cholesterol: Starting at age 20, a minimum of every 5 years.

Blood glucose: Starting at age 45, a minimum of every 3 years.

Visual acuity: Age 40 and under: every 3 to 5 years. Every 2 years ages 40 and 65. Every year after age 65.

Hearing acuity: Periodic hearing checks as needed; more frequently if hearing loss is noted.

Skin assessment: Every 3 years by a skin specialist for age 20 to 40; annually over age 40 years.

Digital rectal exam: During routine physical examination or annually if have at least a 10-year life expectancy. Consult with the provider if screen should continue after age 76.

Colorectal screening: Every year between age 50 and 75 for high-sensitivity fecal occult blood testing, or flexible sigmoidoscopy every 5 years, or colonoscopy every 10 years. Consult with the provider if screen should continue after age 76.

Tests specific for women

Cervical cancer screening: Ages 21 to 29: Papanicolaou test (Pap smear) every 3 years; ages 30 to 65: Pap and human papilloma virus test every 5 years.

Breast cancer screening: Ages 20 to 39: clinical breast examination every 3 years, then annually; ages 40 and older: mammogram annually.

Tests specific for men

Clinical testicular examination: At each routine health care visit starting at age 20.

Prostate-specific antigen test, digital rectal examination: Every year starting at age 50. Consult with the provider if screen should continue after age 76.

PREVENTION

Primary, secondary, and tertiary prevention describe the focus of activities and the level of prevention.

PRIMARY

Primary prevention addresses the needs of healthy clients to promote health and prevent disease with specific protections. It decreases the risk of exposure individual/community to disease.
- Immunization programs
- Child car seat education
- Nutrition, fitness activities
- Health education in schools

SECONDARY

Secondary prevention focuses on identifying illness, providing treatment, and conducting activities that help prevent a worsening health status.
- Communicable disease screening, case finding
- Early detection, treatment of diabetes mellitus
- Exercise programs for older adults who are frail

TERTIARY

Tertiary prevention aims to prevent the long-term consequences of a chronic illness or disability and to support optimal functioning.
- Begins after an injury or illness
- Prevention of pressure ulcers after spinal cord injury
- Promoting independence after traumatic brain injury
- Referrals to support groups
- Rehabilitation center

HEALTHY PEOPLE 2020

The Healthy People 2020 provides a list of national objectives to promote health and prevent disease among the national population. The objectives are updated every 10 years and involve a collaborative effort for implementation by the local governments, voluntary and professional organizations, businesses, and individuals.
- Improve health priorities
- Improve awareness and understanding of the progress involving health, disease, and disability.
- Apply measurable health goals at the local, state, and national level
- Apply best practice to strengthen polices and improve health practice
- Identify the need for research, evaluation and data collection of health disparities

NURSING INTERVENTIONS

Examine risk factors to identify modifications, adopt mutually agreeable goals, and identify support systems.
- Refer clients to educational/community/support resources. Help clients recognize benefits (not smoking reduces the risk of lung cancer) and overcome barriers (not smoking covers expenses for healthful pursuits).
- Advocate for changes in the community.

Use behavior-change strategies.
- Identify clients' readiness to receive and apply health information.
- Identify acceptable interventions.
- Help motivate change by setting realistic timelines.
- Reinforce steps toward change
- Assist the client to recognize his personal perceived barriers that can hinder commitment to adopting and maintaining the plan for a healthy lifestyle change.
- Encourage clients to maintain the change.
- Model healthy behaviors.

Promote healthy lifestyle behaviors by instructing clients to do the following.
- Use stress management strategies.
- Get adequate sleep and rest.
- Eat a nutritious diet to achieve and maintain a healthy weight.
- Avoid saturated fats.
- Participate in regular physical activity most days.
- While outdoors, wear protective clothing, use sunscreen, and avoid sun exposure between 10 a.m. and 4 p.m.
- Wear safety gear (bike helmets, knee and elbow pads) when participating in physical activity. Q⟞
- Avoid tobacco products, alcohol, and illegal drugs.
- Practice safe sex.
- Seek medical care when necessary, get routine screenings, and perform recommended self-examinations (breast, testicular).

Application Exercises

1. A nurse is caring for a 20-year-old client who is sexually active and has come to the college health clinic for a first-time checkup. Which of the following interventions should the nurse perform first to determine the client's need for health promotion and disease prevention?

    A. Measure vital signs.

    B. Encourage HIV screening.

    C. Determine risk factors.

    D. Instruct the client to use condoms.

2. A nurse in a clinic is planning health promotion and disease prevention strategies for a client who has multiple risk factors for cardiovascular disease. Which of the following interventions should the nurse include? (Select all that apply.)

    A. Help the client see the benefits of her actions.

    B. Identify the client's support systems.

    C. Suggest and recommend community resources.

    D. Devise and set goals for the client.

    E. Teach stress management strategies.

3. A nurse in a health clinic is caring for a 21-year-old client who reports a sore throat. The client tells the nurse that he has not seen a doctor since high school. Which of the following health screenings should the nurse expect the provider to perform for this client?

    A. Testicular examination

    B. Blood glucose

    C. Fecal occult blood

    D. Prostate-specific antigen

4. A nurse is talking with a client who recently attended a cholesterol screening event and a heart-healthy nutrition presentation at a neighborhood center. The client's total cholesterol was 248 mg/dL. After seeing the provider, the client started taking medication to lower his cholesterol level. The client was later hospitalized for severe chest pain, and subsequently enrolled in a cardiac rehabilitation program. Which of the following activities for the client is an example of primary prevention?

    A. Cholesterol screening

    B. Nutrition presentation

    C. Medication therapy

    D. Cardiac rehabilitation

5. A nurse at a provider's office is talking about routine screenings with a 45-year-old female client who has no specific family history of cancer or diabetes mellitus. Which of the following client statements indicates that the client understands how to proceed?

    A. "So I don't need the colon cancer procedure for another 2 or 3 years."

    B. "For now, I should continue to have a mammogram each year."

    C. "Because the doctor just did a Pap smear, I'll come back next year for another one."

    D. "I had my blood glucose test last year, so I won't need it again till next year."

PRACTICE Active Learning Scenario

A nurse is caring for a client in a spinal cord injury rehabilitation center following head and neck injuries sustained while riding a bicycle. The client had surgery during the acute phase of treatment to relieve intracranial pressure and to stabilize his cervical spine. Now, the client and his partner are learning essential self-management strategies. Use the ATI Active Learning Template: Basic Concept to complete this item.

RELATED CONTENT: List each of the three levels of prevention with an example of each level from this client's history or from what this client might have done to prevent this injury and its life-altering consequences.

1. A. The nurse should take vital signs when determining the client's need for health promotion and disease prevention. However, there is another action the nurse should take first.

   B. The nurse may suggest for the client to have a HIV screening when determining health promotion and disease prevention. However, there is another action the nurse should take first.

   C. **CORRECT:** The first action the nurse should take using the nursing process is assessment. The nurse should talk with the client first to determine what risk factors the client might have before initiating the appropriate health promotion and disease prevention measures.

   D. The nurse may provide for the client the use of condoms to decrease sexual health risk when determining the client's need for health promotion and disease prevention. However, there is another action the nurse should take first.

   Ⓝ *NCLEX® Connection: Health Promotion and Maintenance, Health Screening*

2. A. **CORRECT:** The nurse should assist the client to recognize the benefits of her health-promoting actions while also overcoming barriers to implementing actions.

   B. **CORRECT:** The nurse should collect information about who can help the client change unhealthful behaviors, and then suggest steps to have friends and family to become involved and supportive.

   C. **CORRECT:** The nurse should promote the client's use of any available community or online resources that can help the client progress toward meeting set goals.

   D. The nurse and the client should work together to devise and set mutually agreeable goals that are also realistic and achievable.

   E. **CORRECT:** The nurse should teach that stress is a contributing factor to cardiovascular disease, as well as many other specific and systemic disorders.

   Ⓝ *NCLEX® Connection: Health Promotion and Maintenance, Health Promotion/Disease Prevention*

3. A. **CORRECT:** Starting at age 20, the client should have examinations for testicular cancer, along with blood pressure and body mass index measurements and cholesterol determinations.

   B. Blood glucose testing begins at age 45.

   C. Testing for fecal occult blood usually begins at age 50.

   D. Testing for prostate-specific antigen usually begins at age 50.

   Ⓝ *NCLEX® Connection: Health Promotion and Maintenance, Health Screening*

4. A. A cholesterol screening is an example of secondary prevention.

   B. **CORRECT:** Primary prevention encompasses strategies that help prevent illness or injury. This level of prevention includes health information about nutrition, exercise, stress management, and protection from injuries and illness.

   C. Starting medication therapy to lower cholesterol is an example of secondary prevention.

   D. Starting cardiac rehabilitation is an example of tertiary prevention.

   Ⓝ *NCLEX® Connection: Health Promotion and Maintenance, Health Promotion/Disease Prevention*

5. A. The female client who has no specific family or personal history of colorectal cancer should begin screening procedures at age 50.

   B. **CORRECT:** The female client who is between the ages of 40 and 50 should have a mammogram annually.

   C. The female client who is between the ages of 30 and 65, with no family or personal history of cervical cancer, should have a Pap smear and human papilloma virus test every 5 years.

   D. The client who is age 45 should have a blood glucose test at least every 3 years. Unless there is a specific family or personal history of diabetes mellitus, annual blood glucose determinations are not necessary.

   Ⓝ *NCLEX® Connection: Health Promotion and Maintenance, Health Promotion/Disease Prevention*

PRACTICE Answer

Using the ATI Active Learning Template: Basic Concept

RELATED CONTENT

- Primary: take various courses, read about bicycle safety (wear a helmet, use reflective accessories and lights for visibility to drivers, follow the rules of the road for cyclists)
- Secondary: emergency care, surgery
- Tertiary: rehabilitative care, learning self-management procedures, strategies

Ⓝ *NCLEX® Connection: Health Promotion and Maintenance, Health Promotion/Disease Prevention*

CHAPTER 17 *Client Education*

Teaching is goal-driven and interactive. It involves purposeful actions to help individuals acquire knowledge, modify attitudes and behavior, and learn new skills.

Learning is the intentional gain of new information, attitudes, or skills, and it promotes behavioral change.

Motivation influences how much and how quickly a person learns. The desire to learn and the ability to learn and understand the content affect motivation.

Information technology increases access to and delivery of knowledge.

NURSING AND CLIENT EDUCATION

- Nurses provide health education to individuals, families, and communities. Q**PCC**
- Some of the most common factors influencing clients' educational needs are health, educational level, socioeconomic status, and cultural and family influences.
- Emotional status, spiritual factors, health perception, willingness to participate, and developmental level are also important to consider when providing client education.
- Client education provides clients with information and skills to:
  - Maintain and promote health and prevent illness (immunizations, lifestyle changes, prenatal care).
  - Restore health (self-administration of insulin).
  - Adapt to permanent illness or injury (ostomy care, swallowing techniques, speech therapy).

DOMAINS OF LEARNING

Cognitive learning requires intellectual behaviors and focuses on thinking. It involves knowledge (learning the new information), comprehension (understanding the new information), application (using the new information in a concrete way), analysis (organizing the new information), synthesis (using the knowledge for a new outcome), and evaluation (determining the effectiveness of learning the new information). For example, cognitive learning takes place when clients learn the manifestations of hypoglycemia and then can verbalize when to notify the provider.

Affective learning involves feelings, beliefs, and values. Hearing the instructor's words, responding verbally and nonverbally, valuing the content, creating a method for identifying values and resolving differences, and employing values consistently in decision-making are all characteristics of affective learning. For example, affective learning takes place when clients learn about the life changes necessary for managing diabetes mellitus and then discuss their feelings about having diabetes.

Psychomotor learning is gaining skills that require mental and physical activity. Psychomotor learning relies on perception (or sensory awareness), set (readiness to learn), guided response (task performance with an instructor), mechanism (increased confidence allowing for more complex learning), adaptation (the ability to alter performance when problems arise), and origination (use of skills to perform complex tasks that require creating new skills). For example, psychomotor learning takes place when clients practice preparing insulin injections.

ASSESSMENT/DATA COLLECTION

- Assess/monitor learning needs.
- Evaluate the learning environment.
- Identify learning style (auditory, visual, kinesthetic).
- Identify areas of concern (low literacy levels, pain, distractions). Q**PCC**
- Identify available resources (financial, social, community).
- Identify developmental level.
- Determine physical and cognitive ability.
- Identify specific needs (visual impairment, decreased manual dexterity, learning challenges).
- Determine motivation and readiness to learn.

PLANNING

- Identify mutually agreeable outcomes.
- Prioritize the learning objectives with clients' needs in mind.
- Use methods that emphasize the learning style.
- Select age-appropriate teaching methods and materials.
- Speak and provide print materials at or below the sixth-grade reading level.
- Avoid nursing terminology (administer, monitor, implement, assess).
- Speak and write in the second person, not the third ("your leg," not "the leg").
- Avoid using all capital letters, minimal white space, and small type in print materials.
- Speak and write in active voice ("take the medication," not "the medication should be taken").
- Provide electronic educational resources (CDs, DVDs, software programs, mobile applications).
- Use reliable Internet sources to access information and support services.
- Organize learning activities to move from simple to more complex tasks and known to unknown concepts.
- Incorporate active participation in the learning process.
- Schedule teaching sessions at optimal times for learning (teaching ostomy care while replacing the pouch).

IMPLEMENTATION

- Create an environment that promotes learning (minimal distractions and interruptions, privacy).
- Use therapeutic communication (active listening, empathy) to develop trust and promote sharing of concerns.
- Review previous knowledge and experiences. Qᴘᴄᴄ
- Explain the therapeutic regimen or procedure.
- Present steps that build toward more complex tasks.
- Demonstrate psychomotor skills.
- Allow time for return demonstrations.
- Provide positive reinforcement.

EVALUATION

- Ask clients to explain the information in their own words.
- Observe return demonstrations (psychomotor learning).
- Use written tools to measure the accuracy of information.
- Ask clients to evaluate their own progress.
- Observe nonverbal communication.
- Reevaluate learning during follow-up telephone calls or contacts, such as home health visits or appointments with the provider.
- Revise the care plan accordingly.

FACTORS AFFECTING LEARNING

FACTORS THAT ENHANCE LEARNING

- Perceived benefit
- Cognitive and physical ability
- Health and cultural beliefs
- Active participation
- Age- and educational level-appropriate methods

BARRIERS TO LEARNING

- Fear, anxiety, depression
- Physical discomfort, pain, fatigue
- Environmental distractions
- Health and cultural beliefs
- Sensory and perceptual deficits
- Psychomotor deficits

Application Exercises

1. A nurse is observing a client drawing up and mixing insulin. Which of the following findings should the nurse identify as an indication that psychomotor learning has taken place?

   A. The client is able to discuss the appropriate technique.

   B. The client is able to demonstrate the appropriate technique.

   C. The client states that he understands.

   D. The client is able to write the steps on a piece of paper.

2. A nurse in a provider's office is collecting data from the mother of a 12-month-old infant. The client states that her son is old enough for toilet training. Following an educational session with the nurse, the client now states that she will postpone toilet training until her son is older. Learning has occurred in which of the following domains?

   A. Cognitive

   B. Affective

   C. Psychomotor

   D. Kinesthetic

3. A nurse is providing preoperative education for a client who will undergo a mastectomy the next day. Which of the following statements should the nurse identify as an indication that the client is ready to learn?

   A. "I don't want my spouse to see my incision."

   B. "Will you give me pain medicine after the surgery?"

   C. "Can you tell me about how long the surgery will take?"

   D. "My roommate listens to everything I say."

4. A nurse is preparing an instructional session for an older adult about managing stress incontinence. Which of the following actions should the nurse take first when meeting with the client?

   A. Encourage the client to participate actively in learning.

   B. Select instructional materials appropriate for the older adult.

   C. Identify goals the nurse and the client agree are reasonable.

   D. Determine what the client knows about stress incontinence.

5. A nurse is evaluating how well a client learned the information he presented in an instructional session about following a heart-healthy diet. The client states that she understands what to do now. Which of the following actions should the nurse take to evaluate the client's learning?

   A. Encourage the client to ask questions.

   B. Ask the client to explain how to select or prepare meals.

   C. Encourage the client to fill out an evaluation form.

   D. Ask the client if she has resources for further instruction on this topic.

PRACTICE Active Learning Scenario

A nurse is preparing a presentation at a community center for a group of parents who want to learn how to prevent childhood obesity. Use the ATI Active Learning Template: Basic Concept to complete this item.

RELATED CONTENT

List at least three factors the nurse should consider when incorporating ways to enhance learning.

List at least three barriers the nurse might encounter among the attendees.

Application Exercises Key

1. A. Discussing the appropriate technique demonstrates learning, but it does not involve the use of motor skills.

   B. **CORRECT:** Demonstrating the appropriate technique indicates that psychomotor learning has taken place.

   C. Verbalizing understanding demonstrates learning, but it does not involve the use of motor skills.

   D. Writing steps on paper demonstrates learning, but it does not involve the motor skills essential for performing the procedure.

   Ⓝ *NCLEX® Connection: Health Promotion and Maintenance, Health Promotion/Disease Prevention*

2. A. An example of cognitive learning is stating the behavior the child will demonstrate when ready to toilet train.

   B. **CORRECT:** Affective learning has taken place because the client's ideas about toilet training changed.

   C. An example of psychomotor learning is performing the proper techniques for introducing the child to toilet training.

   D. Kinesthetic learning is a learning style, not a domain of learning.

   Ⓝ *NCLEX® Connection: Health Promotion and Maintenance, Health Promotion/Disease Prevention*

3. A. The client's concern about her spouse seeing the incision could indicate anxiety or depression.

   B. The client's request for pain medicine could indicate fear and anxiety.

   C. **CORRECT:** Asking a concrete question about the surgery indicates that the client is ready to discuss the surgery. The client's new diagnosis of cancer can cause anxiety, fear, or depression, all of which can interfere with the learning process.

   D. The lack of privacy due to the presence of a roommate can be a barrier to learning.

   Ⓝ *NCLEX® Connection: Reduction of Risk Potential, Therapeutic Procedures*

4. A. Active participation in the learning process is essential for the success of the session. However, this is not the priority action.

   B. It is essential for the nurse to prepare and select instructional materials appropriate for the client's age, developmental level, and other parameters. However, this is not the priority action.

   C. Establishing mutually agreeable goals is essential for the success of the session. However, this is not the priority action.

   D. **CORRECT:** The first action the nurse should take using the nursing process is to assess or collect data from the client. The nurse should determine how much the client knows about stress incontinence, the accuracy of this knowledge, and what the client needs to learn to manage this problem before instructing the client.

   Ⓝ *NCLEX® Connection: Health Promotion and Maintenance, Health Promotion/Disease Prevention*

5. A. The client stated that she understood the content, so she might not ask any questions that would help the nurse evaluate learning.

   B. **CORRECT:** A useful strategy for evaluating learning is to ask the client to explain in her own words how she will implement what she learned.

   C. An evaluation form usually gives the client a means of evaluating the teaching. It might not offer clues about what the client has learned.

   D. The nurse should identify the client's resources early in the instructional process. At this point, the exploration of resources does not help the nurse evaluate the client's learning.

   Ⓝ *NCLEX® Connection: Health Promotion and Maintenance, Health Promotion/Disease Prevention*

PRACTICE Answer

Using the ATI Active Learning Template: Basic Concept

RELATED CONTENT

Factors that enhance learning
- Perceived benefit
- Cognitive and physical ability
- Health and cultural beliefs
- Active participation
- Age
- Educational level-appropriate methods

Barriers to learning
- Fear
- Anxiety
- Depression
- Physical discomfort
- Pain
- Fatigue
- Environmental distractions
- Health and cultural beliefs
- Sensory and perceptual deficits
- Psychomotor deficits

Ⓝ *NCLEX® Connection: Health Promotion and Maintenance, Health Promotion/Disease Prevention*

CHAPTER 18 *Infants (2 Days to 1 Year)*

EXPECTED GROWTH AND DEVELOPMENT FOR NEWBORNS

PHYSICAL DEVELOPMENT

- Lose 5% to 10% body birth weight in first few days, but should regain it by the second week.
- Weight gain is about 150 to 210 g (5 to 7 oz) per week in the first 6 months
- Measurements of crown-to-rump length, head-to-heel length, head circumference and chest circumference are key indicators of appropriate growth.
- Lanugo (soft hair) present on the back.
- Head molding (overlapping of skull bones) present; fontanels are palpable.

REFLEXES

- Include startling, sucking, rooting, grasping, yawning, coughing, plantar and palmar grasp, and Babinski.
- Confirm presence or absence of expected reflexes to monitor for appropriate neurological development.

BODY POSITION

- Generally flexed at rest.
- Movement should involve all four extremities equally, but can be sporadic.

SLEEP

- Sleep patterns may be reversed for several months (daytime sleeping and nighttime wakefulness).
- Average 15 hr of sleep time each day.

COGNITIVE DEVELOPMENT

- Learn to respond to visual stimuli.
- Use cry as a form of communication.
- Cry patterns can change to reflect different needs.

PSYCHOSOCIAL DEVELOPMENT

- Interactions with caregivers affect psychosocial development. Positive interactions promote nurturing and attachment. Negative experience or lack of interaction hinders appropriate attachment.
- Most newborns can mimic the smile of the caregiver by 2 weeks of life.

EXPECTED GROWTH AND DEVELOPMENT FOR INFANTS

PHYSICAL DEVELOPMENT

- Posterior fontanel closes by 2 to 3 months of age.
- Anterior fontanel closes by 12 to 18 months of age.

Tracking parameters

WEIGHT: Birth weight should double by 4 to 6 months and triple by the end of the first year.

HEIGHT: Infants grow about 2.5 cm (1 in) per month in the first 6 months, and then about 1.25 cm (0.5 in) per month until the end of the first year.

HEAD CIRCUMFERENCE: Head circumference increases about 1.25 cm (0.5 in) per month in the first 6 months and then about 0.5 cm (0.2 in) between 6 and 12 months.

DENTITION: Six to eight teeth erupt in the infant's mouth by the end of the first year.
- Use cold teething rings, over-the-counter teething gels, and acetaminophen or ibuprofen. Qpcc
- Use a cool, wet washcloth to clean the teeth.
- Do not give infants a bottle when they are falling asleep. Prolonged exposure to milk or juice can cause dental caries (bottle–mouth caries).

18.1 Motor skill development by age

	GROSS MOTOR SKILLS	FINE MOTOR SKILLS
1 MONTH	Demonstrates head lag	Has a strong grasp reflex
2 MONTHS	Lifts head off mattress when prone	Holds hands in an open position Grasp reflex fading
3 MONTHS	Raises head and shoulders off mattress when prone Only slight head lag	No longer has a grasp reflex Keeps hands loosely open
4 MONTHS	Rolls from back to side	Grasps objects with both hands Places objects in mouth
5 MONTHS	Rolls from front to back	Uses palmar grasp dominantly
6 MONTHS	Rolls from back to front	Holds bottle
7 MONTHS	Bears full weight on feet Sits, leaning forward on both hands	Moves objects from hand to hand
8 MONTHS	Sits unsupported	Begins using pincer grasp
9 MONTHS	Pulls to a standing position	Has a crude pincer grasp Dominant hand preference evident
10 MONTHS	Changes from a prone to a sitting position	Grasps rattle by its handle
11 MONTHS	Cruises or walks while holding onto something Walks with one hand held	Places objects into a container Neat pincer grasp
12 MONTHS	Sits down from a standing position without assistance	Tries to build a two-block tower without success Can turn pages in a book

COGNITIVE DEVELOPMENT

Piaget: Sensorimotor stage (birth to 24 months)
- Separation is the sense of being distinct from other objects in the environment.
- Object permanence develops at about 9 months. This is the process of knowing that an object still exists when it is hidden from view.
- Mental representation is the recognition of symbols.

Language development

- Responds to noises
- Vocalizes with "ooos" and "aahs"
- Laughs and squeals
- Turns head to the sound of a rattle
- Begins to comprehend simple commands
- Pronounces single-syllable words
- Begins speaking two- and then three-word phrases

PSYCHOSOCIAL DEVELOPMENT

Erikson: Trust vs. mistrust (birth to 1 year)
- Infants trust that others will meet their feeding, comfort, stimulation, and caring needs.
- Infants' reflexive behavior (attachment, separation recognition/anxiety, and stranger fear) influences their social development.
- Attachment, when infants begin to bond with their parents, develops within the first month, but actually begins before birth. The process is optimal when the infant and parents are in good health, have positive feeding experiences, and receive adequate rest.
- Separation recognition occurs during the first year as infants recognize the boundaries between themselves and others. Learning how to respond to people in their environment is the next phase of development. Positive interactions with parents, siblings, and other caregivers help establish trust.
- Separation anxiety develops between 4 and 8 months of age. Infants protest loudly when separated from parents, which can cause considerable anxiety for the parents.
- Stranger fear becomes evident between ages 6 to 8 months, when infants are less likely to accept strangers.

Self-concept development

By the end of the first year, infants distinguish themselves as separate from their parents.

Body-image changes

- Infants discover that the mouth is a pleasure producer.
- Hands and feet are objects of play.
- Smiling makes others react.

AGE-APPROPRIATE ACTIVITIES

- Infants have a short attention span and do not interact with other children during play (solitary play). Age-appropriate activities can promote cognitive, social, and motor development.
- Appropriate toys and activities that stimulate the senses and encourage development include rattles, mobiles, teething toys, nesting toys, playing pat-a-cake, playing with balls, and reading books.

HEALTH PROMOTION FOR NEWBORNS AND INFANTS

SCREENINGS

- Newborn screenings for metabolism disorders may be repeated in early weeks of life (phenylketonuria, galactosemia).
- Developmental milestone screenings occur ongoing as part of routine well checkups with the provider at 2 weeks, and 2, 4, 6, 9, and 12 months.

IMMUNIZATIONS

Follow the latest Centers for Disease Control and Prevention (CDC) immunization recommendations (see www.cdc.gov) for healthy infants. During the first year, these generally include immunizations against hepatitis B, diphtheria, tetanus, pertussis, rotavirus, polio, influenza, and pneumococcal pneumonia. The recommendations change periodically, so check them often. Ⓠ EBP

NUTRITION

- Breastfeeding provides optimal nutrition during the first 12 months.
- Feeding alternatives
  - Iron-fortified formula is an acceptable alternative to breast milk.
  - Cow's milk is inadequate and should not be given before 1 year of age.
- Weaning from the breast or bottle can begin when infants can drink from a cup (after 6 months).
  - Replace a single bottle- or breast-feeding with breast milk or formula in a cup.
  - Every few days, replace another feeding with a cup.
  - Replace the bedtime feeding last.
- Solid food is appropriate aound 4 to 6 months.
  - Indicators for readiness include voluntary control of the head and trunk and disappearance of the extrusion reflex (pushing food out of the mouth).
  - Introduce iron-fortified rice cereal first.
  - Start new foods one at a time over a 5- to 7-day period to observe for signs of allergy or intolerance (fussiness, rash, vomiting, diarrhea, constipation). Vegetables, fruits, and meats follow, generally in that order.

- Delay milk, eggs, wheat, citrus fruits, peanuts, and peanut butter until the second half of the first year of life, as they can trigger allergies. Do not give honey to infants until after 12 months of age because it can cause infant botulism.
- Appropriate finger foods to introduce around 9 months include ripe bananas, toast strips, graham crackers, cheese cubes, noodles, and peeled chunks of apples, pears, and peaches.
- Remind parents that solid food is not a substitute for breast milk or formula until after 12 months.
- Fluoridated water or supplemental fluoride is recommended after 6 months to protect against dental caries.

INJURY PREVENTION Qs

Aspiration
- Avoid small objects, such as grapes, coins, and candy, which can become lodged in the throat.
- Provide age-appropriate toys.
- Check clothing for safety hazards (loose buttons).

Bodily harm
- Keep sharp objects out of reach.
- Keep infants away from heavy objects they can pull down.
- Do not leave infants alone with animals.
- Monitor for shaken baby syndrome.

Burns
- Check the temperature of bath water.
- Turn down the thermostat on the hot water heater to 49° C (120° F) or below.
- Have smoke detectors in the home and change their batteries regularly.
- Turn handles of pots and pans toward the back of the stove.
- Apply sunscreen when outdoors during daylight hours.
- Cover electrical outlets.

Drowning: Do not leave infants unattended in the bathtub.

Falls
- Keep the crib mattress in the lowest position with the rails all the way up.
- Use restraints in infant seats.
- Place the infant seat on the ground or floor when outside of a vehicle, and do not leave it unattended or on elevated surfaces.
- Use safety gates across stairs.

Poisoning
- Avoid lead paint exposure.
- Keep toxins and plants out of reach.
- Keep safety locks on cabinets that contain cleaners and other household chemicals.
- Keep a poison control number handy or program it into the phone.
- Keep medications in childproof containers and out of reach.
- Have a carbon monoxide detector in the home.

Motor-vehicle injuries: Use an approved rear-facing car seat in the back seat, preferably in the middle, (away from air bags and side impact). Infants should be in rear-facing car seats until age 2 or until they reach the maximum height and weight for the seat (as long as the top of the head is below the top of the seat back). Convertible restraints should have a five-point harness or a T-shield.

Suffocation
- Avoid plastic bags.
- Keep balloons away from infants.
- Be sure the crib mattress is firm and fits tightly.
- Ensure crib slats are no farther apart than 6 cm (2.4 in).
- Remove crib mobiles or crib gyms by 4 to 5 months of age.
- Do not use pillows in the crib.
- Place infants on the back for sleep.
- Keep toys that have small parts out of reach.
- Remove drawstrings from jackets and other clothing.

Application Exercises

1. A nurse is talking with the parents of a 6-month-old infant about gross motor development. Which of the following gross motor skills are expected findings in the next 3 months? (Select all that apply.)

    A. Rolls from back to front

    B. Bears weight on legs

    C. Walks holding onto furniture

    D. Sits unsupported

    E. Sits down from a standing position

2. A nurse is cautioning the mother of an 8-month-old infant about safety. Which of the following statements by the mother indicates an understanding of safety for the infant?

    A. "My baby loved to play with his crib gym, but I took it away from him."

    B. "I just bought a soft mattress so my baby will sleep better."

    C. "My baby really likes sleeping on the fluffy pillow we just got for him."

    D. "I put the baby's car seat out of the way on the table after I put him in it."

3. A nurse is reviewing car seat safety with the parents of a 1-month-old infant. When reviewing car seat use, which of the following instructions should the nurse include?

    A. Use a car seat that has a three-point harness system.

    B. Position the car seat so that the infant is rear-facing.

    C. Secure the car seat in the front passenger seat of the vehicle.

    D. Convert to a booster seat after 12 months.

4. A nurse is assessing from a 2-week-old newborn during a routine checkup. Which of the following findings should the nurse expect?

    A. Sleeps 14 to 16 hr each day

    B. Posterior fontanel closed

    C. Pincer grasp present

    D. Hands remain in a closed position

    E. Current weight same as birth weight

5. The mother of a 7-month-old infant tells the nurse at the pediatric clinic that her baby has been fussy with occasional loose stools since she started feeding him fruits and vegetables. Which of the following responses should the nurse make? (Select all that apply.)

    A. "It might be good to add bananas, as they can help with loose stools."

    B. "Let's make a list of the foods he is eating so we can spot any problems."

    C. "Did the changes begin after you started one particular food?"

    D. "Has he been vomiting since he started these new foods?"

    E. "Most babies react with a little indigestion when you start new foods."

PRACTICE Active Learning Scenario

A nurse is explaining to the parents of a 4-month-old infant what infant milestones to expect during the first year of life, and how to foster infant development. Use the ATI Active Learning Template: Growth and Development to complete this item.

COGNITIVE DEVELOPMENT
- Name the developmental stage Piaget has identified for the first two years of life.
- Identify three essential components that comprise this stage.

AGE-APPROPRIATE ACTIVITIES: Identify at least two toys and two activities the nurse should suggest that the parents provide for their infant.

Application Exercises Key

1. A. **CORRECT:** The infant should be able to roll from back to front by 6 months.

   B. **CORRECT:** The infant should be able to bear weight on legs by 7 months.

   C. The infant should be able to walk while holding furniture until around 11 months.

   D. **CORRECT:** The infant should be able to sit unsupported by 8 months.

   E. The infant should be able to sit down from a standing position until around 12 months.

   Ⓝ *NCLEX® Connection: Health Promotion and Maintenance, Developmental Stages and Transitions*

2. A. **CORRECT:** Parents should remove gyms and mobiles at 4 to 5 months of age to prevent injury can occur from choking or strangulation.

   B. The nurse should remind the parents the infant's crib mattress should be firm and fit tightly to prevent suffocation.

   C. The nurse should remind the parents to remove pillows or stuffed animals from the crib to prevent possible suffocation.

   D. The nurse should remind the parents to place the infant seat on the ground level when not in a vehicle to prevent falls.

   Ⓝ *NCLEX® Connection: Health Promotion and Maintenance, Developmental Stages and Transitions*

3. A. The nurse should instruct the parents to provide a car seat with a five-point harness system.

   B. **CORRECT:** The nurse should instruct the parents to position the infant car seat in a rear-facing position in the center of the vehicle seat, when possible.

   C. The nurse should instruct the parent to place the infant car seat in the back seat to reduce the risk for injury in the event of a crash.

   D. The nurse should instruct the parents to continue using an infant seat until the child reaches age 2, or meets the height and weight limits for the seat.

   Ⓝ *NCLEX® Connection: Safety and Infection Control, Accident/Error/Injury Prevention*

4. A. **CORRECT:** The nurse should expect the newborn to sleep about 15 hr each day.

   B. The nurse should expect the posterior fontanel to close around 2 to 3 months of age.

   C. The nurse should expect the pincer grasp to develop around 8 months of age.

   D. **CORRECT:** The nurse should expect the newborn to keep hands in a closed position until about 2 months of life.

   E. **CORRECT:** The nurse should expect the newborn to have lost 5% to 10% of birth weight in the first few days of life, and to regain the weight by the second week of life.

   Ⓝ *NCLEX® Connection: Health Promotion and Maintenance, Developmental Stages and Transitions*

5. A. This response by the nurse suggests an intervention without first determining the cause of the infant's problem.

   B. **CORRECT:** This response by the nurse is an attempt to assess about the infant's diet to help determine whether a food allergy or intolerance is the cause of the diarrhea and fussiness.

   C. **CORRECT:** This response by the nurse is an attempt to assess the infant's diet to help determine which food triggered the infant's behavior change. Parents should introduce one food at a time to help identify allergies or intolerances.

   D. **CORRECT:** This response by the is an attempt to assess for other changes caused by the infant's diet which could be linked to a food allergy or intolerance, such as vomiting, rash, or constipation.

   E. This response by the nurse is nontherapeutic because it involves stereotyping, and offers false reassurance without any attempt to understand the infant's problem.

   Ⓝ *NCLEX® Connection: Basic Care and Comfort, Nutrition and Oral Hydration*

PRACTICE Answer

Using the ATI Active Learning Template: Growth and Development

COGNITIVE DEVELOPMENT

Piaget's sensorimotor stage (first 2 years)
- Separation
- Object permanence
- Mental representation

AGE-APPROPRIATE ACTIVITIES
- Toys and activities
- Rattles
- Mobiles
- Teething toys
- Nesting toys
- Playing pat-a-cake
- Playing with balls
- Reading books

Ⓝ *NCLEX® Connection: Health Promotion and Maintenance, Developmental Stages and Transitions*

CHAPTER 19 *Toddlers (1 to 3 Years)*

EXPECTED GROWTH AND DEVELOPMENT

PHYSICAL DEVELOPMENT

The anterior fontanel closes by 18 months.

WEIGHT: At 24 months, toddlers should weigh four times their birth weight.

HEIGHT: Toddlers grow by 6.2 cm (2.5 in) per year.

CONTRIBUTION TO SELF-CARE ACTIVITIES: dressing, feeding, toilet-training

19.1 Motor skills by age

AGE	GROSS MOTOR SKILLS	FINE MOTOR SKILLS
15 months	Walks without help Creeps up stairs	Uses cup well Builds tower of two blocks
18 months	Assumes standing position Jumps in place with both feet	Manages spoon without rotation Turns pages in book two or three at a time
2 years	Walks up and down stairs	Builds a tower with six or seven blocks
2.5 years	Jumps with both feet Stands on one foot momentarily	Draws circles Has good hand-finger coordination

COGNITIVE DEVELOPMENT

Piaget: Sensorimotor transitions to preoperational
- The concept of object permanence is fully developed.
- Toddlers have and demonstrate memories of events that relate to them.
- Domestic mimicry is evident (playing house).
- Preoperational thought does not allow toddlers to understand other viewpoints, but it does allow them to symbolize objects and people in order to imitate activities they have seen.

Language development
- Language increases to about 400 words, with toddlers speaking in two- to three-word phrases.
- Ability to comprehend speech outweighs the number of words and phrases spoken.

PSYCHOSOCIAL DEVELOPMENT

Erikson: autonomy vs. shame and doubt
- Independence is paramount as toddlers attempt to do everything for themselves.
- Separation anxiety continues when parents leave.
- A toddler might show regression (bed-wetting, thumb sucking) as a response to anxiety or separation.
- Engages in parallel play, but by age 3 begins to play and communicate with others.

Moral development
- Moral development parallels cognitive development.
- Egocentric: Toddlers are unable to see another's perspective; they can only view things from their point of view.
- Punishment and obedience orientation begins with a sense that others reward good behavior and punish bad behavior.

Self-concept development: Toddlers progressively see themselves as separate from their parents and increase their explorations away from them.

Body-image changes: Toddlers appreciate the usefulness of various body parts.

AGE-APPROPRIATE ACTIVITIES Qpcc

- Solitary play evolves into parallel play where toddlers observe other children and then engage in activities nearby.
- Temper tantrums result when toddlers are frustrated with restrictions on independence. Providing consistent, age-appropriate expectations helps them work through their frustration.
- Offer choices, such as juice or milk, instead of providing an opportunity for a yes/no response from the toddler.
- Toilet training can begin with awareness of the sensation of needing to urinate or defecate. The toddler should show indications of readiness and parents should demonstrate patience, consistency, and a nonjudgmental attitude with toilet training. Nighttime control can develop last.
- Discipline should be consistent with well-defined boundaries that help develop acceptable social behavior.

Appropriate activities
- Filling and emptying containers
- Playing with blocks
- Looking at books
- Playing with push and pull toys
- Tossing a ball

HEALTH PROMOTION

IMMUNIZATIONS

Follow the latest Centers for Disease Control and Prevention immunization recommendations (see www.cdc.gov) for healthy toddlers 12 months to 3 years of age. These generally include immunizations against hepatitis A and B, diphtheria, tetanus, pertussis, measles, mumps, rubella, varicella, polio, influenza, haemophilus influenza type B, and pneumococcal pneumonia. Recommendations change periodically, so check them often. Q EBP

NUTRITION

- Toddlers are picky eaters with repeated requests for favorite foods.
- Toddlers should consume 2 to 3 cups (16 to 24 oz) per day and can switch from drinking whole milk to drinking low-fat or fat-free milk at 2 years of age.
- Limit juice to 4 to 6 oz a day.
- Food serving size is 1 tbsp for each year of age.
- Toddlers can be reluctant to try or accept foods new to them.
- If there is a family history of allergy, introduce cow's milk, chocolate, citrus fruits, egg whites, seafood, and nut butters gradually while monitoring for reactions.
- As toddlers become more autonomous, they tend to prefer finger foods.
- Regular meal times and nutritious snacks best meet nutrient needs.
- Avoid snacks and desserts that are high in sugar, fat, or sodium.
- Avoid foods that pose choking hazards (nuts, grapes, hot dogs, peanut butter, raw carrots, tough meats, popcorn).
- Supervise toddlers during snacks and mealtimes.
- Cut food into small, bite-sized pieces to make it easier to swallow and to prevent choking.
- Do not allow toddlers to eat or drink during play activities or while lying down.
- Do not use food as a reward or punishment
- Suggest that parents follow U.S. Department of Agriculture nutrition recommendations (www.choosemyplate.gov).
- Brush teeth and begin dental visits. Do not allow child to use a bottle during naps or bedtime to reduce the risk for dental caries.

INJURY PREVENTION Qs

Aspiration
- Avoid small objects (grapes, coins, candy) that can lodge in the throat.
- Keep toys with small parts out of reach.
- Provide age-appropriate toys.
- Check clothing for safety hazards, such as loose buttons.
- Keep balloons away from toddlers.

Bodily harm
- Keep sharp objects out of reach.
- Keep firearms in a locked box or cabinet.
- Do not leave toddlers unattended with animals present.
- Teach stranger safety.

Burns
- Check the temperature of bath water.
- Turn down the thermostat on the water heater.
- Have smoke detectors in the home and replace their batteries regularly.
- Turn pot handles toward the back of the stove.
- Cover electrical outlets.
- Use sunscreen when outside.

Drowning
- Do not leave toddlers unattended in the bathtub.
- Keep toilet lids closed.
- Closely supervise toddlers at the pool or any other body of water.
- Teach toddlers to swim.

Falls
- Keep doors and windows locked.
- Keep the crib mattress in the lowest position with the rails all the way up.
- Use safety gates across stairs.

Motor-vehicle injuries
- Use an approved car seat in the back seat, away from air bags.
- Toddlers should be in a rear-facing car seat until age 2 or until they exceed the height and weight limit of the car seat. They can then sit in an approved forward-facing car seat in the back seat, using a five-point harness or T-shield until they exceed the manufacturer's recommended height and weight for the car seat.
- Prior to instillation, read all car seat safety guidelines.
- Teach toddler not to run or ride a tricycle into the street.
- Never leave a toddler alone in a car, especially in warm weather.

Poisoning
- Avoid exposure to lead paint.
- Place safety locks on cabinets that contain cleaners and other chemicals.
- Keep plants out of reach.
- Keep a poison control number handy or program it into the phone.
- Keep medications in childproof containers out of the child's reach.
- Have a carbon monoxide detector in the home.

Suffocation
- Avoid plastic bags.
- Be sure the crib mattress fits tightly.
- Ensure crib slats are no further apart than 6 cm (2.4 in).
- Keep pillows out of the crib.
- Remove drawstrings from jackets and other clothing.

Application Exercises

1. A nurse is giving a presentation about accident prevention to a group of parents of toddlers. Which of the following accident-prevention strategies should the nurse include? (Select all that apply.)

   A. Store toxic agents in locked cabinets.

   B. Keep toilet seats up.

   C. Turn pot handles toward the back of the stove.

   D. Place safety gates across stairways.

   E. Make sure balloons are fully inflated.

2. A nurse is planning diversionary activities for toddlers on an inpatient unit. Which of the following activities should the nurse include? (Select all that apply.)

   A. Building models

   B. Working with clay

   C. Filling and emptying containers

   D. Playing with blocks

   E. Looking at books

3. A nurse is teaching the parents of a toddler about discipline. Which of the following actions should the nurse suggest?

   A. Establish consistent boundaries for the toddler.

   B. Place the toddler in a room with the door closed.

   C. Inform the toddler how you feel when he misbehaves. .

   D. Use favorite snacks to reward the toddler.

4. A mother tells the nurse that her 2-year-old toddler has temper tantrums and says "no" every time the mother tries to help her get dressed. The nurse should recognize, the toddler is manifesting which of the following stages of development?

   A. Trying to increase her independence

   B. Developing a sense of trust

   C. Establishing a new identity

   D. Attempting to master a skill

5. A nurse is reviewing nutritional guidelines with the parents of a 2-year-old toddler. Which of the following parent statements should indicate to the nurse an understanding of the teaching?

   A. "I should keep feeding my son whole milk until he is 3 years old."

   B. "It's okay for me to give my son a cup of apple juice with each meal."

   C. "I'll give my son about 2 tablespoons of each food at mealtimes."

   D. "My son loves popcorn, and I know it is better for him than sweets."

PRACTICE Active Learning Scenario

A nurse is explaining to the parents of a 14-month-old toddler what physical and cognitive development they can expect from now until their child is 3 years old. Use the ATI Active Learning Template: Growth and Development to complete this item.

PHYSICAL DEVELOPMENT: Identify at least four gross or fine motor skills the parents can expect at specific ages.

COGNITIVE DEVELOPMENT: Describe at least three parameters the parents can expect to observe during the toddler stage.

Application Exercises Key

1. A. **CORRECT:** Parents must prevent toddlers from accessing dangerous substances.

   B. Easy access to the water in the toilet bowl could result in aspiration or drowning.

   C. **CORRECT:** Turn pot handles toward the back of the stove to prevent the toddler from reaching and pulling its contents down on themselves.

   D. **CORRECT:** Safety gates at the bottom of a staircase prevent toddlers from climbing stairs and falling backward. Safety gates placed at the top of a staircase prevent toddlers from falling down the stairs.

   E. Toddlers should not have access to balloons. Balloons can easily burst and toddlers can put fragments of the balloon or the entire deflated balloon in their mouth and asphyxiate.

   Ⓝ *NCLEX® Connection: Safety and Infection Control, Accident/Error/Injury Prevention*

2. A. Toddlers are not cognitively or physically capable of building models. This play activity is acceptable for school-age children.

   B. Toddlers put small objects into their mouths and can easily swallow bits of clay. This activity is unacceptable for a toddler.

   C. **CORRECT:** This activity can help a toddler develop fine motor skills and coordination.

   D. **CORRECT:** This activity can help a toddler develop fine motor skills.

   E. **CORRECT:** This activity can help a toddler prepare to learn to read.

   Ⓝ *NCLEX® Connection: Health Promotion and Maintenance, Developmental Stages and Transitions*

3. A. **CORRECT:** Toddlers need consistent boundaries for discipline to be effective.

   B. Placing a toddler in a room with the door closed can cause anxiety and fear.

   C. A toddler is unable to understand how another person is feeling.

   D. Using favorite foods as rewards can promote unhealthy eating habits.

   Ⓝ *NCLEX® Connection: Health Promotion and Maintenance, Developmental Stages and Transitions*

4. A. **CORRECT:** Toddlers express a drive for independence by opposing the desires of those in authority and attempting to do everything themselves.

   B. Developing trust is a developmental task for infants.

   C. Establishing a new identity is the developmental task of an adolescent.

   D. Mastering a skill is a developmental task of school-age children.

   Ⓝ *NCLEX® Connection: Health Promotion and Maintenance, Developmental Stages and Transitions*

5. A. When toddlers turn 2 years old, the parents should give them low-fat or fat-free milk, not whole milk. This reduces fat and cholesterol intake and helps prevent childhood obesity.

   B. Toddlers should have 4 to 6 oz of juice per day. Juices do not have the whole fiber that fruit has, and they contain sugar, so parents should limit their use.

   C. **CORRECT:** Serving sizes for toddlers should be about 1 tbsp of solid food per year of age, so 2-year-olds should have about 2 tbsp per serving.

   D. Popcorn poses a choking hazard to toddlers.

   Ⓝ *NCLEX® Connection: Health Promotion and Maintenance, Developmental Stages and Transitions*

PRACTICE Answer

Using the ATI Active Learning Template: Growth and Development

PHYSICAL DEVELOPMENT
- At 15 months, gross motor skills: walks without help, creeps up stairs
- At 15 months, fine motor skills: uses cup well, builds tower of two blocks
- At 18 months, gross motor skills: assumes standing position, jumps in place with both feet
- At 18 months, fine motor skills: manages spoon without rotation, turns pages in book two or three at a time
- At 2 years, gross motor skills: walks up and down stairs
- At 2 years, fine motor skills: builds a tower with six or seven blocks
- At 2.5 years, gross motor skills: jumps with both feet, stands on one foot momentarily
- At 2.5 years, fine motor skills: draws circles, has good hand-finger coordination

COGNITIVE DEVELOPMENT: During toddler stage: object permanence, memories of events that relate to them, domestic mimicry (playing house), symbolization of objects and people, use of 400 words, use of two- to three-word phrases

Ⓝ *NCLEX® Connection: Health Promotion and Maintenance, Developmental Stages and Transitions*

CHAPTER 20 *Preschoolers (3 to 6 Years)*

EXPECTED GROWTH AND DEVELOPMENT

PHYSICAL DEVELOPMENT

- Occurs at a more gradual rate than cognitive and psychosocial development.
- Preschoolers evolve from the characteristically unsteady wide stance and protruding abdomen of toddlers to the more graceful, posturally erect, and sturdy physicality of this age group.
- Boys have a tendency to appear larger with more muscle mass.

WEIGHT: Preschoolers gain about 2.3 kg (5 lb) per year.

HEIGHT: Preschoolers grow about 6.2 to 7.5 cm (2.5 to 3 in) per year.

FINE AND GROSS MOTOR SKILLS: Preschoolers show an improvement in fine motor skills, such as copying figures on paper, scribbling, drawing, and dressing themselves.

20.1 Gross motor skills by age

3-YEAR-OLD	4-YEAR-OLD	5-YEAR-OLD
Ride a tricycle	Skip and hop on one foot	Jump rope
Jump off bottom step	Throw ball overhead	Walk backward with heel to toe
Stand on one foot for a few seconds		Move up and down stairs easily

COGNITIVE DEVELOPMENT

Piaget: preoperational phase
- Preschoolers are still in the preoperational phase of cognitive development. They participate in preconceptual thought (from 2 to 4 years of age) and intuitive thought (from 4 to 7 years of age).
- **Preconceptual thought:** Preschoolers make judgments based on visual appearances. Misconceptions in thinking during this stage include:
  - **Artificialism:** Everything is made by humans.
  - **Animism:** Inanimate objects are alive.
  - **Imminent justice:** A universal code exists that determines law and order.
- **Intuitive thought:** Preschoolers can classify and begin to question information and become aware of cause-and-effect relationships.

Time concepts: Preschoolers begin to understand the concepts of past, present, and future. By the end of the preschool years, they can comprehend days of the week.

Language development: Vocabulary continues to increase, and by age 6 contains 8,000 to 14,000 words. Desires and frustrations are more verbally articulated and a need to learn information is expressed through questioning. Phonetically similar words (*eye* and *I*) are difficult to comprehend at this age. Preschoolers speak in sentences, identify colors, and enjoy talking.

PSYCHOSOCIAL DEVELOPMENT

Erikson: Initiative vs. guilt: Preschoolers take on many new experiences, despite not having all of the physical abilities necessary to be successful at everything. When children are unable to accomplish a task, they can feel guilty and believe they have misbehaved. Guide preschoolers to attempt activities within their capabilities while setting limits.

Moral development: Preschoolers continue in the good-bad orientation of the toddler years but begin to understand behavior in terms of what is socially acceptable.

Self-concept development: Preschoolers feel good about themselves for mastering skills, such as dressing and feeding, that allow independence. During stress, insecurity, or illness, they tend to regress to previous immature behavior or develop habits such as nose picking, bed wetting, or thumb sucking.

Body-image changes
- Mistaken perceptions of reality coupled with misconceptions in thinking lead to active fantasies and fears. Preschoolers fear bodily harm, the dark, ghosts, animals, inclement weather, and medical personnel.
- Sex-role identification is typical.

Social development
- During the preschool time period, children generally do not exhibit stranger anxiety and have less separation anxiety. This leads to exploring their neighborhood environment, and making new friends. However, prolonged separation, such as during hospitalization, can provoke anxiety. Favorite toys and play help ease fears.
- Pretend play is healthy and allows children to determine the difference between reality and fantasy.
- Sleep disturbances are common during early childhood, and problems range from difficulties going to bed to night terrors. Advise parents to:
  - Assess whether the bedtime is too early for children who still take naps. Preschoolers average about 12 hr of sleep a day. Some still require a daytime nap.
  - Keep a consistent bedtime routine, and help children slow down in preparation for bedtime.
  - Use a night light.
  - Reassure children who are frightened.

AGE-APPROPRIATE ACTIVITIES

Parallel play shifts to associative play during the preschool years. Play is not highly organized, and preschoolers do not cooperate during play. Activities include the following.
- Playing ball
- Putting puzzles together
- Riding tricycles
- Pretend and dress-up activities
- Musical toys
- Painting, drawing, and coloring
- Sewing cards
- Cooking and housekeeping toys
- Looking at illustrated books
- Technology, such as video and computer programs, to support development and learn new skills

HEALTH PROMOTION

IMMUNIZATIONS

Follow the latest Centers for Disease Control and Prevention immunization recommendations (www.cdc.gov) for healthy preschoolers. Q_{EBP}
- These generally include immunizations against diphtheria, tetanus, pertussis, measles, mumps, rubella, varicella, seasonal influenza, and polio.
- Recommendations change periodically, so check them often.

HEALTH SCREENINGS

Vision screening is routine in the preschool population as part of the prekindergarten physical examination. It is essential to detect and treat myopia and amblyopia before poor visual acuity impairs the learning environment.

NUTRITION

- Preschoolers consume about half the amount of energy that adults do (1,800 calories).
- Picky eating remains a problem for some preschoolers, but often by age 5 they become a bit more willing to sample different foods.
- Preschoolers need 3 to 5 oz complete protein in addition to adequate calcium, iron, folate, and vitamins A and C.
- Parents should provide a balance of nutrients. See www.choosemyplate.gov for nutritional guidelines for preschoolers.

INJURY PREVENTION Q_s

Bodily harm
- Keep firearms in a locked cabinet or container.
- Teach stranger safety.
- Wear helmets when riding a bicycle or tricycle and during any other activities that increase head-injury risk.
- Wear protective equipment (helmet and pads) during physical activity.
- Remove doors from unused refrigerators or other equipment.
- Teach preschoolers not to walk in front of swings.

Burns
- Reduce the temperature setting on the water heater.
- Have smoke detectors in the home and replace the batteries regularly.
- Use sunscreen while outdoors.
- Teach preschoolers not to play with matches.

Drowning
- Do not leave children unattended in the bathtub.
- Closely supervise children at a pool or any body of water.
- Teach children to swim.

Motor-vehicle injuries
Preschoolers must sit in a forward-facing car seat with a harness in the back seat away from airbags for as long as possible, at least to 4 years of age. Children who outgrow the seat before age 4 should use a seat with a harness approved for higher weights and heights. Preschoolers whose weight or height exceed the forward-facing limit for their car seat should use a belt-positioning booster seat until the vehicle's seat belt fits properly, typically beyond the preschooler stage.

Poisoning
- Avoid exposure to lead paint.
- Keep plants out of reach.
- Place safety locks on cabinets with cleaners and other chemicals.
- Keep a poison control number handy or program it into the phone.
- Keep medications in childproof containers out of reach.
- Have a carbon monoxide detector in the home.

Application Exercises

1. A nurse is talking with the parent of a 4-year-old child who states that his child is waking up at night with nightmares. Which of the following interventions should the nurse suggest?

   A. Offer the child a large snack before bedtime.

   B. Allow the child to watch an extra 30 min of TV in the evening.

   C. Have the child take an afternoon nap.

   D. Increase physical activity before bedtime.

2. A nurse is planning diversionary activities for preschoolers on an inpatient pediatric unit. Which of the following activities should the nurse include? (Select all that apply.)

   A. Assembling puzzles

   B. Pulling wheeled toys

   C. Using musical toys

   D. Playing with puppets

   E. Coloring with crayons

3. A nurse is preparing to administer medications to a preschooler. Which of the following strategies should the nurse implement to increase the child's cooperation in taking medications? (Select all that apply.)

   A. Reassure the child an injection will not hurt.

   B. Mix oral medications in a large glass of milk.

   C. Offer the child choices when possible.

   D. Have the parents bring in a favorite toy from home.

   E. Engage the child in pretend play with a toy medical kit.

4. A nurse is reviewing the Centers for Disease Control and Prevention's (CDC) immunization recommendations with the parents of preschoolers. Which of the following vaccines should the nurse include in this discussion? (Select all that apply.)

   A. *Haemophilus influenzae* type B

   B. Varicella

   C. Polio

   D. Hepatitis A

   E. Seasonal influenza

5. A nurse is talking with a parent who is concerned about several issues with her preschooler. Which of the following issues should the nurse identify as the priority?

   A. "My son mimics my husband getting dressed."

   B. "My son has temper tantrums every time we tell him to do something he doesn't want to do."

   C. "I think my son truly believes that his toys have personalities and talk to him."

   D. "I feel bad when I see my son trying so hard to button his shirt."

PRACTICE Active Learning Scenario

A nurse is making safety recommendations to the parents of a two preschoolers. Use the ATI Active Learning Template: Growth and Development to complete this item.

INJURY PREVENTION: List at least four key areas of safety and age-appropriate instructions for addressing each area.

Application Exercises Key

1. A. Eating a large snack, especially one that is heavy or has a high sugar content, is likely to provide stimulation that will make it more difficult for the child to fall asleep. This will not alleviate the child's nightmares.

   B. Watching TV is likely to provide stimulation that will make it more difficult for the child to fall asleep. This will not alleviate the child's nightmares.

   C. **CORRECT:** The nurse should encourage the parent to have the child take an afternoon nap and to empty her bladder before bedtime to alleviate nightmares and night terrors.

   D. Increasing physical activity is likely to provide stimulation that will make it more difficult for the child to fall asleep. This will not alleviate the child's nightmares.

   Ⓝ *NCLEX® Connection: Basic Care and Comfort, Rest and Sleep*

2. A. **CORRECT:** Putting puzzles together helps a preschooler develop fine motor and cognitive skills.

   B. Pulling or pushing toys helps toddlers develop large muscles and coordination.

   C. **CORRECT:** Playing with musical toys helps a preschooler develop fine motor skills and coordination.

   D. **CORRECT:** Playing with puppets helps a preschooler develop oral language and actively use his imagination.

   E. **CORRECT:** Using crayons to color on paper or in coloring books helps a preschooler develop fine motor skills and coordination.

   Ⓝ *NCLEX® Connection: Health Promotion and Maintenance, Developmental Stages and Transitions*

3. A. Telling the preschooler the injection will not hurt will cause the child to distrust the nurse.

   B. Oral medications should be mixed in a small amount of fluid to increase the chance of the child taking the entire dosage.

   C. Offer the child choices when possible gives the child some control and helps reduce the child's fears.

   D. **CORRECT:** Having familiar and cherished objects nearby is therapeutic for children during their hospitalization and is useful as a distraction during uncomfortable procedures.

   E. **CORRECT:** Pretend play helps children determine the difference between reality and fantasy (imagined fears), especially with the assistance of the nurse during hospitalization.

   Ⓝ *NCLEX® Connection: Health Promotion and Maintenance, Developmental Stages and Transitions*

4. A. The CDC recommends *Haemophilus influenzae* type B immunizations during infancy, but not generally beyond 18 months of age.

   B. **CORRECT:** The CDC recommends a varicella (chickenpox) immunization during the preschool years.

   C. **CORRECT:** The CDC recommends a polio immunization during the preschool years.

   D. The CDC recommends hepatitis A immunizations during infancy, but not generally beyond 24 months of age.

   E. **CORRECT:** The CDC recommends seasonal influenza immunizations during the preschool years.

   Ⓝ *NCLEX® Connection: Health Promotion and Maintenance, Health Promotion/Disease Prevention*

5. A. The identification of the son with his father through imitation is nonurgent because it is an expected response for a preschooler. It is common for preschoolers to identify with the parent of the same sex and to mimic that parent's behavior.

   B. **CORRECT:** When using the urgent vs. nonurgent approach to client care, the priority issue is the problem that reflects a lack of completion of the previous stage of development and progression to the current stage of development. According to Erikson, it is a task of the toddler stage to develop autonomy vs. shame and doubt. This preschooler is still acting out with negativism, which is a persistent negative response to requests, often manifested in tantrums. He is still struggling with this task and needs assistance in working through that stage.

   C. The strong imagination of a preschooler is nonurgent because it is expected for preschoolers to have an active imagination as well as an imaginary friend. It is common for preschoolers to manifest misperceptions in thinking, such as animism (the belief that inanimate objects are alive).

   D. Attempting to master activities such as dressing themselves is nonurgent because it is an expected activity for a preschooler. It is common for preschoolers, who are in the stage Erikson describes as initiative vs. guilt, to face the challenge of mastering activities they can perform independently, such as dressing themselves.

   Ⓝ *NCLEX® Connection: Health Promotion and Maintenance, Developmental Stages and Transitions*

PRACTICE Answer

Using the ATI Active Learning Template: Growth and Development

INJURY PREVENTION

Bodily harm
- Keep firearms in a locked cabinet or container.
- Teach stranger safety.
- Wear helmets when riding a bicycle or tricycle and during any other activities that increase head-injury risk.
- Wear protective equipment (helmet and pads) during physical activity.
- Remove doors from unused refrigerators or other equipment.
- Teach preschoolers not to walk in front of swings.

Burns
- Reduce the temperature setting on the water heater.
- Have smoke detectors in the home and replace the batteries regularly.
- Use sunscreen while outdoors.
- Teach preschoolers not to play with matches.

Drowning
- Do not leave children unattended in the bathtub.
- Closely supervise children at a pool or any other body of water.
- Teach children to swim.
- Motor-vehicle injuries
- Use a forward-facing car seat with a harness in the back seat.
- If weight or height exceeds the forward-facing limit, use a belt-positioning booster seat.

Poisoning
- Avoid exposure to lead paint.
- Keep plants out of reach.
- Place safety locks on cabinets with cleaners and other chemicals.
- Keep a poison control number handy or program it into the phone.
- Keep medications in childproof containers out of reach.
- Have a carbon monoxide detector in the home.

Ⓝ *NCLEX® Connection: Health Promotion and Maintenance, Developmental Stages and Transitions*

CHAPTER 21   *School-Age Children (6 to 12 Years)*

EXPECTED GROWTH AND DEVELOPMENT

PHYSICAL DEVELOPMENT

WEIGHT: Gain about 1.8 to 3.2 kg (4 to 7 lb) per year.

HEIGHT: Grow about 5 cm (2 in) per year.

FINE AND GROSS MOTOR DEVELOPMENT: coordination continues to improve and movements become more refined.

- Girls can exceed the height and weight of boys near the end of school-age years.
- Permanent teeth erupt.
- Visual acuity improves to 20/20.
- Auditory acuity and sense of touch fully develop.

CHANGES RELATED TO PUBERTY BEGIN:
- **Girls**
  - Budding of breasts.
  - Appearance of pubic hair
  - Menarche
- **Boys**
  - Enlargement of testicles with changes in the scrotum
  - Appearance of pubic hair

COGNITIVE DEVELOPMENT

Piaget: Concrete Operations
- See weight and volume as unchanging.
- Understand simple analogies and relationships between things and ideas.
- Understand time (days, seasons).
- Classify more complex information.
- Understand various emotions.
- Become self-motivated.
- Solve problems and understand cause and effect.

Language development
- Define many words and understands rules of grammar.
- Understand that a word can have multiple meanings.
- Increased ability to connect words into phrases.
- Reason about a word's meaning rather than the literal translation.
- Understands jokes and riddles.

PSYCHOSOCIAL DEVELOPMENT

Erikson: industry vs. inferiority
School-age children's stage of psychosocial development, according to Erikson, is industry vs. inferiority.
- School-age children develop a sense of industry through advances in learning.
- Tasks that increase self-worth motivate them.
- Stress is increasingly common in this age group from parental and peer expectations, their environment, or observed violence.
- Fears of ridicule by peers and teachers over school-related issues are common. Some children manifest nervous behavior to deal with stress, such as nail biting.

Moral development
- Early on, school-age children might not understand the reasoning behind many rules and will try to find ways around them. Instrumental exchange is in place ("I'll help you if you help me."). They want to make the best deal and do not consider elements of loyalty, gratitude, or justice when making decisions.
- In the latter part of the school years, they move into a law-and-order orientation, placing more emphasis on justice.

Self-concept development
- Strive to develop healthy self-respect by finding out in what areas they excel.
- Need parents to encourage them in educational or extracurricular successes.
- Self-esteem develops based on interactions with peers and perceived self-concept.

Body-image changes
- Body image solidifies.
- Education should address curiosity about sexuality, sexual development, and the reproductive process.
- School-age children are more modest than preschoolers and place more emphasis on privacy.
- Develop concern about appearance and hygiene

Social development
- Social environment can expand to include school, community, and church.
- Peer groups play an important part in social development. However, peer pressure begins to take effect.
- Friendships begin to form among same-gender peers. Clubs and best friends are popular.
- Most relationships come from school associations.
- Children at this age can rival the same-gender parent.
- Conformity becomes evident.
- Become more independent from parents

AGE-APPROPRIATE ACTIVITIES

Competitive and cooperative play predominates.

6- TO 9-YEAR-OLDS
- Play board, video, and number games.
- Play hopscotch.
- Jump rope.
- Collect rocks, stamps, cards, coins, or stuffed animals.
- Ride bicycles.
- Build simple models.
- Artistic activities such as painting and drawing.
- Play team sports: skill building.

9- TO 12-YEAR-OLDS
- Make crafts.
- Read books.
- Build models.
- Develop in hobbies.
- Assemble jigsaw puzzles.
- Play video games.
- Play team sports.
- Learn to play musical instruments

HEALTH PROMOTION

IMMUNIZATIONS

Follow the latest Centers for Disease Control and Prevention immunization recommendations (see www.cdc.gov) for healthy school-age children. These generally include immunizations against diphtheria, tetanus, pertussis, human papillomavirus, hepatitis A and B, measles, mumps, rubella, varicella, seasonal influenza, polio, meningococcal infections, and for some high-risk individuals, pneumococcal infections. Recommendations change periodically, so check them often.

HEALTH SCREENINGS

- Scoliosis: Screening for idiopathic scoliosis, a lateral curvature of the spine with no apparent cause, is essential, especially for girls, during the school-age stage.
- Health promotion and maintenance education is essential to promote healthy choices and prevent illness.

NUTRITION

- By the end of the school-age stage, children eat adult servings of food and also need nutritious snacks.
- Obesity predisposes school-age children to low self-esteem, diabetes mellitus, heart disease, and high blood pressure. Advise parents to:
  - Not use food as a reward.
  - Emphasize physical activity.
  - Provide a balanced diet. See www.choosemyplate.gov for nutritional guidelines for school-age children.
  - Teach children to make healthy food selections for meals and snacks.
  - Avoid eating meals at fast-food restaurants.
  - Avoid skipping meals.

DENTAL HEALTH

- Brush and floss daily.
- Get regular check-ups.

INJURY PREVENTION Qs

Bodily harm
- Keep firearms in a locked cabinet or box.
- Assist with identifying safe play areas.
- Teach stranger safety.
- Teach children to wear helmets and pads when roller skating, skateboarding, bicycling, riding scooters, skiing, and during any other activities that increase injury risk.
- Teach children to wear light reflective clothing at night.

Burns
- Teach fire safety and elimination of potential burn hazards.
- Have working smoke and carbon monoxide detectors in the home.
- Promote sunscreen use.

Drowning
- Supervise children when swimming or near a body of water.
- Teach swimming skills and safety.

Motor-vehicle injuries
- Have children use a car or booster seat until adult seat belts fit correctly.
- Children younger than 13 years of age are safest in the back seat.

Substance abuse/poisoning
- Keep cleaners and chemicals in locked cabinets or out of reach.
- Teach children to say "no" to illegal drugs and alcohol.
- Teach children about the dangers of smoking.

Application Exercises

1. A nurse is talking with parents of a 12-year-old child. Which of the following issues verbalized by the parents should the nurse identify as the priority?

   A. "We just don't understand why our son can't keep up with the other kids in simple activities like running and jumping."

   B. "Our son keeps trying to find ways around our household rules. He always wants to make deals with us."

   C. "We think our son is trying too hard to excel in math just to get the top grades in his class."

   D. "Our son is always afraid the kids in school will laugh at him because he likes to sing."

2. A nurse is planning diversionary activities for school-age children on an inpatient pediatric unit. Which of the following activities should the nurse include? (Select all that apply.)

   A. Building models

   B. Playing video games

   C. Reading books

   D. Using toy carpentry tools

   E. Playing board games

3. A nurse is evaluating teaching about nutrition with the parents of an 11-year-old child. Which of the following statements should indicate to the nurse an understanding of the teaching?

   A. "She wants to eat as much as we do, but we're afraid she'll soon be overweight."

   B. "She skips lunch sometimes, but we figure it's okay as long as she has a healthy breakfast and dinner."

   C. "We limit fast-food restaurant meals to three times a week now."

   D. "We reward her school achievements with a point system instead of a pizza or ice cream."

4. A nurse is talking with the parents of a 10-year-old child who is concerned that their son is becoming secretive, such as closing the door when he showers, and dresses. Which of the following responses should the nurse make?

   A. "Perhaps you should try to find out what he is doing behind those closed doors."

   B. "Suggest that he leave the door ajar for his own safety."

   C. "At this age, children tend to become modest and value their privacy."

   D. "You should establish a disciplinary plan to stop this behavior."

5. A nurse is planning a health promotion and primary prevention class for the parents of school-age children. Which of the following information should the nurse include? (Select all that apply.)

   A. Provide information about the risk of childhood obesity.

   B. Discuss the danger of substance use disorders.

   C. Promote discussion about sexual issues.

   D. Recommend the school-age child sit in the front seat of the car.

   E. Reinforce stranger awareness.

PRACTICE Active Learning Scenario

A nurse is explaining to a group of parents in a community center what cognitive development characteristics they should expect of their school-age children. Use the ATI Active Learning Template: Growth and Development to complete this item.

COGNITIVE DEVELOPMENT: List at least eight cognitive and language development expectations during young adulthood.

Application Exercises Key

1. A. **CORRECT:** When using the urgent vs. nonurgent approach to client care, the priority issue is the delay in motor skills, which could indicate an illness and requires further investigation.

   B. The failure to understand rules is nonurgent because it is common for school-age children to fail to understand the reasoning behind many rules and to try to find ways around them.

   C. The self-motivation to excel is nonurgent because it is common for school-age children, who are in the stage Erikson describes as industry vs. inferiority, to strive to develop a sense of industry through advances in learning.

   D. The fear of disapproval from peers is nonurgent because it is common for school-age children, who are in the stage Erikson describes as industry vs. inferiority, to face the challenge of acquiring new skills and achieving success socially.

   Ⓝ *NCLEX® Connection: Health Promotion and Maintenance, Developmental Stages and Transitions*

2. A. **CORRECT:** Building simple models helps the school-age child develop fine motor and cognitive skills.

   B. **CORRECT:** Playing video games, especially educational and nonviolent ones, helps school-age children develop fine motor and cognitive skills.

   C. **CORRECT:** Reading books helps the school-age child develop cognitive and communication skills.

   D. Using toy carpentry tools helps preschoolers develop imagination and fine motor skills.

   E. CORRECT: Playing board games builds cognitive skills and promotes social interaction.

   Ⓝ *NCLEX® Connection: Health Promotion and Maintenance, Developmental Stages and Transitions*

3. A. By the end of the school-age stage, parents should expect children to eat adult-size portions of food.

   B. Skipping meals can lead to unhealthful snacking and overeating later in the day.

   C. Parents should avoid fast-food restaurants completely to keep children from eating food high in sugar, fat, and starches.

   D. **CORRECT:** Parents should avoid rewarding children with food for good behavior or achievements. Associations between food and feeling good can lead to weight problems.

   Ⓝ *NCLEX® Connection: Basic Care and Comfort, Nutrition and Oral Hydration*

4. A. This response implies that the child is doing something wrong.

   B. A toddler requires constant supervision. This response suggests that the school-age child has something to fear in his own home, or that the child requires constant supervision.

   C. **CORRECT:** School-age children develop a need for privacy. It is important for the parents to show trust in the child and respect the child's need for privacy.

   D. This suggestion sounds like a punishment, and the parents have not presented any evidence that the child is doing anything wrong.

   Ⓝ *NCLEX® Connection: Health Promotion and Maintenance, Developmental Stages and Transitions*

5. A. **CORRECT:** Parents of school-age children need to be aware of nutritional strategies for preventing childhood obesity.

   B. **CORRECT:** Parents of school-age children need to know how to teach children to say no to illegal drugs, alcohol, and all other harmful or addictive substances.

   C. **CORRECT:** Parents should discuss sexual issues with school-age children to promote healthy behavior.

   D. The nurse should instruct the parents of school-age children to keep children under 13 years in the back seat of the car to reduce the risk of injury. .

   E. **CORRECT:** Parents should reinforce stranger safety as soon as their children are old enough to understand it, and throughout all stages of childhood.

   Ⓝ *NCLEX® Connection: Health Promotion and Maintenance, Health Promotion/Disease Prevention*

PRACTICE Answer

Using the ATI Active Learning Template: Growth and Development

COGNITIVE DEVELOPMENT

- See weight and volume as unchanging.
- Understand simple analogies and relationships between things and ideas.
- Understand time (days, seasons).
- Classify more complex information.
- Understand various emotions people experience.
- Become self-motivated.
- Solve problems and understand cause and effect.
- Define many words and understands rules of grammar.
- Understand that a word can have multiple meanings.

Ⓝ *NCLEX® Connection: Health Promotion and Maintenance, Developmental Stages and Transitions*

UNIT 2   HEALTH PROMOTION
SECTION: NURSING THROUGHOUT THE LIFESPAN

CHAPTER 22 *Adolescents*
(12 to 20 Years)

EXPECTED GROWTH AND DEVELOPMENT

PHYSICAL DEVELOPMENT

- Adolescents gain the final 20% to 25% of height during puberty.
- Sleep habits change with puberty due to increased metabolism and rapid growth during the adolescent years. Adolescents stay up late, sleep later in the morning, and perhaps sleep longer than they did during the school-age years.

GIRLS

- Grow 5 to 20 cm (2 to 8 in) and gain 7 to 25 kg (15.5 to 55 lb) during the prepuberty growth spurt
- Stop growing around 16 to 17 years of age
- Mature sexually in the following order
  - Appearance of breast buds
  - Growth of pubic hair (can have hair growth prior to breast bud development)
  - Onset of menstruation

BOYS

- Grow 10 to 30 cm (4 to 12 in) and gain 7 to 29 kg (15 to 65 lb) during the prepuberty growth spurt
- Stop growing at around 18 to 20 years of age
- Mature in the following order
  - Increase in the size of the testes and scrotum
  - Appearance of pubic hair
  - Rapid growth of genitalia
  - Growth of axillary hair
  - Appearance of downy hair on upper lip
  - Change in voice

COGNITIVE DEVELOPMENT

Piaget: Formal operations
- Think at an adult level.
- Think abstractly and deal with principles and hypothetical situations.
- Evaluate the quality of their own thinking.
- Have a longer attention span.
- Are highly imaginative and idealistic.
- Make decisions through logical operations.
- Are future-oriented.
- Are capable of deductive reasoning.
- Understand how actions of an individual influence others.

Language development
Adolescents communicate one way with the peer group and another way with adults. Use open-ended questions to communicate and discuss sensitive issues.

PSYCHOSOCIAL DEVELOPMENT

Erikson: identity vs. role confusion
- They develop a sense of personal identity that family expectations influence.
- Adolescents strive for independence from parents and identify with peers.

Group identity: They become part of a peer group that greatly affects behavior.

Vocationally: Work habits and plans for college and career begin to solidify.

Sexuality: Sexual identity develops during adolescence, with increasing interest in the opposite gender, the same gender, or both genders, according to self-identification with heterosexuality, homosexuality, or bisexuality. Self-identification can shift as sexual maturity progresses.

Health perceptions: Adolescents often feel invincible to bad outcomes of risky behaviors.

Moral development: conventional law and order. Adolescents do not see rules as absolutes, instead looking at each situation and adjusting the rules. Not all adolescents attain this level of moral development during these years.

Self-concept development: Adolescents develop a healthy self-concept by having healthy relationships with peers, family, and teachers while striving for emotional independence. Identifying a skill or talent helps them maintain a healthy self-concept. Participation in sports, hobbies, or the community can have a positive outcome.

Body-Image changes: Adolescents seem particularly concerned with the body images the media portray. Changes during puberty result in comparisons between adolescents and peers. Parents also give their input for hair styles, dress, and activity. Adolescents require interventions if depression or eating disorders result from poor body image.

Social development
- Group relationships are important, as they lead to personal acceptance, approval, and learned behaviors.
- Peer relationships develop as a support system.
- Best-friend relationships are more stable and long-lasting than in previous years.
- Parent-child relationships change to allow more independence.

AGE-APPROPRIATE ACTIVITIES

- Nonviolent video games, music, movies
- Sports, social events
- Caring for a pet
- Career-training programs
- Reading

HEALTH PROMOTION

IMMUNIZATIONS

Follow the latest Centers for Disease Control and Prevention (CDC) immunization recommendations (see www.cdc.gov) for healthy adolescents. These generally include immunizations against diphtheria, tetanus, pertussis, human papillomavirus, hepatitis A and B, measles, mumps, rubella, varicella, seasonal influenza, meningococcal and polio, and for some high-risk individuals, pneumococcal infections. The recommendations change periodically, so check them often.

HEALTH SCREENINGS

Provide health promotion and maintenance education related to illness prevention.

SCOLIOSIS: Screening for idiopathic scoliosis, a lateral curvature of the spine with no apparent cause, is essential, especially for girls, during the adolescent growth spurt because it is most evident at that time.

NUTRITION

- Rapid growth and high metabolism require increases in high-quality nutrients. Nutrients that tend to be deficient during this stage of life are iron, calcium, and vitamins A and C.
- Eating disorders commonly develop during adolescence (more in girls than in boys) due to a fear of being overweight, fad diets, or as a mechanism of maintaining control over some aspect of life.
  - Anorexia nervosa
  - Bulimia nervosa
  - Overeating
- Advise parents to:
  - Not use food as a reward.
  - Emphasize physical activity.
  - Provide a balanced diet. See www.choosemyplate.gov for nutritional guidelines for adolescents.
  - Teach adolescents to make healthy food selections for meals and snacks.

DENTAL HEALTH

- Brush daily.
- Floss daily.
- Get regular check-ups.

INJURY PREVENTION Qs

Bodily harm
- Keep firearms in a locked cabinet or box.
- Teach proper use of sporting equipment prior to use.
- Insist on helmet use and/or pads when roller skating, skateboarding, bicycling, riding scooters, skiing, and during any other activities that increase injury risk.
- Avoid trampolines.
- Be aware of changes in mood and monitor for self-harm in at-risk adolescents. Watch for the following.
  - Poor school performance
  - Lack of interest in things of previous interest
  - Social isolation
  - Disturbances in sleep or appetite
  - Expression of suicidal thoughts

Burns
- Teach fire safety.
- Promote sunscreen use.

Drowning: Teach swimming skills and safety.

Motor-vehicle injury
- Encourage attendance at drivers' education courses.
- Emphasize seat belt use.
- Discourage use of cell phones, including texting, while driving.
- Teach the dangers of combining substance use with driving.

Substance use
- Monitor at-risk adolescents.
- Teach adolescents about the dangers of smoking
- Teach adolescents to say "no" to drugs and alcohol.
- Present a no-tolerance attitude.

Sexually transmitted infections (STIs)
- Identify risk factors through the assessment and interview process.
- Provide education about prevention of STIs, and resources for treatment.

Pregnancy prevention
- Provide education.
- For pregnant adolescents, provide resources for supervision of pregnancy, nutrition, and psychological support.

1. A nurse is teaching the father of a 12-year-old boy about manifestations of puberty. The nurse should explain that which of the following physical changes occurs first?

   A. Appearance of downy hair on the upper lip

   B. Hair growth in the axillae

   C. Enlargement of the testes and scrotum

   D. Deepening of the voice

2. A nurse on a pediatric unit is caring for an adolescent who has multiple fractures. Which of the following interventions should the nurse take? (Select all that apply.)

   A. Suggest that his parents bring in video games for him to play.

   B. Provide a television and DVDs for the adolescent to watch.

   C. Limit visitors to the adolescent's immediate family.

   D. Involve the adolescent in treatment decisions when possible.

   E. Allow the adolescent to perform his own morning care.

3. A nurse is reviewing the CDC's immunization recommendations with the parents of an adolescent. Which of the following recommendations should the nurse include in this discussion? (Select all that apply.)

   A. Rotavirus

   B. Varicella

   C. Herpes zoster

   D. Human papilloma virus

   E. Seasonal influenza

4. A nurse is talking with an adolescent who is having difficulty dealing with several issues. Which of the following issues should the nurse identify as the priority?

   A. "I kind of like this boy in my class, but he doesn't like me back."

   B. "I want to hang out with the kids in the science club, but the jocks pick on them."

   C. "I am so fat, I skip meals to try to lose weight."

   D. "My dad wants me to be a lawyer like him, but I just want to dance."

5. A nurse is preparing a wellness presentation for families about health screening for adolescents. Which of the following information should the nurse include? (Select all that apply.)

   A. Obtain a periodic mental status evaluation.

   B. Discuss prevention of sexually transmitted infections.

   C. Regularly screen for tuberculosis.

   D. Provide education about drug and alcohol use.

   E. Teach monthly breast examinations for girls.

PRACTICE Active Learning Scenario

A nurse on a pediatric unit is reviewing with a group of newly licensed nurses the cognitive developmental milestones to expect from adolescent clients. Use the ATI Active Learning Template: Growth and Development to complete this item.

COGNITIVE DEVELOPMENT: List at least five cognitive development expectations during adolescence.

Application Exercises Key

1. A. The nurse should identify emerging facial hair is a pubescent change. However, evidence-based practice indicates that another change occurs first.

   B. The nurse should identify hair growth in nongenital areas is a pubescent change. However, evidence-based practice indicates that another change occurs first.

   C. **CORRECT:** Using evidence-based practice, the first prepubescent change in boys is an increase in the size of the testicles and scrotum, and growth of pubic hair.

   D. The nurse should identify changing vocal quality is a pubescent change. However, evidence-based practice indicates that another change occurs first.

   Ⓝ *NCLEX® Connection: Health Promotion and Maintenance, Developmental Stages and Transitions*

2. A. **CORRECT:** Nonviolent video games are suitable diversional activities for an adolescent.

   B. **CORRECT:** Nonviolent DVDs are suitable diversional activities for an adolescent.

   C. An adolescent client forms a strong attachment to peers. Allowing friends to visit should reduce the adolescent's feelings of isolation.

   D. **CORRECT:** The adolescent is capable of thinking through problems. Involving the adolescent in decisions helps promote independence and control.

   E. **CORRECT:** Allowing the adolescent to perform his own morning care helps promote a sense of independence and shows respect for his privacy.

   Ⓝ *NCLEX® Connection: Health Promotion and Maintenance, Developmental Stages and Transitions*

3. A. The CDC recommends rotavirus immunizations during infancy and not generally beyond 8 months of age.

   B. **CORRECT:** The CDC recommends varicella (chickenpox) immunizations during adolescence.

   C. The CDC recommends herpes zoster (shingles) immunizations during middle adulthood, typically one dose at age 60 or beyond.

   D. **CORRECT:** The CDC recommends human papilloma virus (genital warts) immunizations during adolescence.

   E. **CORRECT:** The CDC recommends seasonal influenza immunizations during adolescence.

   Ⓝ *NCLEX® Connection: Health Promotion and Maintenance, Health Promotion/Disease Prevention*

4. A. The client is at risk for developing an altered self-esteem due to rejection from his peers. However, another issue is the priority. It is common for adolescents, who are in the stage Erikson describes as identity vs. role confusion, to face the challenge of forming peer relationships and dating relationships.

   B. The client is at risk for developing an altered self-esteem due to rejection from his peers. However, another issue is the priority. It is common for adolescents, who are in the stage Erikson describes as identity vs. role confusion, to face the challenge of becoming part of a peer group and establishing a group identity.

   C. **CORRECT:** The greatest risk to the client is injury due to an eating disorder. The priority issue is to provide counseling to promote body image and ensure proper nutrition.

   D. The client is at risk for developing an altered self-identity due to pressure from a parent;. However, another issue is the priority. It is common for adolescents, who are in the stage Erikson describes as identity vs. role confusion, to face the challenge of forming an identity that will lead to higher education and a career.

   Ⓝ *NCLEX® Connection: Health Promotion and Maintenance, Developmental Stages and Transitions*

5. A. **CORRECT:** Obtain an occasional mental status evaluation is important for the adolescent to reduce the risk for suicide, eating disorders, or substance use disorder.

   B. **CORRECT:** Discuss prevention of sexually transmitted infections is important for the adolescent to reduce the risk for developing a sexually transmitted disease.

   C. **CORRECT:** Periodically screen for tuberculosis is important for the adolescent to reduce the risk for developing or spreading tuberculosis.

   D. **CORRECT:** Providing education about drug and alcohol use is important for the adolescent to reduce the risk for the use of alcohol and recreational drugs.

   E. Young adult women should begin monthly breast examinations to screen for early breast cancer.

   Ⓝ *NCLEX® Connection: Health Promotion and Maintenance, Health Screening*

PRACTICE Answer

Using the ATI Active Learning Template: Growth and Development

Cognitive Development
- Think at an adult level
- Think abstractly and deal with principles
- Evaluate the quality of their own thinking
- Have a longer attention span
- Are highly imaginative and idealistic
- Make decisions through logical operations
- Are future-oriented
- Are capable of deductive reasoning
- Understand how actions of an individual influence others

Ⓝ *NCLEX® Connection: Health Promotion and Maintenance, Developmental Stages and Transitions*

CHAPTER 23 *Young Adults (20 to 35 Years)*

EXPECTED GROWTH AND DEVELOPMENT

PHYSICAL DEVELOPMENT

- Growth has concluded around age 20.
- Physical senses peak.
- Cardiac output and efficiency peak.
- Muscles function optimally at ages 25 to 30.
- Metabolic rate decreases 2% to 4% every decade after age 20.
- Libido is high for men.
- Libido for women peaks during the latter part of this stage.
- Time for childbearing is optimal.
- Pregnancy-related changes occur.

COGNITIVE DEVELOPMENT

Piaget: Formal operations
The young adult years are an optimal time for education, both formal and informal. Qpcc
- Critical thinking skills improve.
- Memory peaks in the 20s.
- Ability for creative thought increases.
- Values/norms of friends (social groups) are relevant.
- Decision-making skills are flexible with increased openness to change.

PSYCHOSOCIAL DEVELOPMENT

According to Erikson, young adults must achieve intimacy vs. isolation.
- Young adults can take on more adult commitments and responsibilities.
- Young adults' occupational choices relate to:
  ○ High goals/dreams
  ○ Exploration/experimentation

Moral development
- Young adults can personalize values and beliefs.
- They can base reasoning on ethical fairness principles, such as justice.

Self-concept development: Influences on the formation of a healthy self-concept during the young adult years include:
- Avoidance of substance use disorders
- Formation of a family
- Frequency interactions with family and friends
- Personal choice and response to ethical situations

Body-image changes
- Affected by diet and exercise patterns.
- Pregnancy-related body image changes can also occur.

Social development
Young adults might:
- Leave home and establish independent living situation.
- Establish close friendships (intimacy).
- Transition from being single to being a member of a new family.
- Question their ability to parent.
- Experience increased anxiety and/or depression, especially after the birth of a child.

HEALTH PROMOTION

Young adults are especially at risk for alterations in health from:
- Substance use disorders
- Periodontal disease due to poor oral hygiene
- Unplanned pregnancies: a source of high stress
- Sexually transmitted infections (STIs)
- Infertility
- Work-related injuries or exposures
- Violent death and injury

IMMUNIZATIONS

Follow the latest Centers for Disease Control and Prevention (CDC) immunization recommendations (see www.cdc.gov). Primary vaccinations for young adults include annual influenza, as well as tetanus, diphtheria, and pertussis. Other vaccines are given to "catch up" the young adult for incomplete immunization series, or to provide additional protection to high-risk individuals. These include immunizations against hepatitis A and B, measles, mumps, rubella, varicella, human papillomavirus, and pneumococcal and meningococcal infections. The recommendations change periodically, so check them often. Qebp

HEALTH SCREENINGS

- Young adults should follow age-related guidelines for screening.
- Encourage selecting a primary care provider for ongoing, routine medical care.
- Provide education about contraception and regular physical activity.

ROUTINE HEALTH CARE VISITS

Should include obtaining height, weight, vital signs, and family history; screening for stress; education related to STIs and substance use disorders; and encouragement of good nutrition.

NUTRITION

- Monitor for adequate nutrition and proper physical activity.
- Monitor calcium intake in women.
- See choosemyplate.gov for nutritional recommendations.

INJURY PREVENTION Qs

- Avoiding drugs, including alcohol, which can lead to substance use disorders
- Avoiding driving a vehicle during or after drinking alcohol or taking drugs that impair sensory and motor functions
- Wearing a seat belt when operating a vehicle
- Wearing a helmet while bike riding, skiing, and other recreational activities that increase head-injury risk
- Installing smoke and carbon monoxide detectors in the home
- Securing firearms in a safe location

Application Exercises

1. A nurse is teaching a young adult client about health promotion and illness prevention. Which of the following statements by the client indicates an understanding of the teaching?

   A. "I already had my immunizations as a child, so I'm protected in that area."

   B. "It is important to schedule routine health care visits even if I am feeling well."

   C. "I will just go to an urgent care center for my routine medical care."

   D. "There's no reason to seek help if I am feeling stressed because it's just part of life."

2. A nurse is reviewing CDC immunization recommendations with a young adult client. Which of the following vaccines should the nurse recommend as routine, rather than catch-up, during young adulthood? (Select all that apply.)

   A. Influenza

   B. Measles, mumps, rubella

   C. Pertussis

   D. Tetanus

   E. Polio

3. A charge nurse is explaining the various stages of the lifespan to a group of newly licensed nurses. Which of the following examples should the charge nurse should include as a developmental task for a young adult?

   A. Becoming actively involved in providing guidance to the next generation

   B. Adjusting to major changes in roles and relationships due to losses

   C. Devoting a great deal of time to establishing an occupation

   D. Finding oneself "sandwiched" between and being responsible for two generations

4. A nurse is counseling a young adult who describes having difficulty dealing with several issues. Which of the following client statements should the nurse identify as the priority to assess further?

   A. "I have my own apartment now, but it's not easy living away from my parents."

   B. "It's been so stressful for me to even think about having my own family."

   C. "I don't even know who I am yet, and now I'm supposed to know what to do."

   D. "My girlfriend is pregnant, and I don't think I have what it takes to be a good father."

5. A nurse is reviewing safety precautions with a group of young adults at a community health fair. Which of the following recommendations should the nurse include to address common health risks for this age group? (Select all that apply.)

   A. Install bath rails and grab bars in bathrooms.

   B. Wear a helmet while skiing.

   C. Install a carbon monoxide detector.

   D. Secure firearms in a safe location.

   E. Remove throw rugs from the home.

PRACTICE Active Learning Scenario

A nurse at a community center is teaching a group of young adults what physical and cognitive development characteristics they should expect at this stage of life. Use the ATI Active Learning Template: Growth and Development to complete this item.

PHYSICAL DEVELOPMENT: List at least five physical development expectations.

COGNITIVE DEVELOPMENT: List at least three cognitive development expectations during young adulthood.

Application Exercises Key

1. A. For protection against a wide variety of communicable illnesses, the nurse should encourage adults to obtain CDC-recommended immunizations throughout the lifespan.

    B. **CORRECT:** Despite being in relatively good health, young adult clients should plan to participate in routine screenings and health care visits.

    C. Urgent care centers offer limited services, typically for acute injuries or problems that cannot wait until a primary care provider is available. The nurse should encourage clients to establish a relationship with a primary care provider to consult for nonurgent health problems.

    D. Although it is true that stress is inevitable, chronic stress can lead to severe health alterations. Young adults who have stress that is recurrent or escalating should seek medical care.

    Ⓝ *NCLEX® Connection: Health Promotion and Maintenance, Health Promotion/Disease Prevention*

2. A. **CORRECT:** The CDC recommends annual influenza immunization during adulthood.

    B. The CDC recommends obtaining the measles, mumps, and rubella vaccines routinely during childhood. The series can be administered during adulthood for individuals who meet certain criteria.

    C. **CORRECT:** The CDC recommends a booster dose of pertussis vaccine during adulthood.

    D. **CORRECT:** The CDC recommends ongoing booster doses of tetanus and diphtheria vaccines during adulthood.

    E. The CDC recommends the polio vaccine to be administered routinely during childhood. The series can be administered during adulthood for individuals who meet certain criteria.

    Ⓝ *NCLEX® Connection: Health Promotion and Maintenance, Health Promotion/Disease Prevention*

3. A. The nurse should identify active involvement in the next generation as a developmental task for middle adults.

    B. The nurse should identify adjusting to major role changes associated with loss as a developmental task for older adults.

    C. **CORRECT:** The nurse should identify exploring career options and then establishing oneself in a specific occupation as a major developmental task for a young adult.

    D. The nurse should identify assuming responsibility for the previous as well as the next generation as a developmental task for middle adults.

    Ⓝ *NCLEX® Connection: Health Promotion and Maintenance, Developmental Stages and Transitions*

4. A. Living away from home and establishing independent living is nonurgent because it is an expected challenge during a young adulthood. There is another statement the nurse should identify as the priority.

    B. Transitioning from being single to being a member of a new family is nonurgent because it is an expected challenge during young adulthood. There is another statement the nurse should identify as the priority.

    C. **CORRECT:** When using the urgent vs. nonurgent approach to client care, the nurse determines that the counseling priority is the problem that reflects a lack of completion of the previous stage of development and progression to the current stage. According to Erikson, it is a task of adolescence to develop identity vs. role confusion. The nurse should recognize this young adult is still struggling with this task and needs assistance in working through that dilemma.

    D. Considering childbearing and parenting is nonurgent because it is an expected challenge during young adulthood. There is another statement the nurse should identify as the priority.

    Ⓝ *NCLEX® Connection: Health Promotion and Maintenance, Developmental Stages and Transitions*

5. A. Although bath rails and grab bars add a measure of safety to bathing activities, this recommendation addresses health risks common to the older adult population due to their risk for falls.

    B. **CORRECT:** The nurse should encourage the client to wear a helmet while skiing to reduce the risk of head injury. Although it applies to other age groups, many young adults engage in winter sports. Therefore, this is an age-appropriate recommendation for this developmental group.

    C. **CORRECT:** The nurse should remind the client to install a carbon monoxide detector in the home. This is an essential safety precaution for young adults as well as for all other developmental stages.

    D. **CORRECT:** The nurse should warn the client to secure firearms in a safe location to reduce the risk of accidental gunshot injuries. Although it applies to all age groups, many young adults own firearms, so this is an age-appropriate recommendation for this developmental group.

    E. Although throw rugs can pose a safety hazard, this recommendation addresses health risks common to the older adult population due to their risk for falls.

    Ⓝ *NCLEX® Connection: Health Promotion and Maintenance, Developmental Stages and Transitions*

PRACTICE Answer

Use the ATI Active Learning Template: Growth and Development

PHYSICAL DEVELOPMENT

- Completion of growth
- Peak in physical senses
- Peak in cardiac output, efficiency
- Optimal muscle function
- Gradual decline in metabolic rate

- High libido (men)
- Eventual peak in libido (women)
- Optimal childbearing
- Pregnancy-related changes

COGNITIVE DEVELOPMENT

- Improvement in critical thinking
- Peak in memory
- Increased ability for creative thought
- Relevance of values/ norms of friends

Ⓝ *NCLEX® Connection: Health Promotion and Maintenance, Developmental Stages and Transitions*

CHAPTER 24 *Middle Adults
(35 to 65 Years)*

EXPECTED GROWTH AND DEVELOPMENT

PHYSICAL DEVELOPMENT

Decreases in the following:
- Skin turgor and moisture
- Subcutaneous fat
- Melanin in hair (graying)
- Hair
- Visual acuity, especially for near vision
- Auditory acuity, especially for high-pitched sounds
- Sense of taste
- Skeletal muscle mass
- Height
- Calcium/bone density
- Blood vessel elasticity
- Respiratory vital capacity
- Large intestine muscle tone
- Gastric secretions
- Decreased glomerular filtration rate
- Estrogen/testosterone
- Glucose tolerance

COGNITIVE DEVELOPMENT

Piaget: Formal operations
- Reaction time and speed of performance slow slightly.
- Memory is intact.
- Crystallized intelligence remains (stored knowledge).
- Fluid intelligence (how to learn and process new information) declines slightly.

PSYCHOSOCIAL DEVELOPMENT

According to Erikson, middle adults must achieve generativity vs. stagnation.
Middle adults strive for generativity.
- Use life as an opportunity for creativity and productivity.
- Have concern for others.
- Consider parenting an important task.
- Contribute to the well-being of the next generation.
- Strive to do well in one's own environment.
- Adjust to changes in physical appearance and abilities.

Moral development
- Religious maturity
- Spiritual beliefs and religion can take on added importance.
- Middle adults can become more secure in their convictions.
- Middle adults often have advanced moral development.

Self-concept development: Some middle adults have issues related to:
- Menopause
- Sexuality
- Depression
- Irritability
- Difficulty with sexual identity
- Job performance and ability to provide support
- Marital changes with the death of a spouse or divorce

Body image changes
- Sex drive can decrease as a result of declining hormones, chronic disorders, or medications.
- Changes in physical appearance can raise concerns about desirability.
- WOMEN: Symptoms of menopause can represent as:
  ○ Loss of the reproductive role or femininity.
  ○ New interest in intimacy.
- MEN: Decreasing strength can be frustrating or frightening.

Social development
- Need to maintain and strengthen intimacy.
- Empty nest syndrome: experiencing sadness when children move away from home.
- Provide assistance to aging parents, adult children, and grandchildren, giving this stage of life the name "sandwich generation."

HEALTH PROMOTION

Especially at risk for alterations in health due to:
- Obesity, type 2 diabetes mellitus
- Cardiovascular disease
- Cancer
- Substance use disorders (alcohol use disorder)
- Psychosocial stressors

IMMUNIZATIONS

Follow the latest Centers for Disease Control and Prevention (CDC) immunization recommendations (see www.cdc.gov). Primary vaccinations for young adults include annual influenza immunization, as well as tetanus, diphtheria, zoster, pneumococcal, and pertussis. Other vaccines are given to "catch-up" the young adult for incomplete immunization series, or to provide additional protection to high-risk individuals. These include immunizations against hepatitis A and B, measles, mumps, rubella, varicella, and pneumococcal and meningococcal infections. The recommendations change periodically, so check them often. Q℗

HEALTH SCREENINGS

Middle adults should follow age-related guidelines for screening.
- Dual-energy x-ray absorptiometry (DXA) screening for osteoporosis
- Eye examination for glaucoma and other disorders every 2 to 3 years or annually depending on provider.
- Mental health screening for anxiety and depression

NUTRITION

Nutrition counseling for middle adults generally includes:
- Obtaining adequate protein.
- Increasing the consumption of whole grains and fresh fruits and vegetables.
- Limiting fat and cholesterol.
- Increasing vitamin D and calcium supplementation (especially for women).

> See www.choosemyplate.gov for nutritional recommendations.

INJURY PREVENTION Qs

- Avoid drugs, including alcohol, that can lead to substance use disorders.
- Avoid driving a vehicle during or after drinking alcohol or taking drugs that impair sensory and motor functions.
- Wear a seat belt when operating a vehicle.
- Wear a helmet while bike riding, skiing, and other recreational activities that increase head-injury risk.
- Install smoke and carbon monoxide detectors in the home.
- Secure firearms in a safe location.

Application Exercises

1. A nursing instructor is explaining the various stages of the lifespan to a group of nursing students. Which of the following examples should the nurse include as a developmental task for middle adulthood?

    A. The client evaluates his behavior after a social interaction.

    B. The client states he is learning to trust others.

    C. The client wishes to find meaningful friendships.

    D. The client expresses concerns about the next generation.

2. A nurse is collecting data to evaluate a middle adult's psychosocial development. The nurse should expect middle adults to demonstrate which of the following developmental tasks? (Select all that apply.)

    A. Develop an acceptance of diminished strength and increased dependence on others.

    B. Spend time focusing on improving job performance.

    C. Welcome opportunities to be creative and productive.

    D. Commit to finding friendship and companionship.

    E. Become involved with community issues and activities.

3. A nurse is collecting history and physical examination data from a middle adult. The nurse should expect to find decreases in which of the following physiologic functions? (Select all that apply.)

    A. Metabolism

    B. Ability to hear low-pitched sounds

    C. Gastric secretions

    D. Far vision

    E. Glomerular filtration

4. A nurse is preparing a health promotion course for a group of middle adults. Which of the following strategies should the nurse recommend? (Select all that apply.)

    A. Eye examination every 1 to 3 years

    B. Decrease intake of calcium supplements

    C. DXA screening for osteoporosis

    D. Increase intake of carbohydrate in the diet

    E. Screening for depressive disorders

5. A nurse is counseling a middle adult client who describes having difficulty dealing with several issues. Which of the following client statements should the nurse identify as the priority to assess further?

    A. "I am struggling to accept that my parents are aging and need so much help."

    B. "It's been so stressful for me to think about having intimate relationships."

    C. "I know I should volunteer my time for a good cause, but maybe I'm just selfish."

    D. "I love my grandchildren, but my son expects me to relive my parenting days."

PRACTICE Active Learning Scenario

A nurse in a community health center is explaining to a group of middle adults what moral and cognitive development characteristics they should expect at this stage of life. Use the ATI Active Learning Template: Growth and Development to complete this item.

COGNITIVE DEVELOPMENT
- List at least two moral development expectations during middle adulthood.
- List at least four cognitive development expectations during middle adulthood.

Application Exercises Key

1. A. The nurse should identify evaluating behavior after a social interaction as a developmental task that begins during the preschool years.

   B. The nurse should identify learning to trust others as a developmental task of infancy during Erickson's trust vs. mistrust stage.

   C. The nurse should identify finding meaningful friendships as a developmental task for school-aged children.

   D. **CORRECT:** Erickson's task for a middle adult as generativity vs. stagnation. The nurse should include showing concern for the next generation as an example for this age group.

   Ⓝ *NCLEX® Connection: Health Promotion and Maintenance, Developmental Stages and Transitions*

2. A. The nurse should identify acceptance of diminished strength and increased dependence as a developmental task for older adulthood.

   B. **CORRECT:** Psychosocially healthy middle adults strive to do well in their environment as part of achieving Erikson's stage of generativity vs. stagnation.

   C. **CORRECT:** Psychosocially healthy middle adults accept life's opportunities for creativity and productivity and use these opportunities for achieving Erikson's stage of generativity vs. stagnation.

   D. The nurse should identify seeking and forming friendships as a developmental task of young adulthood.

   E. **CORRECT:** Psychosocially healthy middle adults work to contribute to future generations through community involvement and parenting as part of achieving Erikson's stage of generativity vs. stagnation.

   Ⓝ *NCLEX® Connection: Health Promotion and Maintenance, Health Screening*

3. A. **CORRECT:** The nurse should expect metabolism to decline, causing weight gain during middle adulthood.

   B. The nurse should expect a decline in the ability to hear high-pitched sounds during middle adulthood.

   C. **CORRECT:** In middle adulthood, decreases in secretions of bicarbonate and gastric mucus begin and persist into older age. This increases the risk of peptic ulcer disease.

   D. The nurse should expect a decline in near vision (presbyopia) during middle adulthood.

   E. **CORRECT:** Middle adults begin to lose nephron units, which results in a decline in glomerular filtration rates.

   Ⓝ *NCLEX® Connection: Health Promotion and Maintenance, Health Promotion/Disease Prevention*

4. A. **CORRECT:** The nurse should recommend middle adult clients have an eye examination every 1 to 3 years to screen for glaucoma and other disorders.

   B. The nurse should recommend that middle adult clients, especially women, increase intake of vitamin D and calcium to prevent osteoporosis.

   C. **CORRECT:** The nurse should recommend middle adult client have a DXA scan to screen for osteoporosis.

   D. **CORRECT:** The nurse should recommend middle adult clients obtain adequate protein, and consume more fresh fruits, vegetables and whole grains.

   E. **CORRECT:** The nurse should recommend screening for anxiety and depression during middle adulthood.

   Ⓝ *NCLEX® Connection: Basic Care and Comfort, Nutrition and Oral Hydration*

5. A. Adjusting to and caring for aging parents is nonurgent because it is an expected challenge during middle adulthood. There is another statement that the nurse should identify as the priority.

   B. **CORRECT:** When using the urgent vs. nonurgent approach to client care, the counseling priority is the problem that reflects a lack of completion of the previous stage and progression to the current stage of development. According to Erikson, developing intimacy vs. isolation is a task of young adulthood. This middle adult is still struggling with this task and needs assistance in working through searching for and developing intimate relationships with others.

   C. Contributing to the community is nonurgent because it is an expected challenge during middle adulthood. There is another statement that the nurse should identify as the priority.

   D. Questioning the ability to contribute to future generations is nonurgent because it is an expected challenge during middle adulthood. There is another statement that the nurse should identify as the priority.

   Ⓝ *NCLEX® Connection: Health Promotion and Maintenance, Developmental Stages and Transitions*

PRACTICE Answer

Using the ATI Active Learning Template: Growth and Development

COGNITIVE DEVELOPMENT
Moral development
- Spiritual beliefs and religion can take on added importance.
- Middle adults can become more secure in their convictions.
- Middle adults often have advanced moral development.
Cognitive development
- Reaction time and speed of performance slow slightly.
- Memory is intact.
- Crystallized intelligence remains (stored knowledge).
- Fluid intelligence (how to learn and process new information) declines slightly.

Ⓝ *NCLEX® Connection: Safety and Infection Control, Accident/Error/Injury Prevention*

CHAPTER 25   *Older Adults (65 Years and Older)*

EXPECTED GROWTH AND DEVELOPMENT

PHYSICAL DEVELOPMENT

Integumentary
- Decreased skin turgor, subcutaneous fat, and connective tissue (dermis), which leads to wrinkles and dry, transparent skin
- Loss of subcutaneous fat, which makes it more difficult for older adults to adjust to cold temperatures
- Thinning and graying of hair, as well as a more sparse distribution
- Thickening of fingernails and toenails

Cardiovascular/pulmonary
- Decreased chest wall movement, vital capacity, and cilia, which increases the risk for respiratory infections
- Reduced cardiac output
- Decreased peripheral circulation
- Increased blood pressure

Neurosensory
- Slower reaction time
- Decreased touch, smell, and taste sensations
- Decreased production of saliva
- Decline in visual acuity
- Decreased ability for eyes to adjust from light to dark, leading to night blindness, which is especially dangerous when driving
- Inability to hear high-pitched sounds (presbycusis)
- Reduced spatial awareness

Gastrointestinal
- Decreased digestive enzymes
- Decreased intestinal motility, which can lead to increased risk of constipation
- Increased dental problems

Neuromuscular
- Decreased height due to intervertebral disk changes
- Decreased muscle strength and tone
- Decalcification of bones
- Degeneration of joints

Genitourinary
- Decreased bladder capacity
- Prostate hypertrophy in men
- Decline in estrogen or testosterone production
- Atrophy of breast tissue in women

Endocrine
- Decline in triiodothyronine (T3) production, yet overall function remains effective
- Decreased sensitivity of tissue cells to insulin

COGNITIVE DEVELOPMENT

Piaget: Formal operations
- Many older adults maintain their cognitive function. There is some decline in speed of the cognitive function versus cognitive ability.
- A number of factors influence older adults' abilities to function, such as overall health, the number of stressors, and lifelong mental well-being.
- Slowed neurotransmission, vascular circulation impairment, disease states, poor nutrition, and structural brain changes can result in the following cognitive disorders.
  - **Delirium:** Acute, temporary, and can have a physiologic source, such as infection, sleep deprivation, or pain, or related to a change in surroundings, such as being in an unfamiliar or new environment. Delirium is often the first manifestation of infection (such as urinary tract infection) in older adults.
  - **Dementia:** Chronic, progressive, and possibly with an unknown cause (Alzheimer's disease, vascular dementia).
  - **Depression:** Chronic, acute, or gradual onset (present for at least 6 weeks). Often due to loss of a loved one, feelings of isolation, or chronic disease.

PSYCHOSOCIAL DEVELOPMENT

Erikson: Integrity vs. despair
Older adults need to:
- Adjust to lifestyle changes related to retirement (decrease in income, living situation, loss of work role).
- Adapt to changes in family structure (can be role reversal in later years).
- Adapt to changes in living environment.
- Deal with multiple losses (death of a spouse, friends, siblings).
- Face death.

Self-concept development: Older adults face difficulties in the area of self-concept.
- Seeing oneself as an aging person
- Finding ways to maintain a good quality of life
- Becoming more dependent on others for activities of daily living

Body image changes: An adjustment to decreases in physical strength and endurance is often difficult, especially for older adults who are cognitively active and engaged. Many older adults feel frustrated that their bodies are limiting what they desire to do.

Social development
- Find ways to remain socially active and to overcome isolation.
- Maintain sexual health.

HEALTH PROMOTION

HEALTH RISKS

Cardiovascular diseases
- Coronary artery disease
- Hypertension

Factors affecting mobility
- Arthritis
- Osteoporosis
- Falls

Mental health disorders
- Depression
- Dementia
- Suicide
- Alcohol use disorder
- Tobacco use disorder

Other disorders
- Stroke
- Diabetes mellitus
- Cancer
- Incontinence
- Abuse and neglect
- Cataracts
- Chronic pain
- Issues related to poor dental hygiene (gingivitis, missing teeth, gum disease)

IMMUNIZATIONS Q̲EBP

Follow the latest Centers for Disease Control and Prevention (CDC) immunization recommendations (www.cdc.gov) for healthy older adults. These generally include:
- Immunizations against diphtheria, tetanus, pertussis, varicella, seasonal influenza, herpes zoster, and pneumococcal infections
- Immunizations against, hepatitis A and B, haemophilus influenzae type b, and meningococcal infections for high-risk individuals

HEALTH SCREENINGS

Older adults should follow age-related guidelines for screening.

ANNUAL SCREENINGS
- Hearing
- Fecal occult blood test
- Digital rectal and prostate-specific antigen (men)
- Dual-energy x-ray absorptiometry (DXA) scanning for osteoporosis
- Eye examination for glaucoma and other disorders

PERIODIC SCREENING
- Mental health screening for depression
- Cholesterol and diabetes screening every 3 years

NUTRITION

- In addition to gastrointestinal alterations, other factors influence nutrition in older adults.
  - Difficulty getting to and from the supermarket to shop for food
  - Low income
  - Impaired mobility
  - Depression or dementia
  - Social isolation (preparing meals for one person, eating alone)
  - Medications that alter taste or appetite
  - Prescribed diets that are unappealing
  - Incontinence that can cause the person to limit fluid intake
  - Constipation
- Metabolic rates and activity decline as individuals age, so total caloric intake should decrease to maintain a healthy weight. With the reduction of total calorie intake, it becomes even more important that the calories older adults consume be of good nutritional value.

Go to www.choosemyplate.gov for nutritional recommendations.

NUTRITIONAL RECOMMENDATIONS
- Increase intake of vitamins D, B_{12}, E, folate, fiber, and calcium.
- Increase fluid intake to minimize the risk of dehydration and prevent constipation.
- Take a low-dose multivitamin along with mineral supplementation.
- Limit sodium, fat, refined sugar, and alcohol intake.

PSYCHOSOCIAL INTERVENTIONS

To improve self-concept and alleviate social isolation
- Therapeutic communication
- Touch
- Reality orientation
- Validation therapy
- Reminiscence therapy
- Attending to physical appearance
- Assistive devices (canes, walkers, hearing aids)

INJURY PREVENTION Qs

- Install bath rails, grab bars, and handrails on stairways.
- Remove throw rugs.
- Eliminate clutter from walkways and hallways.
- Remove extension and phone cords from walkways and hallways.
- Instruct clients about how to properly use ambulation-assistive devices (walkers, canes).
- Teach clients about safe medication use.
- Ensure adequate lighting.
- Remind clients to wear eyeglasses and hearing aids.

- Prevent substance use disorders.
- Avoid driving a vehicle during or after drinking alcohol or taking substances that impair sensory and motor functions.
- Wear a seat belt when operating a vehicle.
- Wear a helmet while bike riding, skiing, and other recreational activities that increase the risk of head injury.
- Install smoke and carbon monoxide detectors in the home.
- Secure firearms in a safe location.

> **PRACTICE** Active Learning Scenario
>
> A nurse is reviewing safety precautions for older adults with a group of home health care assistive personnel. Use the ATI Active Learning Template: Growth and Development to complete this item.
>
> **INJURY PREVENTION:** List at least 10 safety recommendations for older adults.

Application Exercises

1. A nurse is counseling an older adult who describes having difficulty dealing with several issues. Which of the following problems verbalized by the client should the nurse identify as the priority?

   A. "I spent my whole life dreaming about retirement, and now I wish I had my job back."

   B. "It's been so stressful for me to have to depend on my son to help around the house."

   C. "I just heard my friend Al died. That's the third one in 3 months."

   D. "I keep forgetting which medications I have taken during the day."

2. A nurse is providing teaching for an older adult client who has lost 4.5 kg (9.9 lb) since his last admission 6 months ago. Which of the following instructions should the nurse include in the teaching? (Select all that apply.)

   A. "Eat three large meals a day."

   B. "Eat your meals in front of the television."

   C. "Eat foods that are easy to eat, such as finger foods."

   D. "Invite family members to eat meals with you."

   E. "Exercise every day to increase appetite."

3. A nurse is planning a presentation for a group of older adults about health promotion and disease prevention. Which of the following interventions should the nurse plan to recommend? (Select all that apply.)

   A. Human papilloma virus (HPV) immunization

   B. Pneumococcal immunization

   C. Yearly eye examination

   D. Periodic mental health screening

   E. Annual fecal occult blood test

4. A nurse is talking with an older adult client about improving her nutritional status. Which of the following interventions should the nurse recommend? (Select all that apply.)

   A. Increase protein intake to increase muscle mass.

   B. Decrease fluid intake to prevent urinary incontinence.

   C. Increase calcium intake to prevent osteoporosis.

   D. Limit sodium intake to prevent edema.

   E. Increase fiber intake to prevent constipation.

5. A nurse is collecting data from an older adult client as part of a comprehensive physical examination. Which of the following findings should the nurse expect as associated with aging? (Select all that apply.)

   A. Skin thickening

   B. Decreased height

   C. Increased saliva production

   D. Nail thickening

   E. Decreased bladder capacity

Application Exercises Key

1. A. The client is at risk for social isolation and loss of independence because of retirement. However, another issue is the priority.

    B. The client is at risk for loss of independence and reduced self-esteem due to dependence upon his son. However, another issue is the priority.

    C. The client is at risk for social isolation due to the loss of a friend. However, another issue is the priority.

    D. **CORRECT:** The greatest risk to this client is injury from overdosing or underdosing medications due to loss of short-term memory. The priority issue for the nurse is to assist the client to implement safe medication strategies. The nurse should assist the client to use a pill organizer to help him remember to take his medications and to keep a list of all current medications.

    N *NCLEX® Connection: Health Promotion and Maintenance, Developmental Stages and Transitions*

2. A. The client should eat small frequent meals to increase nutritional intake.

    B. The client should avoid distractions during meals to increase nutritional intake.

    C. **CORRECT:** The nurse should encourage the client to eat finger foods because finger foods are easier for the older adult client to eat.

    D. **CORRECT:** The nurse should encourage the client to involve family members with meals. Socialization during meals promotes nutritional intake.

    E. **CORRECT:** The nurse should encourage the client to exercise daily to increase appetite.

    N *NCLEX® Connection: Health Promotion and Maintenance, Health Screening*

3. A. The HPV vaccine is recommended for female clients from age 11 to 26 and male clients from age 9 to 26. It is not a recommendation for older adults.

    B. **CORRECT:** The pneumococcal vaccine is recommended for older adult clients.

    C. **CORRECT:** A yearly eye examination to screen for glaucoma and vision changes is recommended for older adults.

    D. **CORRECT:** Periodic mental health assessments are recommended for older adult clients to screen for depression.

    E. **CORRECT:** An annual fecal occult blood test is recommended for older adults.

    N *NCLEX® Connection: Health Promotion and Maintenance, Health Promotion/Disease Prevention*

4. A. **CORRECT:** Older adults should increase protein intake to increase muscle mass and improve would healing.

    B. Older adults should increase fluid intake to prevent dehydration and constipation.

    C. **CORRECT:** Older adults should increase calcium intake to reduce the risk for osteoporosis.

    D. **CORRECT:** Older adults should limit sodium intake to reduce the risk for edema and hypertension.

    E. **CORRECT:** Older adults should increase fiber intake to prevent constipation.

    N *NCLEX® Connection: Basic Care and Comfort, Nutrition and Oral Hydration*

5. A. Physiological changes that occur with aging can include decreased skin turgor, subcutaneous fat, and connective tissue (dermis), which can cause wrinkles and dry, thin, transparent skin.

    B. **CORRECT:** Physiological changes that occur with aging can include loss in height due to the thinning of intervertebral disks.

    C. Physiological changes that occur with aging can include decreased saliva production, making xerostomia (dry mouth) a common problem.

    D. **CORRECT:** Physiological changes that occur with aging can include thickening of the nails of the fingers and toes.

    E. **CORRECT:** Physiological changes that occur with aging can include a reduced bladder capacity. While young adults have a bladder capacity of about 500 to 600 mL, older adults have a capacity of about 250 mL.

    N *NCLEX® Connection: Health Promotion and Maintenance, Developmental Stages and Transitions*

PRACTICE Answer

Using the ATI Active Learning Template: Growth and Development

INJURY PREVENTION

- Install bath rails, grab bars, and handrails on stairways.
- Teach clients about safe medication use.
- Remove throw rugs.
- Eliminate clutter from walkways and hallways.
- Remove extension and phone cords from walkways and hallways.
- Instruct about how to use ambulation-assistive devices (walkers, canes).
- Ensure adequate lighting.
- Remind clients to wear eyeglasses and hearing aids.
- Prevent substance use disorders.
- Avoid driving a vehicle during or after drinking alcohol or taking substances that impair sensory and motor functions.
- Wear a seat belt when operating a vehicle.
- Wear a helmet while bike riding, skiing, and other recreational activities that increase head-injury risk.
- Install smoke and carbon monoxide detectors in the home.
- Secure firearms in a safe location.

N *NCLEX® Connection: Safety and Infection Control, Accident/Error/Injury Prevention*

When reviewing the following chapters, keep in mind the relevant topics and tasks of the NCLEX outline, in particular:

Client Needs: Health Promotion and Maintenance

AGING PROCESS: Provide care and education for the adult client ages 18 through 64 years.

DEVELOPMENTAL STAGES AND TRANSITIONS: Compare client development to expected age/developmental stage and report any deviations.

HEALTH PROMOTION/DISEASE PREVENTION: Assist the client in maintaining an optimum level of health.

Client Needs: Management of Care

CONFIDENTIALITY/INFORMATION SECURITY: Maintain client confidentiality and privacy.

Client Needs: Reduction of Risk Potential

CHANGES/ABNORMALITIES IN VITAL SIGNS: Apply knowledge needed to perform related nursing procedures and psychomotor skills when assessing vital signs.

SYSTEM SPECIFIC ASSESSMENT: Perform focused assessment.

Client Needs: Health Promotion/Disease Prevention

HEALTH SCREENING: Perform health history/health and risk assessments.

TECHNIQUES OF PHYSICAL ASSESSMENT: Apply knowledge of nursing procedures and psychomotor skills to techniques of physical assessment.

CHAPTER 26

CHAPTER 26 ## Data Collection and General Survey

Data collection includes obtaining subjective and objective information from clients. The health history provides subjective data. The physical examination and diagnostic tests provide objective data.

INTERVIEWING TECHNIQUES

Standardized formats are a framework for obtaining information about clients' physical, developmental, emotional, intellectual, social, and spiritual dimensions.

Therapeutic techniques for health assessment foster communication and create an environment that promotes an optimal health assessment/data collection experience.

THERAPEUTIC COMMUNICATION

Therapeutic communication helps develop rapport with clients. The techniques encourage a trusting relationship, whereby clients feel comfortable telling their story. Begin with the purpose of the interview, gather information, and then conclude the interview by summarizing the findings. **(26.1)**

- Introduce yourself and the various parts of the assessment.
- Determine what the client wants you to call him.
- Allow more time for responses from older adults. Ⓒ
- Make sure the client is comfortable (room temperature, chair).
- When possible, start by asking for the health history, performing the general survey, and measuring vital signs to build rapport prior to moving on to more sensitive parts of the examination.
- Reduce environmental noises (TV, radio, visitors talking) to enhance communication and eliminate distractions.
- Ensure understanding by obtaining interpretive services for clients who have language or other communication barriers.
- Note the client's nonverbal communication (body language, eye contact, tone of voice).
- Avoid using medical or nursing jargon, giving advice, ignoring feelings, and offering false reassurance.

HEALTH HISTORY COMPONENTS

The health history provides subjective data about health status.

DEMOGRAPHIC INFORMATION: Identifying data include:
- Name, address, contact information
- Birth date, age
- Gender
- Race, ethnicity
- Relationship status
- Occupation, employment status
- Insurance
- Emergency contact information
- Family, others living at home
- Advance directives

SOURCE OF HISTORY
- Client, family members or close friends, other medical records, other providers
- Reliability of the historian

CHIEF CONCERN: A brief statement in the client's own words of why he is seeking care

HISTORY OF PRESENT ILLNESS
- A detailed, chronological description of why the client seeks care
- Details about the manifestation(s), such as location, quality, quantity, setting, timing (onset and duration), precipitating factors, alleviating or aggravating factors, associated phenomena (concomitant manifestations)

PAST HEALTH HISTORY AND CURRENT HEALTH STATUS
- Childhood illnesses, both communicable and chronic
- Medical, surgical, obstetrical, gynecological, psychiatric history, including time frames, diagnoses, hospitalizations, treatments
- Current immunization status, dates and results of any screening tests
- Allergies to medication, environment, food
- Current medications including prescription, over-the-counter, vitamins, supplements, herbal remedies, time of last dose(s)
- Habits and lifestyle patterns (alcohol, tobacco, caffeine, recreational drugs)

26.1 Therapeutic communication techniques

ACTIVE LISTENING: Show clients that they have your undivided attention.

OPEN-ENDED QUESTIONS: Use initially to encourage clients to tell their story in their own way. Use terminology clients can understand.

CLARIFYING: Question clients about specific details in greater depth or direct them toward relevant parts of their history.

BACK CHANNELING: Use active listening phrases such as "Go on" and "Tell me more" to convey interest and to prompt disclosure of the entire story.

PROBING: Ask more open-ended questions such as "What else would you like to add to that?" to help obtain comprehensive information.

CLOSED-ENDED QUESTIONS: Ask questions that require yes or no answers to clarify information, such as "Do you have any pain when you cannot sleep?"

SUMMARIZING: Validate the accuracy of the story.

FAMILY HISTORY
- Health information of grandparents, parents, siblings, children, grandchildren
- Family structure, interaction, support system, function
- Current ages or age at death, acute and chronic disorders of family members

PSYCHOSOCIAL HISTORY: Relationships, support systems, concerns about living or work situations, financial status, ability to perform activities of daily living, spiritual health

HEALTH PROMOTION BEHAVIORS
- Exercise/activity, diet, sun exposure, wearing of safety equipment, substance use, environmental exposures, home environment, resources, stress, sleep patterns, coping measures
- Awareness of risks for heart disease, cancer, diabetes mellitus, stroke

REVIEW OF SYSTEMS

An extensive review of systems ascertains information about the functioning of all body systems and health problems

QUESTIONS TO ASK

Integumentary system
- Do you have any skin diseases?
- Do you have any itching, bruising, lumps, hair loss, nail changes, or sores?
- Do you have any allergies?
- How do you care for your hair, skin, and nails?
- Do you use lotions, soaps, or sunscreen or wear protective clothing?

Head and neck
- Do you get headaches? If so, how often? (Ask about and note onset, precipitating factors, duration, character, pattern, and concomitant manifestations.)
- What do you do to relieve the pain?
- Have you ever had a head injury?
- Can you move your head and shoulders with ease?
- Are any of your lymph nodes swollen? (If so, ask about recent colds or viral infections.)
- Have you noticed any unusual facial movements?
- Does anyone in your family have thyroid disease?

Eyes
- How is your vision?
- Have you noticed any changes in your vision?
- Do you ever have any fluid draining from your eyes?
- Do you wear eyeglasses? Contact lenses?
- When was your last eye examination?
- Does anyone in your family have any eye disorders?
- Do you have diabetes?

Ears, nose, mouth, and throat
- How well do you hear?
- Have you noticed any changes in your hearing?
- Have other people commented that you aren't hearing what they say?
- Do you wear hearing aids?
- Do you ever have ringing or buzzing in your ears, drainage, dizziness, or pain?
- Have you had ear infections?
- How do you clean your ears?
- Are you having any pain, stuffiness, or fluid draining from your nose?
- Do you have nosebleeds?
- Do you have any difficulty breathing through your nose?
- Have you noticed any change in your sense of smell or taste?
- How often do you go to the dentist?
- Do you have dentures or retainers?
- Do you have any problems with your gums, like bleeding or soreness?
- Do you have any difficulty swallowing or problems with hoarseness or a sore throat?
- Do you have allergies?
- Do you use nasal sprays?
- Do you know if you snore?

Breasts
- Do you perform breast self-examinations? For women: What time of the month do you perform them?
- Do you have any tenderness, lumps, thickening, pain, drainage, distortion, or change in breast size, or any retraction or scaling of the nipples?
- Has anyone in your family had breast cancer?
- Are you aware of breast cancer risks?
- For clients over 40: How often do you get a mammogram?

Respiratory system
- Do you have any difficulties breathing?
- Do you breathe easier in any particular position?
- Are you ever short of breath?
- Have you recently been around anyone who has a cough, cold, or influenza?
- Do you receive an influenza vaccine every year?
- Have you had the pneumonia vaccine?
- Do you smoke? If yes, for how long and how much? Are you interested in quitting?
- Are you around second-hand smoke?
- Do you have environmental allergies?
- Has anyone in your family had lung cancer or tuberculosis?
- Have you ever been around anyone who has tuberculosis?
- Have you had a tuberculosis test?

Cardiovascular system
- Do you have any problems with your heart?
- Do you take any medications for your heart?
- Do you ever have pain in your chest? Do you also feel it in your arms, neck, or jaw?
- Do you know if you have high cholesterol or high blood pressure?
- Do you have any swelling in your feet and ankles?
- Do you cough frequently?
- Are you familiar with the risk factors for heart disease?

Gastrointestinal system
- Do you have any problems with your stomach, such as nausea, vomiting, heartburn, or pain?
- Do you have any problems with your bowels, such as diarrhea or constipation?
- When was your last bowel movement?
- Do you ever use laxatives or enemas?
- Have you had any black or tarry stools?
- Do you take aspirin or ibuprofen? If so, how often?
- Do you have any abdominal or lower back pain or tenderness?
- Have you had any recent weight changes?
- Do you have any swallowing difficulties?
- Do you drink alcohol? If so, how much?
- For clients over 50: Have you had a colonoscopy? If so, when was your last one? Ⓖ
- Do you know the signs and symptoms of colon cancer?
- What is your typical day's intake of food and fluid?
- Do you have any dietary restrictions, food intolerances, or special practices?

Genitourinary system
- Do you have any difficulties with urination, such as burning, leakage or loss of urine, urgency, frequency, waking up at night to urinate, or hesitancy?
- Have you noticed any change in the color of your urine?
- For women: Have you noticed any changes in your menstrual cycle?
- Have you had pain during intercourse?
- Have you had any sexual problems?
- For men: Have you had any pain in your scrotum or testes?

Musculoskeletal system
- Have you noticed any pain in your joints or muscles?
- Do you have any weakness or twitching?
- Have you had any recent falls?
- Are you able to care for yourself?
- Do you exercise or participate in sports?
- For postmenopausal women: What was your maximum height? Ⓖ
- For postmenopausal women: Do you take calcium supplements? Ⓖ

Neurological system
- Have you noticed any change in your vision, speech, ability to think clearly, or loss of or change in memory?
- Do you have any dizziness or headaches?
- Do you ever have seizures? If so, what triggers them?
- Do you ever have any weakness, tremors, numbness, or tingling anywhere? If so, where?

Mental health
- Is there anything stressful going on at work or at home?
- Are you having any problems with depression or changes in mood?
- Have you had any recent losses?
- Are you having any problems concentrating?

Endocrine system
- Have you noticed any change in urination patterns?
- Have you noticed any change in your energy level?
- Have you noticed any change in your ability to handle stress?
- Have you had any change in weight or appetite?
- Have you had any visual disturbances?
- Have you had any palpitations?

Allergic/immunologic system
- Do you have any allergies to medications, foods, or environmental substances?
- Have you ever received a blood transfusion? If so, did you have any adverse reactions?

PHYSICAL ASSESSMENT TECHNIQUES

During a physical examination

- Make sure there is adequate lighting.
- Maintain a quiet and comfortable environment.
- Provide privacy, using a gown or draping the client with a sheet and visualizing only one section of the body at a time.
- Explain the various assessment/data collection techniques you will use.
- Look and observe before touching.
- Keep nails short, and hands and stethoscope warm.
- Do not feel or listen through clothing. (Clothing can obscure or create sounds.)
- Have necessary equipment ready.
- Use standard precautions when in contact with body fluids, wound drainage, and open lesions.

ADDITIONAL GUIDELINES FOR OLDER ADULT CLIENTS Ⓖ
- Allow enough time for position changes.
- Perform assessments/data collection in several shorter segments to avoid overtiring older adults. Organize the examination, finishing all techniques requiring the same position before moving on to the next position.
- Make sure older adults who use sensory aids (eyeglasses, hearing aids) have them available for use.
- Invite the client to use the bathroom before beginning the physical examination. Collect urine or fecal specimens at this time.

INSPECT, PALPATE, PERCUSS, AUSCULTATE

Inspect, palpate, percuss, and auscultate in that order.

> The exception is the abdomen; inspect, auscultate, percuss, and palpate in that order to avoid altering bowel sounds.

Inspection

Inspection begins with the first interaction and continues throughout the examination.

- A penlight, an otoscope, an ophthalmoscope, or another lighted instrument can enhance the process.
- Inspection involves using the senses of vision, smell (olfaction), and hearing to observe and detect any expected or unexpected findings. Inspect for size, shape, color, symmetry (comparing both sides of the body), and position.
- Validate findings with the client.

Palpation

Palpation is the use of touch to determine the size, consistency, texture, temperature, location, and tenderness of the skin, underlying tissues, an organ, or a body part. Palpate tender areas last.

- Use light palpation (less than 1 cm [0.4 in]) for most body surfaces. Use deeper palpation (4 cm [1.6 in]) to evaluate abdominal organs or masses.
- Various parts of your hands detect different sensations.
  - The **dorsal surface** is the most sensitive to temperature.
  - The **palmar surface and base of the fingers** are sensitive to vibration.
  - **Fingertips** are sensitive to pulsation, position, texture, turgor, size, and consistency.
  - The **fingers and thumb** are useful for grasping an organ or mass.
- Starting with light palpation, be systematic, calm, and gentle. Proceed to deep palpation if necessary.

Percussion

Percussion involves tapping body parts with fingers, fists, or small instruments to vibrate underlying tissues and evaluate size, location, tenderness, and presence or absence of fluid or air in body organs, and to detect any abnormalities. The denser the tissue, the quieter the sound. An understanding of the effect of various densities on sound can help you locate organs or masses, find their edges, and estimate their size.

TECHNIQUES FOR PERCUSSION

- **Direct** percussion, which involves striking the body to elicit sounds.
- **Indirect** percussion, which involves placing your hand flatly on the body, as the striking surface, for sound production.
- **Fist** percussion, which helps identify tenderness over the kidneys, liver, and gallbladder.

Auscultation

Auscultation is the process of listening to sounds the body produces to identify unexpected findings. Some sounds are loud enough to hear unaided (speech and coughing), but most sounds require a stethoscope or a Doppler technique (heart sounds, air moving through the respiratory tract, blood moving through blood vessels). Learn to isolate the various sounds to collect data accurately.

- Evaluate sounds for amplitude or intensity (loud or soft), pitch or frequency (high or low), duration (time the sound lasts), and quality (what it sounds like).
- Use the diaphragm of the stethoscope to listen to high-pitched sounds (heart sounds, bowel sounds, lung sounds).

> Place the diaphragm firmly on the body part.

- Use the bell of the stethoscope to listen to low-pitched sounds (unexpected heart sounds, bruits).

> Place the bell lightly on the body part.

EQUIPMENT FOR SCREENING EXAMINATION

- Gown
- Drapes
- Scale with height measurement
- Thermometer
- Stethoscope with diaphragm and bell
- Sphygmomanometer
- Reading/eye chart
- Otoscope, ophthalmoscope, nasal speculum
- Penlight or ophthalmoscope
- Cotton balls
- Sharp and dull objects
- Tuning fork
- Glass of water
- Items to test smell and taste
- Clean gloves
- Tongue depressor
- Reflex hammer
- Pulse oximeter
- Marking pen
- Measuring tape and clear, flexible ruler with measurements in centimeters
- Watch or clock to measure time in seconds

26.2 Sample documentation

Client: 16-year-old male, alert and oriented x 3. No distress. Personal hygiene and grooming slightly unkempt but appropriate for age. Weight appropriate for height, erect posture, and steady gait. Full range of motion. Does not maintain eye contact. Volunteers no information but answers questions appropriately. No gross abnormalities.

GENERAL SURVEY

The general survey is a written summary or appraisal of overall health. Gather this information from the first encounter with the client and continue to make observations throughout the assessment process. **(26.2)**

Assess/collect data about the following.

PHYSICAL APPEARANCE
- Age
- Gender
- Race and/or ethnicity
- Level of consciousness
- Color of skin
- Facial features
- Signs of distress (pallor, labored breathing, guarding, anxiety)
- Signs of possible physical abuse or neglect
- Signs of substance use disorders

BODY STRUCTURE
- Body build, stature, height, and weight
- Nutritional status
- Symmetry of body parts
- Posture and usual position
- Gross abnormalities (skin lesions, amputations)

MOBILITY
- Gait
- Movements (purposeful, tremulous)
- Range of motion
- Motor activity

BEHAVIOR
- Facial expression and mannerisms
- Mood and affect
- Speech
- Dress, hygiene, grooming, and odors (body, breath)

VITAL SIGNS
- Temperature
- Pulse
- Respirations
- Blood pressure
- Oxygen saturation

PRACTICE Active Learning Scenario

A nurse is reviewing the data to collect from a client for a comprehensive health history prior to the systems review. Use the ATI Active Learning Template: Basic Concept to complete this item.

RELATED CONTENT: List at least six general categories to cover and the essential data to include in each category.

Application Exercises

1. A nurse is introducing herself to a client as the first step of a comprehensive physical examination. Which of the following strategies should the nurse use with this client? (Select all that apply.)

   A. Address the client with the appropriate title and her last name.

   B. Use a mix of open- and closed-ended questions.

   C. Reduce environmental noise.

   D. Have the client complete a printed history form.

   E. Perform the general survey before the examination.

2. A nurse in a provider's office is documenting his findings following an examination he performed for a client new to the practice. Which of the following parameters should he include as part of the general survey? (Select all that apply.)

   A. Posture

   B. Skin lesions

   C. Speech

   D. Allergies

   E. Immunization status

3. A nurse is collecting data for a client's comprehensive physical examination. After the nurse inspects the client's abdomen, which of the following skills of the physical examination process should she perform next?

   A. Olfaction

   B. Auscultation

   C. Palpation

   D. Percussion

4. A nurse is performing a comprehensive physical examination of an older adult client. Which of the following interventions should the nurse use in consideration of the client's age? (Select all that apply.)

   A. Collect the data in one continuous session.

   B. Plan to allow plenty of time for position changes.

   C. Make sure the client has any essential sensory aids in place.

   D. Tell the client to take her time answering questions.

   E. Invite the client to use the bathroom before beginning the examination.

5. A nurse in a family practice clinic is performing a physical examination of an adult client. Which part of her hands should she use during palpation for optimal assessment of skin temperature?

   A. Palmar surface

   B. Fingertips

   C. Dorsal surface

   D. Base of the fingers

Application Exercises Key

1. A. The nurse should ask the client what she wants the nurse to call her.

   B. **CORRECT:** Open-ended questions help the client tell her story in her own way. Closed-ended questions are useful for clarifying and verifying information the nurse gathers from the client's story.

   C. **CORRECT:** A quiet, comfortable environment eliminates distractions and helps the client focus on the important aspects of the interview.

   D. Having the client fill out a printed history form might deter the establishment of a therapeutic relationship. When the nurse asks about her history, the client might feel they are wasting time because she already wrote that information on the form.

   E. **CORRECT:** The general survey is noninvasive and, along with the health history and vital sign measurement, can help put the client at ease before the more sensitive parts of the process, such as the examination.

   Ⓝ *NCLEX® Connection: Health Promotion and Maintenance, Techniques of Physical Assessment*

2. A. **CORRECT:** Posture is part of the body structure or general appearance portion of the general survey.

   B. **CORRECT:** Skin lesions are part of the body structure or general appearance portion of the general survey.

   C. **CORRECT:** Speech is part of the behavior portion of the general survey.

   D. Allergies are part of the health history, not the general survey.

   E. Immunization status is part of the health history, not the general survey.

   Ⓝ *NCLEX® Connection: Health Promotion and Maintenance, Techniques of Physical Assessment*

3. A. Olfaction is the use of the sense of smell to detect any unexpected findings that the nurse cannot detect via other means, such as a fruity breath odor. Unless there is an open lesion on the client's abdomen, this is not the next step in an abdominal examination.

   B. **CORRECT:** Because palpation and percussion can alter the frequency and intensity of bowel sounds, the nurse should auscultate the abdomen next and before using those two techniques.

   C. Palpation is the next step in examining other areas of the body, but not the abdomen.

   D. Percussion is important for detecting gas, fluid, and solid masses in the abdomen, but it is not the next step in an abdominal assessment.

   Ⓝ *NCLEX® Connection: Reduction of Risk Potential, System Specific Assessments*

4. A. The nurse should perform the various parts of the assessment in several shorter segments to avoid overtiring the client.

   B. **CORRECT:** Because many older adults have mobility challenges, the nurse should plan to allow extra time for position changes.

   C. **CORRECT:** The nurse should make sure clients who use sensory aids have them available for use. The client has to be able to hear the nurse and see well enough to avoid injury.

   D. **CORRECT:** Some older clients need more time to collect their thoughts and answer questions, but most are reliable historians. Feeling rushed can hinder communication.

   E. **CORRECT:** This is a courtesy for all clients, to avoid discomfort during palpation of the lower abdomen for example, but this is especially important for older clients who have a smaller bladder capacity.

   Ⓝ *NCLEX® Connection: Health Promotion and Maintenance, Techniques of Physical Assessment*

5. A. The palmar surface of the hands is especially sensitive to vibration, not temperature.

   B. The fingertips are sensitive to pulsation, position, texture, size, and consistency, not temperature.

   C. **CORRECT:** The dorsal surface of the hand is the most sensitive to temperature.

   D. The base of the fingers is especially sensitive to vibration, not temperature.

   Ⓝ *NCLEX® Connection: Reduction of Risk Potential, System Specific Assessments*

PRACTICE Answer

Using the ATI Active Learning Template: Basic Concept

RELATED CONTENT

- Demographic information
  - Name, address, contact information
  - Birth date, age
  - Gender
  - Race, ethnicity
  - Relationship status
  - Occupation, employment status
  - Insurance
  - Emergency contact information
  - Family, others living at home
  - Advance directives
- Source of history
  - Client, family members or close friends, other medical records, other providers
  - Reliability of the historian
- Chief concern: Brief statement in the client's own words of why he is seeking care

- History of present illness
  - Detailed, chronological description of why the client seeks care
  - Details about the manifestation(s), such as location, quality, quantity, setting, timing (onset and duration), precipitating factors, alleviating or aggravating factors, associated phenomena (concomitant manifestations)
- Past health history and current health status
  - Childhood illnesses, both communicable and chronic
  - Medical, surgical, obstetrical, gynecological, psychiatric history including time frames, diagnoses, hospitalizations, treatments
  - Current immunization status, dates and results of any screening tests
  - Allergies to medication, environment, food
  - Current medications including prescription, over-the-counter, vitamins, supplements, herbal remedies, time of last dose(s)
  - Habits and lifestyle patterns (alcohol, tobacco, caffeine, recreational drugs)

- Family history
  - Health information of grandparents, parents, siblings, children, grandchildren
  - Family structure, interaction, support system, function
  - Current ages or age at death, acute and chronic disorders in family members
- Psychosocial history: Relationships, support systems, concerns about living or work situations, financial status, ability to perform activities of daily living, spiritual health
- Health promotion behavior
  - Exercise/activity, diet, sun exposure, wearing of safety equipment, substance use, environmental exposures, home environment, resources, stress, coping measures
  - Awareness of risks for heart disease, cancer, diabetes mellitus, and cerebrovascular accident

Ⓝ *NCLEX® Connection: Health Promotion and Maintenance, Techniques of Physical Assessment*

CHAPTER 27   *Vital Signs*

Vital signs are measurements of the body's most basic functions and include temperature, pulse, respiration, and blood pressure. Many facilities also consider pain level and oxygen saturation vital signs. **(SEE CHAPTER 41: PAIN MANAGEMENT AND CHAPTER 53: AIRWAY MANAGEMENT.)**

Temperature reflects the balance between heat the body produces and heat lost to the environment.

Pulse is the measurement of heart rate and rhythm. Pulse corresponds to the bounding of blood flowing through various points in the circulatory system. It provides information about circulatory status.

Respiration is the body's mechanism for exchanging oxygen and carbon dioxide between the atmosphere and the blood and cells of the body, which is accomplished through breathing and recorded as the number of breaths per minute.

Blood pressure (BP) reflects the force the blood exerts against the walls of the arteries during contraction (systole) and relaxation (diastole) of the heart. Systolic blood pressure (SBP) occurs during ventricular systole of the heart, when the ventricles force blood into the aorta and pulmonary artery, and it represents the maximum amount of pressure exerted on the arteries when ejection occurs. Diastolic blood pressure (DBP) occurs during ventricular diastole of the heart, when the ventricles relax and exert minimal pressure against arterial walls, and represents the minimum amount of pressure exerted on the arteries. Q̇EBP

Temperature

PHYSIOLOGIC RESPONSES

- The neurological and cardiovascular systems work together to regulate body temperature. Disease or trauma of the hypothalamus or spinal cord will alter temperature control.
- The rectum, tympanic membrane, temporal artery, pulmonary artery, esophagus, and urinary bladder are core temperature measurement sites.
- The skin, mouth, and axillae are surface temperature measurement sites.

HEAT PRODUCTION AND LOSS

Heat production results from increases in basal metabolic rate, muscle activity, thyroxine output, testosterone, and sympathetic stimulation, which increases heat production.

Heat loss from the body occurs through:
- **Conduction:** Transfer of heat from the body directly to another surface (when the body is immersed in cold water).
- **Convection:** Dispersion of heat by air currents (wind blowing across exposed skin).
- **Evaporation:** Dispersion of heat through water vapor (perspiration).
- **Radiation:** Transfer of heat from one object to another object without contact between them (heat lost from the body to a cold room).
- **Diaphoresis:** Visible perspiration on the skin.

ASSESSMENT/DATA COLLECTION

EXPECTED TEMPERATURE RANGES

- An **oral** temperature range of 36° to 38° C (96.8° to 100.4° F) is acceptable. The average is 37° C (98.6° F).
- **Rectal** temperatures are usually 0.5° C (0.9° F) higher than oral and tympanic temperatures.
- **Axillary** temperatures are usually 0.5° C (0.9° F) lower than oral and tympanic temperatures
- **Temporal** temperatures are close to rectal, but they are nearly 0.5° C (1° F) higher than oral, and 1° C (2° F) higher than axillary temperatures.
- A client's usual temperature serves as a baseline for comparison.

CONSIDERATIONS

Newborns have a large surface-to-mass ratio, so they lose heat rapidly to the environment. A newborn's temperature should be between 36.5° and 37.5° C (97.7° and 99.5° F).

Older adult clients experience a loss of subcutaneous fat that results in lower body temperatures and feeling cold. Their average body temperature is 36° C (96.8° F). Older adult clients are more likely to develop adverse effects from extremes in environmental temperatures (heat stroke, hypothermia). It also takes longer for body temperature to register on a thermometer due to changes in temperature regulation. Ⓖ

Hormonal changes can influence temperature. In general, temperature rises slightly with ovulation and menses. With menopause, intermittent body temperature can increase by up to 4° C (7.2° F).

Exercise, activity, and dehydration can contribute to the development of hyperthermia.

Illness and injury can cause elevations in temperature. Fever is the body's response to infectious and inflammatory processes. Fever causes an increase in the body's immune response by:
- Increasing WBC production.
- Decreasing plasma iron concentration to reduce bacteria growth.
- Stimulating interferon to suppress virus production.

Recent food or fluid intake and smoking can interfere with accurate oral measurement of body temperature, so it is best to wait 20 to 30 min before measuring oral temperature.

Circadian rhythm, stress, and environmental conditions can also affect body temperature.

NURSING INTERVENTIONS

EQUIPMENT

Electronic thermometers use a probe to measure oral, rectal, or axillary temperature. Place a disposable probe cover on the probe, insert the probe, and when you hear the signal, note the digital reading then discard the probe cover. Tympanic temperatures require a device specifically for measuring temperature at the tympanic membrane (eardrum).

Disposable, single-use thermometers are for oral or axillary temperature measurement. They reduce the risk of cross-infection.

PROCEDURES FOR TAKING TEMPERATURE

Perform hand hygiene, provide privacy, and apply clean gloves.

Oral

- Gently place the thermometer (with an oral probe) under the tongue in the posterior sublingual pocket lateral to the center of the lower jaw.
- Leave it in place until you hear the signal.

AGE-SPECIFIC: Use this site for clients who are 4 years of age and older.

> Note: Do not use this site for clients who breathe through their mouth or have experienced trauma to the face or mouth. Qs

Rectal

- Assist the client to Sims' position with the upper leg flexed. Wearing gloves, expose the anal area while keeping other body areas covered. Spread the buttocks to expose the anal opening.
- Ask the client to breathe slowly and relax when placing a lubricated thermometer (with a rectal probe) into the anus in the direction of the umbilicus 2.5 to 3.5 cm (1 to 1.5 in) for an adult. If you encounter resistance, remove it immediately. Once inserted, hold the thermometer in place until you hear the signal.
- Clean the anal area to remove feces or lubricant.
- Use the rectal site to obtain a second measurement if the temperature is above 37.2° C (99° F).

SAFETY MEASURE: Do not use for clients who have diarrhea, are on bleeding precautions (such as those who have a low platelet count), or have rectal disorders. Qs

AGE-SPECIFIC: A rectal measurement of temperature is more accurate than axillary. However, because of the risk of rectal perforation, the American Academy of Pediatrics recommends screening infants 3 months old and younger by measuring axillary temperature initially.

> Note: Stool in the rectum can cause inaccurate readings.

Axillary

- Place the thermometer (with an oral probe) in the center of the client's clean, dry axilla. Lower the arm over the probe.
- Hold the arm down, keeping the thermometer in position until you hear the signal.

Tympanic

- Pull the ear up and back (for an adult) or down and back (for a child who is younger than 3 years old).
- Place the thermometer probe snugly into the client's outer ear canal and press the scan button.
- Leave it in place until you hear the signal.
- Carefully remove the thermometer from the ear canal and read the temperature.
- Ambient temperature can affect readings.

AGE-SPECIFIC: The American Academy of Pediatrics advises against the use of electronic ear thermometers for infants 3 months old and younger due to the inaccuracy of readings.

> Note: Excess earwax can alter the reading. If noted, use the other ear or select another site for temperature assessment.

Temporal

- Remove the protective cap and wipe the lens of the scanning device with alcohol to make sure it is clean.
- While pressing the scan button, hold the probe flat against the forehead while moving it gently across the forehead over the temporal artery, and then touch the skin behind the earlobe.
- Release the scan button to display the temperature reading.

> Note: Depending on facility policy, either use disposable probe covers or clean the probe with a disinfectant wipe between clients.

COMPLICATIONS

Fever

Usually not harmful unless it exceeds 39° C (102.2° F).

Hyperthermia

Hyperthermia is an abnormally elevated body temperature.

NURSING INTERVENTIONS
- Obtain specimens for blood, urine, sputum, or wound cultures as needed.
- Assess/monitor white blood cell counts, sedimentation rates, and electrolytes.
- Administer antibiotics (after obtaining specimens for culture).
- Provide fluids and rest. Minimize activity. Use a cooling blanket.
- Children and older adults are at particular risk for fluid volume deficit. Ⓖ
- Provide antipyretics (aspirin, acetaminophen, ibuprofen). Do not give aspirin to manage fever for children and adolescents who have a viral illness (influenza, chickenpox) due to the risk of Reye syndrome.
- Prevent shivering, as this increases energy demand.
- Offer blankets during chills and remove them when the client feels warm.
- Provide oral hygiene and dry clothing and linens.
- Keep environmental temperature between 21° and 27° C (70° to 80° F).

Hypothermia

Hypothermia is a body temperature less than 35° C (95° F).

NURSING INTERVENTIONS
- Provide a warm environmental temperature, heated humidified oxygen, warming blanket, and/or warmed oral or IV fluids.
- Keep the head covered.
- Provide continuous cardiac monitoring.
- Have emergency resuscitation equipment on standby.

Pulse

PHYSIOLOGIC RESPONSES

Autonomic nervous system controls the heart rate.

Parasympathetic nervous system lowers the heart rate.

Sympathetic nervous system raises the heart rate.

ASSESSMENT/DATA COLLECTION

Assess the wave-like sensations or impulses you feel in a peripheral arterial vessel or over the apex of the heart as a gauge of cardiovascular status.

Rate: The number of times per minute you feel or hear the pulse.

Rhythm: The regularity of impulses. A premature, late heartbeat or a missed beat can result in an irregular interval between impulses and can indicate altered electrical activity of the heart. Typically, you should detect an impulse at regular intervals.

Strength (amplitude): Reflects the volume of blood ejected against the arterial wall with each heart contraction and the condition of the arterial vascular system. The strength of the impulse should be the same from beat to beat. Grade strength on a scale of 0 to 4.
- 0 = Absent, unable to palpate
- 1+ = Diminished, weaker than expected
- 2+ = Brisk, expected
- 3+ = Increased, strong
- 4+ = Full volume, bounding

Equality: Peripheral pulse impulses should be symmetrical in quality and quantity from the right side of the body to the left. Assess strength and equality to evaluate the adequacy of the vascular system. An inequality or absence of pulse on one side of body can indicate a disease state (e.g., thrombus, aortic dissection).

CONSIDERATIONS

Dysrhythmia: An irregular heart rhythm, generally with an irregular radial pulse.

Pulse deficit: The difference between the apical rate and the radial rate. With dysrhythmias, the heart can contract ineffectively, resulting in a beat at the apical site with no pulsation at the radial pulse point. To determine the pulse deficit accurately, two clinicians should measure the apical and radial pulse rates simultaneously.

Age: For infants, the expected pulse rate is 120 to 160/min. The rate gradually decreases as the child grows older. The average pulse for a 12- to 14-year-old child is 80 to 90/min. The strength of the pulsation can weaken in older adult clients due to poor circulation or cardiac dysfunction, which makes the peripheral pulses more difficult to palpate. Ⓖ

EXPECTED HEART RATE RANGE

The expected reference range for an adult client's pulse is 60 to 100/min at rest.

Tachycardia

A rate greater than the expected range or greater than 100/min.

FACTORS LEADING TO TACHYCARDIA

- Exercise
- Fever, heat exposure
- Medications: epinephrine, levothyroxine beta$_2$–adrenergic agonists (albuterol)
- Changing position from lying down to sitting or standing
- Acute pain
- Hyperthyroidism
- Anemia, hypoxemia
- Stress, anxiety, fear
- Hypovolemia, shock, heart failure, hemorrhage

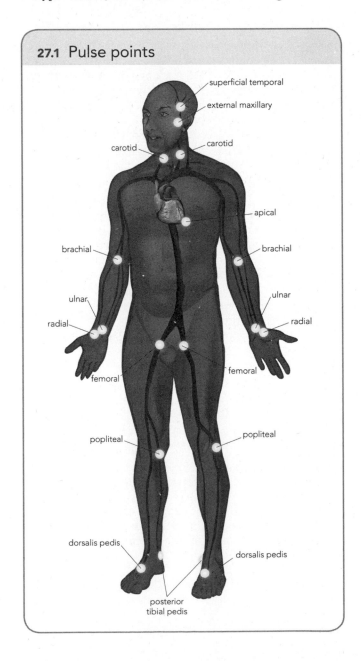

27.1 Pulse points

superficial temporal
external maxillary
carotid
carotid
apical
brachial
brachial
ulnar
ulnar
radial
radial
femoral
femoral
popliteal
popliteal
dorsalis pedis
dorsalis pedis
posterior tibial pedis

Bradycardia

A rate less than the expected range or slower than 60/min.

FACTORS LEADING TO BRADYCARDIA

- Long-term physical fitness
- Hypothermia
- Medications: digoxin, beta-blockers (propranolol), calcium channel blockers (verapamil)
- Changing position from standing or sitting to lying down
- Chronic severe pain
- Hypothyroidism
- Relaxation

NURSING INTERVENTIONS

EQUIPMENT

A watch or clock that allows for counting seconds

Stethoscope

PROCEDURE

- Perform hand hygiene and provide privacy.
- Locate the radial pulse on the radial- or thumb-side of the forearm at the wrist. **(27.1)** Q$_{PCC}$
  - Place the index and middle finger of one hand gently but firmly over the pulse. Assess the pulsation for rate, rhythm, amplitude, and quality.
  - If the peripheral pulsation is regular, count the rate for 30 sec and multiply by 2. If the pulsation is irregular, count for a full minute and compare the result to the apical pulse rate.

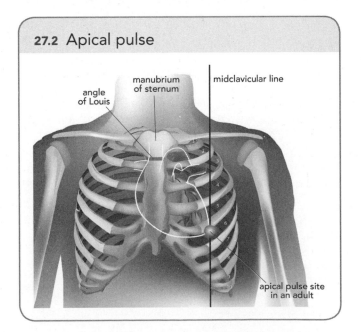

27.2 Apical pulse

angle of Louis
manubrium of sternum
midclavicular line
apical pulse site in an adult

- Locate the apical pulse at the fifth intercostal space at the left midclavicular line. **(27.2)**
  - Use this site for assessing the heart rate of an infant, rapid rates (faster than 100/min), irregular rhythms, and rates prior to the administration of cardiac medications.
  - Place the stethoscope on the chest at the fifth intercostal space at the left midclavicular line. If the rhythm is regular, count for 30 sec and multiply by 2. If the rhythm is irregular or the client is receiving cardiovascular medications, count for 1 full min.

COMPLICATIONS

Tachycardia

NURSING INTERVENTIONS
- Monitor for pain, anxiety, restlessness, fatigue, low blood pressure, and low oxygen saturation.
- Monitor for potential adverse effects of medications.
- Prevent injury. Qs

Bradycardia

NURSING INTERVENTIONS
- Monitor for hypotension, chest pain, syncope, diaphoresis, dyspnea, and altered mental state.
- Monitor for potential adverse effects of medications.
- Prevent injury.

Respirations

PHYSIOLOGICAL RESPONSES

Chemoreceptors in the carotid arteries and the aorta primarily monitor carbon dioxide (CO_2) levels of the blood. Rising CO_2 levels trigger the respiratory center of the brain to increase the respiratory rate. The increased respiratory rate rids the body of excess CO_2. For clients who have chronic obstructive pulmonary disease (COPD), a low oxygen level becomes the primary respiratory drive.

PROCESSES OF RESPIRATION

Ventilation: The exchange of oxygen and carbon dioxide in the lungs. Measure ventilation with the respiratory rate, rhythm, and depth.

Diffusion: The exchange of oxygen and carbon dioxide between the alveoli and the red blood cells. Measure diffusion with pulse oximetry.

Perfusion: The flow of red blood cells to and from the pulmonary capillaries. Measure perfusion with pulse oximetry.

ASSESSMENT/DATA COLLECTION

Accurate assessment of respiration involves observing the rate, depth, and rhythm of chest-wall movement during inspiration and expiration. Do not inform the client that you are measuring respirations.

Rate: The number of full inspirations and expirations in 1 min. Determine this by observing the number of times the client's chest rises and falls. The expected reference range for adults is 12 to 20/min.

Depth: The amount of chest wall expansion that occurs with each breath. Altered depths are deep or shallow.

Rhythm: The observation of breathing intervals. For adults, expect a regular rhythm (eupnea) with an occasional sigh.

PULSE OXIMETRY

This is a noninvasive, indirect measurement of the oxygen saturation (SaO_2) of the blood (the percent of hemoglobin that is bound with oxygen in the arteries is the percent of saturation of hemoglobin). The expected reference range is 95% to 100%, although acceptable levels for some clients range from 91% to 100%. Some illness states can even allow for an SaO_2 of 85% to 89%. Q_EBP

CONSIDERATIONS

Age: Respiratory rate decreases with age. Newborns have rates of 35 to 40/min. School-age children have respiratory rates of 20 to 30/min.

Sex: Men and children are diaphragmatic breathers, and abdominal movements are more noticeable. Women use more thoracic muscles, and chest movements are more pronounced when they breathe.

Pain in the chest wall area can decrease the depth of respirations. At the onset of acute pain, the respiration rate increases but stabilizes over time.

Anxiety increases the rate and depth of respirations.

Smoking causes the resting rate of respirations to increase.

Body position: Upright positions allow the chest wall to expand more fully.

Medications such as opioids, sedatives, bronchodilators, and general anesthetics decrease respiratory rate and depth. Respiratory depression is a serious adverse effect. Amphetamines and cocaine increase rate and depth.

Neurological injury to the brainstem decreases respiratory rate and rhythm.

Illnesses can affect the shape of the chest wall, change the patency of passages, impair muscle function, and diminish respiratory effort. With these conditions, the use of accessory muscles, such as those visible in the neck, and the respiratory rate increase.

Impaired oxygen-carrying capacity of the blood that occurs with anemia or at high altitudes results in increases in the respiratory rate and alterations in rhythm to compensate.

NURSING INTERVENTIONS

Respiratory rate

EQUIPMENT: A watch or clock that allows for counting seconds.

PROCEDURE
- Perform hand hygiene and provide privacy.
- Place the client in semi-Fowler's position, being sure the chest is visible.
- Have the client rest an arm across the abdomen, or place a hand directly on the client's abdomen. Qpcc
- Observe one full respiratory cycle, look at the timer, and then begin counting the rate.
- Count a regular rate for 30 seconds and multiply by 2. Count the rate for 1 min if irregular, faster than 20/min, or slower than 12/min. Note depth (shallow, normal, or deep) and rhythm (regular or irregular).

Oxygen saturation

EQUIPMENT: Pulse oximeter with digit probe, earlobe probe, or disposable sensor pad

PROCEDURE
- Choose an intact, nonedematous site for probe or sensor placement.
- Place the digit probe on the client's finger.
- Use earlobe or bridge of nose for clients who have peripheral vascular disease.
- A disposable sensor pad can be applied to the sole of an infant's foot.
- When the readout on the pulse oximeter is stable, record this value as the oxygen saturation.

Blood pressure

PHYSIOLOGICAL RESPONSES

The principal determinants of blood pressure are cardiac output (CO) and systemic (peripheral) vascular resistance (SVR). QEBP

$$BP = CO \times SVR$$

Cardiac output

- CO is determined by
  - Heart rate
  - Contractility
  - Blood volume
  - Venous return
- Increases in any of these increase CO and BP
- Decreases in any of these decrease CO and BP

Systemic vascular resistance

- SVR reflects the amount of constriction or dilation of the arteries, and diameter of blood vessels.
- Increases in SVR increase BP
- Decreases in SVR decrease BP

ASSESSMENT/DATA COLLECTION

CLASSIFICATIONS OF BLOOD PRESSURE

27.3 BP classifications
according to the Seventh Report of the Joint National Committee on Prevention, Detection, Evaluation, and Treatment of High Blood Pressure

	SYSTOLIC BP (mm Hg)		DIASTOLIC BP (mm Hg)
NORMAL	less than 120	*and*	less than 80
PREHYPERTENSION	120 to 139	*or*	80 to 89
STAGE 1 HYPERTENSION	140 to 159	*or*	90 to 99
STAGE 2 HYPERTENSION	greater than 160	*or*	greater than 100

- Base the classification on the highest reading. A client who has a BP of 124/92 mm Hg has stage 1 hypertension because the DBP places the client in that category. A client who has a BP of 146/82 mm Hg also has stage 1 hypertension because the SBP places the client in that category.
- If the client has a SBP greater than 140 mm Hg and a DBP greater than 90 mm Hg that are averages of two or more BP measurements, he should return for two or more visits for additional readings. If the readings are elevated on at least three separate occasions over several weeks, the client has hypertension. QEBP

Hypotension is a blood pressure below the expected reference range (systolic less than 90 mm Hg) and can be a result of fluid depletion, heart failure, or vasodilation.

Pulse pressure is the difference between the systolic and the diastolic pressure readings.

Orthostatic (postural) hypotension is a blood pressure that decreases when a client changes position from lying to sitting or standing, and it can result from various causes (peripheral vasodilation, medication adverse effects, fluid depletion, anemia, prolonged bed rest).

> Assess orthostatic changes by taking the client's BP and heart rate (HR) in the supine position. Next, have the client change to the sitting or standing position, wait 1 to 3 min, and reassess BP and HR. The client has orthostatic hypotension if the SBP decreases more than 20 mm Hg and/or the DBP decreases more than 10 mm Hg with a 10% to 20% increase in HR. Do not delegate this procedure to an assistive personnel.

CONSIDERATIONS

Age
- Infants have a low BP that gradually increases with age.
- Older children and adolescents have varying BP based on body size. Larger children have a higher BP.
- Adults' BP can increase with age.
- Older adult clients can have a slightly elevated systolic pressure due to decreased elasticity of blood vessels. Ⓖ

Circadian (diurnal) rhythms affect BP, with BP usually lowest in the early morning hours and peaking during the later part of the afternoon or evening.

Stress associated with fear, emotional strain, and acute pain can increase BP.

Ethnicity: African Americans have a higher incidence of hypertension in general and at earlier ages.

Sex: Adolescent to middle-age men have higher blood pressures than their female counterparts. Postmenopausal women have higher blood pressures than their male counterparts.

Medications such as opiates, antihypertensives, and cardiac medications can lower BP. Cocaine, nicotine, cold medications, oral contraceptives, alcohol, and antidepressants can raise BP.

Exercise can cause a decrease in BP for several hours afterward.

Obesity is a contributing factor to hypertension.

Family history of hypertension, lack of exercise, high sodium intake, and continuous stress can increase the risk of hypertension.

NURSING INTERVENTIONS

EQUIPMENT

Auscultatory method
- Sphygmomanometer with a pressure manometer (aneroid or mercury) and a correctly sized cuff
  - The width of the cuff should be 40% of the arm circumference at the point where the cuff is wrapped.
  - The bladder (inside the cuff) should surround 80% of the arm circumference of an adult and the whole arm for a child.
  - Cuffs that are too large give a falsely low reading, and cuffs that are too small give a falsely high reading.
- Stethoscope

Automatic blood pressure devices

Use when available for monitoring clients who require frequent evaluation. Measure BP first using the auscultatory method to make sure the automatic device readings are valid. Q𝐄𝐁𝐏

PROCEDURE (AUSCULTATORY METHOD)
- Perform hand hygiene and provide privacy.
- Initially measure BP in both arms. If the difference is more than 10 mm Hg, use the arm with the higher reading for subsequent measurements. This difference can indicate a vascular problem.
- Apply the BP cuff 2.5 cm (1 in) above the antecubital space with the brachial artery in line with the marking on the cuff.
- Use a lower extremity if the brachial artery is not accessible.
- Estimate systolic pressure by palpating the radial pulse and inflating the cuff until the pulse disappears. Inflate the cuff another 30 mm Hg, and slowly release the pressure to note when the pulse is palpable again (the estimated systolic pressure).
- Deflate the cuff and wait 1 min.
- Position the stethoscope over the brachial artery.
- Close the pressure bulb by turning the valve clockwise until tight.
- Quickly inflate the cuff to 30 mm Hg above the palpated systolic pressure.
- Release the pressure no faster than 2 to 3 mm Hg per second.
- The level at which you hear the first clear sounds is the systolic pressure.
- Continue to deflate the cuff until the sounds muffle and disappear and note the diastolic pressure.
- Record the systolic over the diastolic pressure (110/70 mm Hg).

The client should

- Not use nicotine or drink any caffeine for 30 min prior to measurement.
- Rest for 5 min before measurement.
- Sit in a chair, with the feet flat on floor, the back and arm supported, and the arm at heart level.

The nurse should

- Use the auscultatory method with a properly calibrated and validated instrument.
- Not measure BP in an arm with an IV infusion in progress or on the side where the client had a mastectomy or an arteriovenous shunt or fistula.
- Average two or more readings, taken at least 2 min apart. (If they differ by more than 5 mm Hg, obtain additional readings and average them.)
- After initial readings, measure BP and pulse with the client standing.

UNEXPECTED BP READINGS

- It is helpful to measure the BP again near the end of an encounter with the client. Earlier pressures can be higher due to the stress of the clinical setting.
- Recheck blood pressures when you use an automatic device.
- Deflate the cuff completely between attempts. Wait at least 1 full min before reinflating the cuff. Air trapped in the bladder can cause a falsely high reading.

COMPLICATIONS

Orthostatic (postural) hypotension

NURSING INTERVENTIONS

- Assess/monitor BP.
- Assess for dizziness, weakness, and fainting.
- Instruct the client to activate the call light and not to get out of bed without assistance. Qs
- Have the client sit at the edge of the bed for at least 1 min before standing up.
- Assist with ambulation.

HOME CARE INSTRUCTIONS

- Warn the client that lightheadedness and dizziness can occur.
- Advise the client to sit or lie down if these manifestations occur.
- Suggest that the client get up slowly when lying or sitting and avoid sudden changes in position.

Hypertension

NURSING INTERVENTIONS

- Assess/monitor for tachycardia, bradycardia, pain, and anxiety. Primary hypertension is usually without manifestations.
- Assess for identifiable causes of hypertension (kidney disease, thyroid disease, medication).
- Administer pharmacological therapy.
- Assess for risk factors.
- Encourage the client to follow up with the provider.
- Encourage lifestyle modifications.
  - Cessation of smoking or use of smokeless tobacco
  - Weight control
  - Modification of alcohol intake
  - Physical activity
  - Stress reduction
  - Dietary modifications
    - Dietary Approaches to Stop Hypertension (DASH) diet
    - Restrict sodium intake.
    - Consume adequate potassium, calcium, and magnesium, which help lower BP. QEBP
    - Restrict cholesterol and saturated fat intake.

Application Exercises

1. A nurse is caring for an 82-year-old client in the emergency department who has an oral body temperature of 38.3° C (101° F), pulse rate 114/min, and respiratory rate 22/min. He is restless and his skin is warm. Which of the following interventions should the nurse take? (Select all that apply.)

   A. Obtain culture specimens before initiating antimicrobials.

   B. Restrict the client's oral fluid intake.

   C. Encourage the client to rest and limit activity.

   D. Allow the client to shiver to dispel excess heat.

   E. Assist the client with oral hygiene frequently.

2. A nurse is instructing an assistive personnel (AP) about caring for a client who has a low platelet count as a result of chemotherapy. Which of the following instructions is the priority for measuring vital signs for this client?

   A. "Do not measure the client's temperature rectally."

   B. "Count the client's radial pulse for 30 seconds and multiply it by 2."

   C. "Do not let the client know you are counting her respirations."

   D. "Let the client rest for 5 minutes before you measure her blood pressure."

3. A nurse is instructing a group of nursing students in measuring a client's respiratory rate. Which of the following guidelines should the nurse include? (Select all that apply.)

   A. Place the client in semi-Fowler's position.

   B. Have the client rest an arm across the abdomen.

   C. Observe one full respiratory cycle before counting the rate.

   D. Count the rate for 30 sec if it is irregular.

   E. Count and report any sighs the client demonstrates.

4. A nurse who is admitting a client who has a fractured femur obtains a blood pressure reading of 140/94 mm Hg. The client denies any history of hypertension. Which of the following actions should the nurse take first?

   A. Request a prescription for an antihypertensive medication.

   B. Ask the client if she is having pain.

   C. Request a prescription for an antianxiety medication.

   D. Return in 30 min to recheck the client's blood pressure.

5. A nurse is performing an admission assessment on a client. The nurse determines the client's radial pulse rate is 68/min and the simultaneous apical pulse rate is 84/min. What is the client's pulse deficit?

PRACTICE Active Learning Scenario

A nurse is explaining to a group of nursing students the various factors that can affect a client's heart rate. Use the ATI Active Learning Template: Basic Concept to complete this item.

UNDERLYING PRINCIPLES: List at least five factors that can cause tachycardia and at least five factors that can cause bradycardia.

Application Exercises Key

1. A. **CORRECT:** The provider can prescribe cultures to identify any infectious organisms causing the fever. The nurse should obtain culture specimens before antimicrobial therapy to prevent interference with the detection of the infection.

   B. The nurse should increase oral fluid intake to replace the loss of body fluids from the diaphoresis and increased metabolic rate the fever can cause.

   C. **CORRECT:** Rest helps conserve energy and decreases metabolic rate. Activity can increase heat production.

   D. The nurse should provide interventions to prevent shivering, because shivering increases energy demands.

   E. **CORRECT:** Oral hygiene helps prevent cracking of dry mucous membranes of the mouth and lips.

   Ⓝ *NCLEX® Connection: Reduction of Risk Potential, Changes/Abnormalities in Vital Signs*

2. A. **CORRECT:** The greatest risk to a client who has a low platelet count is an injury that results in bleeding. Using a thermometer rectally poses a risk of injury to the rectal mucosa. The low platelet count contraindicates the use of the rectal route for this client.

   B. The AP should count the radial pulse, unless it is irregular, for 30 seconds and then multiply by 2 to obtain the number of pulsations per minute. However, this is not the highest priority.

   C. The AP should avoid letting the client know about counting respirations as this awareness can sometimes alter the respiratory rate. However, this is not the highest priority.

   D. The AP should let the client rest for 5 min before measuring blood pressure as activity can alter the reading. However, this is not the highest priority.

   Ⓝ *NCLEX® Connection: Reduction of Risk Potential, Changes/Abnormalities in Vital Signs*

3. A. **CORRECT:** Having the client sit upright facilitates full ventilation and gives the students a clear view of chest and abdominal movements.

   B. **CORRECT:** With the client's arm across the abdomen or lower chest, it is easier for the students to see respiratory movements.

   C. **CORRECT:** Observing for one full respiratory cycle before starting to count assists the students in obtaining an accurate count.

   D. The students should count the rate for 1 min if it is irregular.

   E. An occasional sigh is an expected finding in adults and can assist to expand airways. Students do not need to count sighs.

   Ⓝ *NCLEX® Connection: Reduction of Risk Potential, Changes/Abnormalities in Vital Signs*

4. A. The nurse should request a prescription for an antihypertensive medication if the client's blood pressure remains elevated after the nurse implements other interventions to reduce it. However, there is another action the nurse should take first

   B. **CORRECT:** The first action the nurse should take using the nursing process is to assess the client for pain which can cause multiple complications, including elevated blood pressure. Therefore, the nurse's priority is to perform a pain assessment. If the client's blood pressure is still elevated after pain interventions, the nurse should report this finding to the provider.

   C. The nurse should request a prescription for an anti-anxiety medication if the client's blood pressure remains elevated after the nurse implements other interventions to reduce it. However, there is another action the nurse should take first.

   D. The nurse should recheck the client's blood pressure in 30 min and periodically thereafter if it remains elevated after the nurse implements other interventions to reduce it. However, there is another action the nurse should take first.

   Ⓝ *NCLEX® Connection: Reduction of Risk Potential, Changes/Abnormalities in Vital Signs*

5. **16**/min

   The pulse deficit is the difference between the apical and radial pulse rates. It reflects the number of ineffective or nonperfusing heartbeats that do not transmit pulsations to peripheral pulse points. 84-68 = 16

   Ⓝ *NCLEX® Connection: Reduction of Risk Potential, Changes/Abnormalities in Vital Signs*

PRACTICE Answer

Using the ATI Active Learning Template: Basic Concept

UNDERLYING PRINCIPLES

Tachycardia
- Exercise
- Fever
- Medications: epinephrine, levothyroxine, beta₂ adrenergic agonists (albuterol)
- Changing position from lying down to sitting or standing
- Acute pain
- Hyperthyroidism
- Anemia, hypoxemia
- Stress, anxiety, fear
- Hypovolemia, shock, heart failure

Bradycardia
- Long-term physical fitness
- Hypothermia
- Medications: digoxin, beta-blockers (propranolol), calcium channel blockers (verapamil)
- Changing position from standing or sitting to lying down
- Chronic, severe pain
- Hypothyroidism

Ⓝ *NCLEX® Connection: Reduction of Risk Potential, Changes/Abnormalities in Vital Signs*

CHAPTER 28 *Head and Neck*

This examination includes the head, neck, eyes, nose, mouth, and throat.

Head and neck

- This examination includes the skull, face, hair, neck, shoulders, lymph nodes, thyroid gland, trachea position, carotid arteries, and jugular veins.
- Use the techniques of inspection, palpation, and auscultation to examine the head and neck.
- Unexpected findings include palpation of a mass, limited range of motion of the neck, and enlarged lymph nodes.
- Equipment includes a stethoscope.
- Test the following cranial nerves (CN) during the head and neck examination.
  - CN V (trigeminal): Assess the face for strength and sensation.
  - CN VII (facial): Assess the face for symmetrical movement.
  - CN XI (spinal accessory): Assess the head and shoulders for strength.

HEALTH HISTORY: REVIEW OF SYSTEMS

QUESTIONS TO ASK
- Do you get headaches? If so, how often? Would you point to the exact location? Do you have any other manifestations related to your headaches, such as nausea and vomiting? What do you do to relieve the pain?
- Have you ever had a head injury?
- Do you have any pain in your neck?
- Can you move your head and shoulders with ease?
- Have you noticed any unusual facial movements?
- Are any of your lymph nodes swollen?
- Does anyone in your family have thyroid disease?

INSPECTION, PALPATION, AND AUSCULTATION

Skull

EXPECTED FINDINGS
- Size (normocephalic)
- No depressions, deformities, masses, tenderness
- Overall contour and symmetry

Face

EXPECTED FINDINGS
- Symmetry of facial features (If there is asymmetry, note if all features on one side of face are affected, or only some of the features)
- Symmetry of expressions
- No involuntary movements
- Proportionate features (no thickening as with acromegaly)
- **CN V**
  - MOTOR: Test the strength of the muscle contraction by asking the client to clench her teeth while you palpate the masseter and temporal muscles, and then the temporomandibular joint. Joint movement should be smooth.
  - SENSORY: Test light touch by having the client close her eyes while you touch her face gently with a wisp of cotton. Ask her to tell you when she feels the touch.
- **CN VII: MOTOR:** Test facial movement and symmetry by having the client smile, frown, puff out her cheeks, raise her eyebrows, close her eyes tightly, and show her teeth.

Neck

EXPECTED FINDINGS
- Muscles of the neck symmetric.
- Shoulders equal in height and with average muscle mass.
  - RANGE OF MOTION (ROM): Moving her head smoothly and without distress in the following directions:
    - Chin to chest (flexion).
    - Ear to shoulder bilaterally (lateral flexion).
    - Chin up (hyperextension).
  - **CN XI:** Place your hands on the client's shoulders and ask her to shrug her shoulders against resistance; then turn head against resistance of your hand.

Lymph nodes

- Chains of lymph nodes extend from the lower half of the head down into the neck. Palpate each node for enlargement, in the following sequence.
  - **Occipital nodes:** Base of the skull
  - **Postauricular nodes:** Over the mastoid
  - **Preauricular nodes:** In front of the ear
  - **Tonsillar (retropharyngeal) nodes:** Angle of the mandible
  - **Submandibular nodes:** Along the base of the mandible
  - **Submental nodes:** Midline under the chin
  - **Anterior cervical nodes:** Along the sternocleidomastoid muscle
  - **Posterior cervical nodes:** Posterior to the sternocleidomastoid muscle
  - **Supraclavicular nodes:** Above the clavicles
- Lymph nodes are usually difficult to palpate and not tender or visible.
- Use the pads of the index and middle fingers and move the skin over the underlying tissue in a circular motion to try to detect enlarged nodes. Compare from side to side.
- Evaluate any enlarged nodes for location, tenderness, size, shape, consistency, mobility, and warmth.

Thyroid gland

The thyroid gland has two lobes and is fixed to the trachea. It lies in front of the trachea and extends to both sides.

Examine the gland by
- First, inspecting the lower half of the neck to see any enlargement of the gland. An average-size thyroid gland is not visible. Having the client hyperextend the neck helps makes the skin taut and allows better visualization.
- Instructing the client to take a sip of water and feeling the thyroid gland as it moves up with the trachea.
- Palpating the thyroid gland on both sides of the trachea for size, masses, and smoothness.

AUSCULTATION: If the thyroid is enlarged, auscultate the gland using a stethoscope. A bruit indicates an increase in blood flow to the area, possibly due to hyperthyroidism.

Trachea

Inspect and palpate the trachea for any deviation from midline above the suprasternal notch. Masses in the neck or mediastinum and pulmonary abnormalities cause lateral displacement.

Eyes

- This examination includes the external and internal anatomy of the eye, visual pathways, fields, visual acuity, extraocular movements, and reflexes.
- The primary technique for examination of the eyes is inspection, with a limited amount of palpation that requires gloves.
- Unexpected findings include loss of visual fields, asymmetric corneal light reflex, periorbital edema, conjunctivitis, and corneal abrasion.
- Perform the eye examination in the following sequence, using the correct equipment.
  - Visual acuity
    - Distant vision: Snellen and Rosenbaum charts, eye cover, Ishihara test for color blindness
    - Near vision: hand-held card
  - Extraocular movements (EOMs): Penlight or ophthalmoscope light, eye cover
  - Visual fields: Eye cover
  - External structures: Penlight or ophthalmoscope light, gloves
  - Internal structures: Ophthalmoscope
- Test cranial nerves during the eye examination.
  - CN II (optic): visual acuity
  - CN III (oculomotor), CN IV (trochlear), CN VI (abducens): extraocular movements
  - CN II (optic): visual fields
  - CN II (optic), CN III (oculomotor): corneal light reflex, pupillary reaction to light

HEALTH HISTORY: REVIEW OF SYSTEMS

QUESTIONS TO ASK
- How is your vision? Have you noticed any changes?
- Do you ever have blurry or double vision? Do you ever see spots or halos?
- Do you have any eye pain, sensitivity to light, burning, itching, dryness, or excessively watery eyes?
- Do you ever have drainage or crusting from your eyes?
- Do you wear eyeglasses? Contact lenses?
- When was your last eye examination?
- Have you ever been diagnosed with an eye disorder?
- Does anyone in your family have any eye disorders?
- Do you have diabetes mellitus?

INSPECTION

Visual acuity: CN II

- Have the client stand 20 feet from the Snellen (E) chart.
- Evaluate both eyes and then each eye separately with and without correction.
- For each eye, cover the opposite eye.
- Ask the client to read the smallest line of print visible.
- Note the smallest line the client can read correctly.
- The first number is the distance (in feet) the client stands from the chart. The second number is the distance at which a visually unimpaired eye can see the same line clearly.

> For example: A 20/30 vision means a client can read a line from 20 feet away that a person who has unimpaired vision can read from 30 feet away.

Snellen chart: Use to screen for myopia (impaired far vision).

Rosenbaum eye chart: Hold 14 inches from the client's face to screen for presbyopia (impaired near vision or farsightedness). Readings correlate with the Snellen chart.

Color vision: Assess using the Ishihara test. The client should be able to identify the various shaded shapes.

Extraocular movements: CN III, IV, VI

Assess EOMs to determine the coordination of the eye muscles using three different tests (CN III, CN IV, CN VI).
- Assess for parallel eye movement, the position of the upper eyelid, and the presence of abnormal eye movements while the client looks in each direction (28.1).
- Test the corneal light reflex by directing a light onto the eyes and looking to see if the reflection is symmetric on the corneas.
- Screen for strabismus with the cover/uncover test. While covering one eye, ask the client to look in another direction. Remove the cover and expect both eyes to be gazing in the same direction.
- The six cardinal positions of gaze require the client to follow your finger with his eyes without moving his head. Move your finger in a wide "H" pattern about 20 to 25 cm (7.9 to 9.8 in) to from the client's eyes. Expect smooth, symmetric eye movements with no jerky or tremor-like movements (nystagmus).

Visual fields: CN II

Evaluate by facing the client at a distance of 60 cm (2 ft). The client covers one eye while you cover your direct opposite eye (client's right eye and your left eye). Ask the client to look at you and report when she can see the fingers on your outstretched arm coming in from four directions (up, down, temporally, nasally). The expected finding is that the client sees your fingers at the same time you do.

External structures

EXPECTED FINDINGS

- Eyes parallel to each other without bulging (exophthalmos) or crossing (strabismus)
- Eyebrows symmetric from the inner to the outer canthus: can raise and lower symmetrically
- Eyelids closing completely and opening to show the lower border and most of the upper portion of the iris without ptosis (the upper eyelid covering the pupil)
- Eyelashes curving outward with no inflammation around any of the hair follicles
- No edema or redness in the area of the lacrimal glands.
- Conjunctiva
  - Palpebral pink
  - Bulbar transparent
- The sclerae will be white in those who have fair skin and light yellow in clients who have a dark complexion.
- Corneas clear, shiny, and smooth.
- Lenses clear, cloudy with cataracts
- Irises round and illuminating fully when you shine a light across from the side. A partially illuminated iris indicates glaucoma. Note the color of the irises.

PERRLA (CN II, CN III)

- **P:** Pupils clear
- **E:** Equal and between 3 to 7 mm in diameter
- **R:** Round
- **RL:** Reactive to light both directly and consensually when you direct light into one pupil and then the other
- **A:** Accommodation of the pupils when they dilate to look at an object far away and then converge and constrict to focus on a near object

Internal structures

Examine by
- Darken the room.
- Turn on the ophthalmoscope, and use the lens selector disc to find the large white disc.
- The diopter is set at 0. You can change the setting to bring structures into focus during the examination.
- Use your right eye to examine the client's right eye and vice versa.
- Instruct the client to stare at a point somewhere behind you.
- Start slightly lateral and 25 to 30 cm from the client, finding and following the red reflex, to within a distance of 2 to 3 cm of the client's eye.

EXPECTED FINDINGS

- The optic disc is light pink or more yellow than the surrounding retina.
- The retina is without lesions. The color will be dark pink in those with a dark complexion and light pink in those who have fair skin.
- The arteries and veins have a 2:3 ratio with no nicking.
- Without pupil dilation, you might only glimpse the macula briefly when the client looks directly at the light.

PALPATION

Palpate the lacrimal apparatus to assess for tenderness and to express any discharge from the lacrimal duct. Expected findings include no tenderness, no discharge, and clear fluid (tears).

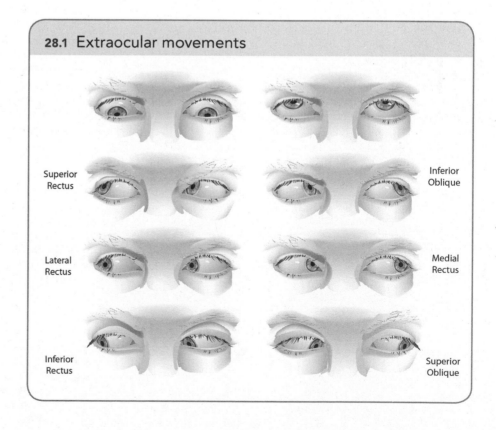

28.1 Extraocular movements

Superior Rectus

Inferior Oblique

Lateral Rectus

Medial Rectus

Inferior Rectus

Superior Oblique

Ears, nose, mouth, and throat

This examination includes the external, middle, and internal ear; evaluation of hearing; the nose and sinuses; and the mouth and throat.

- Use the techniques of inspection and palpation to examine the ears, nose (sinuses), mouth, and throat.
- Unexpected findings include otitis externa, osteoma, polyp, retracted drum, decreased hearing acuity, and lateralization.
- Test the following cranial nerves during the ears, nose, mouth, and throat examination.
  - CN I (olfactory): Assess the nose for smell.
  - CN VII (facial) and CN IX (glossopharyngeal): Assess the mouth for taste.
  - CN VIII (auditory): Assess the ears for hearing.
  - CN IX (glossopharyngeal) and CN X (vagus): Assess the mouth for movement of the soft palate and the gag reflex. Assess swallowing and speech.
  - CN XII (hypoglossal): Assess the tongue for movement and strength.

EQUIPMENT
- Otoscope
- Wristwatch or clock to measure time in seconds
- Tuning fork
- Nasal speculum
- Tongue blade
- Penlight
- Gauze square
- Cotton-tipped applicators

HEALTH HISTORY: REVIEW OF SYSTEMS

QUESTIONS TO ASK
- How well do you hear?
- Have you noticed any changes in your hearing? Do you wear hearing aids?
- Have other people commented that you aren't hearing what they say?
- Do you ever have ringing or buzzing in your ears, drainage, dizziness, itching, or pain? Do you have a history of ear infections?
- Are you routinely exposed to loud noises (work, recreation)?
- How do you clean your ears?
- Do you ever have pain, stuffiness, or fluid draining from your nose?
- Have you ever suffered an injury to your nose?
- Do you ever have nosebleeds?
- Have you noticed any change in your senses of smell or taste?
- Do you use nasal sprays?
- Do you snore or have difficulty breathing through your nose?
- How often do you go to the dentist? Do you have dentures? Retainers? Do you have any problems with your gums?
- Do you have any difficulty swallowing or problems with hoarseness or sore throat?

INSPECTION AND PALPATION

Ears

EXTERNAL EAR EXPECTED FINDINGS
- Alignment: The top of the auricles meeting an imaginary horizontal line that extends from the outer canthus of the eye. The auricles should be of equal size and level with one another.
- Ear color matching face color
- No lesions, deformities, or tenderness
- No foreign bodies or discharge
- Presence of a small amount of cerumen

INTERNAL EAR
Straighten the ear canal by pulling the auricle up and back for adults and older children, and down and back for younger children. Using the otoscope, insert the speculum slightly down and forward 1 to 1.5 cm (0.4 to 0.6 in) following, but not touching, the ear canal to visualize:
- Tympanic membranes that are pearly gray and intact, taut, and free from tears.
- A light reflex that is visible and in a well-defined cone shape.
- Umbo and manubrium landmarks are readily visible.
- Ear canals are pink with fine hairs.

AUDITORY SCREENING TESTS
- **Whisper test (CN VIII)**
  - TECHNIQUE
    - Occlude one ear and test the other to see if the client can hear whispered sounds without seeing your mouth move.
    - Repeat with the other ear.
  - EXPECTED FINDING: The client can hear you whisper softly from 30 to 60 cm (1 to 2 ft) away.
- **Rinne test (28.2)**
  - TECHNIQUE
    - Place a vibrating tuning fork firmly against the mastoid bone. Have the client state when he can no longer hear the sound. Note the length of time that the client heard the sound (bone conduction).
    - Then move the tuning fork in front of the ear canal. When the client can no longer hear the tuning fork sound, note the length of time the sound was heard (air conduction).
  - EXPECTED FINDING: Air conduction (AC) sound longer than bone conduction (BC) sound; 2:1 ratio.
- **Weber test (28.3)**
  - TECHNIQUE: Place a vibrating tuning fork on top of the client's head. Ask whether the client can hear the sound best in the right ear, the left ear, or both ears equally.
  - EXPECTED FINDING: The client hears sound equally in both ears (negative Weber test).

Nose

EXPECTED FINDINGS

- The nose is midline, symmetrical, and the same color as the face. Observe for tenderness, swelling, masses, or deviations.
- Each naris (nostril) is patent without excessive flaring. The structure of the nose is firm and stable.
- To examine internal structures, insert a nasal speculum just barely into each naris as the client tips his head back.
  - Septum is midline and intact.
  - Mucous membranes are deep pink and moist with no discharge or lesions.
- Assess smell (CN I) by asking the client to close his eyes, occlude one naris at a time, and identify a familiar smell with the eyes closed.

Mouth and throat

EXPECTED FINDINGS

- **Lips:** Darker pigmented skin than the face and are moist, symmetric, smooth, soft with no lesions, and nontender.
- **Gums:** Coral pink and tight against the teeth with no bleeding on gloves from palpation.
- **Mucous membranes:** Pink and moist with no lesions.
- **Tongue:** Use a gauze pad to hold the tip and move the tongue from side to side. The dorsal surface is pink, with the presence of papillae, and symmetric. The underside of the tongue is smooth with a symmetric vascular pattern. Assess taste (CN VII, CN IX) by having the client close his eyes and identify foods you place on his tongue. Ask the client to move his tongue up, down, and side to side. Test strength (CN XII) by applying resistance against each cheek while the client sticks his tongue into each cheek. The tongue is midline, moist, free of lesions, and moves freely.

- **Teeth:** Shiny, white, and smooth. Check for malocclusions by asking the client to clench his teeth. Note any missing or loose teeth, as well as any discoloration. Yellow or darkened teeth are common in older adults because of long-term wear.
- **Hard palate:** Whitish, intact, symmetric, firm, and concave.
- **Soft palate:** Light pink, intact, smooth, symmetric, and moves with vocalization (CN IX, CN X).
- **Uvula:** Pink, midline, intact, and moves with vocalization.
- **Tonsils:** The same color as the surrounding mucosa and vary in size and visibility.
  - +1: Barely visible
  - +2: Halfway to the uvula
  - +3: Touching the uvula
  - +4: Touching each other or midline
- **Gag reflex:** Elicit by using a tongue blade to stimulate the back of the throat (CN IX, CN X). Explain the procedure to the client prior to performing this assessment.
- **Speech:** Clear and articulate.

Sinuses

TECHNIQUE

- Palpate the frontal sinuses by pressing upward with the thumbs from just below the eyebrows on either side of the bridge of the nose.
- Palpate the maxillary sinuses by pressing upward at the skin crevices that run from the sides of the nose to the corner of the mouth.

EXPECTED FINDING: Nontender

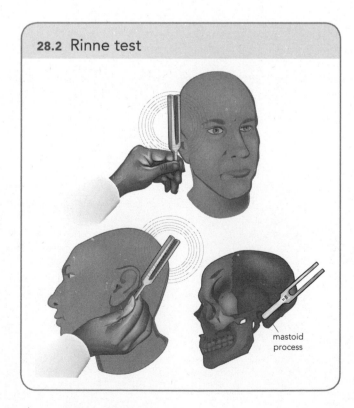

28.2 Rinne test

mastoid process

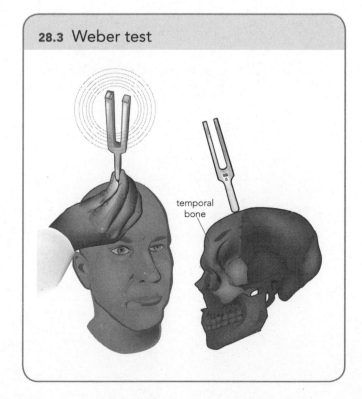

28.3 Weber test

temporal bone

EXPECTED CHANGES WITH AGING

Eyes: Decreased visual acuity, decreased peripheral vision, diminishing ability to see close objects or read small print (presbyopia), decreased ability to accommodate extreme changes in light (glare, darkness), difficulty distinguishing colors, intolerance to glare, delayed pupillary reaction to light, yellowing of the lens, thin gray–white ring surrounding the cornea, loss of lateral third of eyebrows

Ears: Hearing loss, loss of acuity for high-frequency tones (presbycusis), cerumen accumulation in the ear canal, thickening of the tympanic membrane

Mouth: Decreased sense of taste due to reduced number of taste buds, tooth loss, pale gums, gum disease due to inadequate oral hygiene, darkening of teeth, decreased salivation

Voice: Rise in pitch, loss of power and range

Nose: Decreased sense of smell

SAMPLE DOCUMENTATION

Client reports no pain in head or neck region.

Skull normocephalic, symmetrical, and nontender. Symmetric facial features, movements. Trachea midline. Thyroid lobes palpable but not enlarged; no nodules. Neck supple with no palpable lymph nodes. Full range of motion of the neck.

Visual acuity 20/30 in the left eye, 20/20 in the right eye, 20/20 in both eyes without correction. EOMs symmetric with no strabismus or nystagmus. Peripheral fields full bilaterally. Eyebrows evenly distributed. Eyelids close completely with no ptosis. No discharge. Bulbar conjunctiva clear, palpebral conjunctiva pink, sclerae white, irises blue bilaterally. Corneas and lenses clear. PERRLA intact bilaterally. Red reflex bilaterally. Retinas yellowish orange with no nicking or hemorrhaging of vessels.

No lesions or tenderness on external ears. Top of ears align with outer canthus of eyes. Tympanic membranes pearly gray and translucent with well-defined cone of light. Light yellow cerumen in ear canals bilaterally. Auditory acuity intact to whispered voice bilaterally. Negative Weber test and AC > BC bilaterally. Nose midline, symmetrical. Nares patent. Nasal mucosa pink, septum intact and midline, no discharge. No sinus tenderness. Lips darker pink and intact, symmetric. Oral mucosa pink, no dental caries, no missing teeth. Tongue pink and midline. Papillae on dorsum, symmetrical vascular pattern on the underside of the tongue. Gums tight against the teeth with no bleeding. Hard and soft palates intact with no lesions. Uvula midline. Gag reflex present. Tonsils +1 bilaterally. Taste and smell sensations intact. Speech clear. CN I through XII intact.

Application Exercises

1. A nurse in a provider's office is preparing to test a client's cranial nerve function. Which of the following directions should she include when testing cranial nerve V? (Select all that apply.)

   A. "Close your eyes."

   B. "Tell me what you can taste."

   C. "Clench your teeth."

   D. "Raise your eyebrows."

   E. "Tell me when you feel a touch."

2. A nurse is assessing a client's thyroid gland as part of a comprehensive physical examination. Which of the following findings should the nurse expect? (Select all that apply.)

   A. Palpating the thyroid in the lower half of the neck

   B. Visualizing the thyroid on inspection of the neck

   C. Hearing a bruit when auscultating the thyroid

   D. Feeling the thyroid ascend as the client swallows

   E. Finding symmetric extension off the trachea on both sides of the midline

3. A nurse is assessing an adult client's internal ear canals with an otoscope as part of a head and neck examination. Which of the following actions should the nurse take? (Select all that apply.)

   A. Pull the auricle down and back.

   B. Insert the speculum slightly down and forward.

   C. Insert the speculum 2 to 2.5 cm (0.8 to 1 in).

   D. Make sure the speculum does not touch the ear canal.

   E. Use the light to visualize the tympanic membrane in a cone shape.

4. A nurse is caring for a client who asks what her Snellen eye test results mean. The client's visual acuity is 20/30. Which of the following responses should the nurse make?

   A. "Your eyes see at 20 feet what visually unimpaired eyes see at 30 feet."

   B. "Your right eye can see the chart clearly at 20 feet, and your left eye can see the chart clearly at 30 feet."

   C. "Your eyes see at 30 feet what visually unimpaired eyes see at 20 feet."

   D. "Your left eye can see the chart clearly at 20 feet, and your right eye can see the chart clearly at 30 feet."

5. A nurse is performing a head and neck examination for an older adult client. Which of the following age-related findings should the nurse expect? (Select all that apply.)

   A. Reddened gums

   B. Lowered vocal pitch

   C. Tooth loss

   D. Glare intolerance

   E. Thickened eardrums

PRACTICE Active Learning Scenario

A nurse is assessing a client's lymph nodes as part of a comprehensive physical examination. Use the ATI Active Learning Template: Nursing Skill to complete this item.

DESCRIPTION OF SKILL: List the nine chains of lymph nodes and the location of each, in the appropriate sequence for palpating them.

Application Exercises Key

1. A. The first step of testing cranial nerve I, the olfactory nerve, is to have the client close his eyes.

   B. Testing cranial nerve VII, the facial nerve, involves testing the mouth for taste sensations.

   C. **CORRECT:** Testing cranial nerve V, the trigeminal nerve, involves testing the strength of muscle contraction by asking the client to clench his teeth while the nurse palpates the masseter and temporal muscles, and then the temporomandibular joint.

   D. Testing cranial nerve VII, the facial nerve, involves testing for a range of facial expressions by having the client smile, raise his eyebrows, puff out his cheeks, and perform other facial movements.

   E. **CORRECT:** Testing cranial nerve V, the trigeminal nerve, involves testing light touch by having the client tell the nurse when he feels a gentle touch on his face from a wisp of cotton.

   Ⓝ *NCLEX® Connection: Reduction of Risk Potential, Diagnostic Tests*

2. A. **CORRECT:** The thyroid gland lies in the anterior portion of the lower half of the neck, just in front of the trachea.

   B. An average-size thyroid gland is not visible on inspection.

   C. A bruit indicates increased blood flow, possibly due to hyperthyroidism.

   D. **CORRECT:** When the client swallows a sip of water, the nurse should feel the thyroid move upward with the trachea.

   E. **CORRECT:** The thyroid gland lies in front of the trachea and extends symmetrically to both sides of the midline.

   Ⓝ *NCLEX® Connection: Reduction of Risk Potential, System Specific Assessments*

3. A. The nurse should pull the auricle up and back for adults and down and back for children younger than 3 years.

   B. **CORRECT:** Inserting the speculum slightly down and forward follows the natural shape of the ear canal.

   C. The nurse should insert the speculum 1 to 1.5 cm (0.4 to 0.6 in).

   D. **CORRECT:** The lining of the ear canal is sensitive. Touching it with the speculum could cause pain.

   E. **CORRECT:** Due to the angle of the ear canal, the nurse can only visualize the light reflecting off of the tympanic membrane as a cone shape rather than a circle.

   Ⓝ *NCLEX® Connection: Reduction of Risk Potential, Diagnostic Tests*

4. A. **CORRECT:** The first number is the distance (in feet) the client stands from the chart. The second number is the distance at which a visually unimpaired eye can see the same line clearly.

   B. Each eye has its own visual acuity, which includes both numbers.

   C. The numerator of visual acuity results is a constant. It does not change with a client's ability to see clearly.

   D. Each eye has its own visual acuity, which includes both numbers.

   Ⓝ *NCLEX® Connection: Reduction of Risk Potential, Therapeutic Procedures*

5. A. The nurse should expect an older adult's gums to be pale.

   B. The nurse should expect an older adult's vocal pitch to rise.

   C. **CORRECT:** Tooth loss and gum disease are common in older adults.

   D. **CORRECT:** Older adults tend to become intolerant of glaring lights and also lose some ability to distinguish colors.

   E. **CORRECT:** Tympanic membranes (eardrums) thicken in older adults, and they tend to accumulate cerumen in their ear canals.

   Ⓝ *NCLEX® Connection: Physiological Adaptation, Pathophysiology*

PRACTICE Answer

Using the ATI Active Learning Template: Nursing Skill

DESCRIPTION OF SKILL

- Occipital nodes: base of the skull
- Postauricular nodes: over the mastoid
- Preauricular nodes: in front of the ear
- Tonsillar (retropharyngeal) nodes: angle of the mandible
- Submandibular nodes: along the base of the mandible
- Submental nodes: midline under the chin
- Anterior cervical nodes: along the sternocleidomastoid muscle
- Posterior cervical nodes: posterior to the sternocleidomastoid muscle
- Supraclavicular nodes: above the clavicles

Ⓝ *NCLEX® Connection: Health Promotion and Maintenance, Techniques of Physical Assessment*

UNIT 2   HEALTH PROMOTION
SECTION: HEALTH ASSESSMENT/DATA COLLECTION

CHAPTER 29 *Thorax, Heart, and Abdomen*

This examination includes the thorax (breast and lungs), heart, and abdomen.

Breasts

- For clients who have had a mastectomy, breast augmentation, or reconstruction, palpate the incisional lines. Look for lymphedema in clients who have impaired lymphatic drainage on the affected side.
- Instruct clients who do not currently perform monthly breast self-examination (BSE) to inspect their breasts in front of a mirror and palpate them during a shower. The optimal time is right after menstruation ends. Clients who are pregnant or postmenopausal should perform BSE on the same day of each month. Q EBP
- Perform breast examinations on female and male clients.
- Use the techniques of inspection and palpation to examine the breasts.

EQUIPMENT
- Gloves
- Drape
- Small pillow or folded towel

DOCUMENTATION OF NODULES
- Location (quadrant or clock method)
- Size (centimeters)
- Shape
- Consistency (soft, firm, or hard)
- Discreteness (well-defined borders of mass)
- Tenderness
- Erythema
- Dimpling or retraction over the mass
- Lymphadenopathy
- Mobility

HEALTH HISTORY: REVIEW OF SYSTEMS

QUESTIONS TO ASK
- Do you perform breast self-examinations? How often?
- Have you noticed any tenderness or lumps? For women: Does this change with your menstrual cycle?
- Do you have any thickening, pain, drainage, distortion, or change in breast size, or any retraction or scaling of the nipples?
- For clients over 40: How often are you having mammograms?
- Has anyone in your family had breast cancer?
- Are you aware of the risks for breast cancer?

INSPECTION

Position client
- WOMEN: Four positions (sitting or standing)
  - Arms at the side
  - Arms above the head
  - Hands on the hips pressing firmly
  - Leaning forward (arms out in front or on hips)
- MEN: In sitting or lying position (with arms at the side only)

Inspect for
- Size, symmetry (One breast is often slightly larger than the other.)
- Shape (convex, conical, pendulous)
- Symmetric venous patterns and consistency of skin color
- No lesions, edema, erythema (Rashes and ulcerations are unexpected findings.)
- Round or oval shape of areola
- Darker-pigmented areola and nipple
- Direction of nipples (Nipples are usually everted; recent inversion is unexpected.)
- Bleeding or discharge from the nipples
- For women with large breasts, check for excoriation under the breasts.

PALPATION

Palpate axillary and clavicular lymph nodes with the client sitting with her arms at her sides. Expect them to be nonpalpable with no tenderness.

Breast examination

- Wear gloves if skin is not intact. Feel for lumps using the finger pads of your three middle fingers. The best position is for the client to be lying down with the arm up by her head and a small pillow or folded towel under the shoulder of the side you are examining. This position spreads the breast tissue more evenly over the chest wall, allowing for easier palpation.
- Palpate each breast from the sternum to the posterior axillary line, and from the clavicle to the bra line (including the areola, nipple, and tail of Spence) using one of three techniques.
  - Circular pattern
  - Wedge pattern
  - Vertical strip pattern
- Compress the nipples carefully between your thumb and index finger to check for discharge (unexpected in nonlactating women). Note the color, consistency, and odor of any discharge.
- For pendulous breasts, use one hand to support the lower portion of the breast while using your other hand to palpate breast tissue against the supporting hand.

EXPECTED FINDINGS

- WOMEN
  - Breasts firm, dense, elastic, and without lesions or nodules
  - Breast tissue granular or lumpy bilaterally in some women
- MEN
  - No edema, masses, nodules, or tenderness
  - Areolas round and darker pigmented

UNEXPECTED FINDINGS

- WOMEN: Fibrocystic breast disease: tender cysts often more prominent during menstruation
- MEN: Unilateral or bilateral (but asymmetrical) gynecomastia in adolescent boys or bilateral gynecomastia in older adult males

Thorax and lungs

- This examination includes the anterior and posterior thorax and lungs.
- Use the techniques of inspection, palpation, percussion, and auscultation.

EQUIPMENT
- Stethoscope
- Centimeter ruler
- Wristwatch or clock that allows for counting seconds

POSITIONING: Assess the posterior thorax with the client sitting or standing. Assess the anterior thorax with the client sitting, lying, or standing.

ANATOMICAL REMINDER: The right lung has three lobes; the left lung has two lobes. Auscultate the right middle lobe via the axillae.

VERTICAL CHEST LANDMARKS: Use the following landmarks to perform assessments and describe findings.
- The **midsternal line** is through the center of the sternum.
- The **midclavicular line** is through the midpoint of the clavicle.
- The **anterior axillary line** is through the anterior axillary folds.
- The **midaxillary line** is through the apex of the axillae.
- The **posterior axillary line** is through the posterior axillary fold.
- The **right and left scapular lines** are through the inferior angle of the scapula.
- The **vertebral line** is along the center of the spine.

PERCUSSION AND AUSCULTATORY SITES are in the intercostal spaces (ICSs). The number of the ICSs corresponds to the rib above it.
- **Posterior thorax:** The sites are between the scapula and the vertebrae on the upper portion of the back. Below the scapula, the sites are along the right and left scapular lines.
- **Anterior thorax:** The sites are along the midclavicular lines bilaterally, with several sites at the anterior/midaxillary lines bilaterally in the lower portions of the chest wall and on either side of the sternum following along the rib cage. Observe for accessory muscle use.
- Percussing and auscultating in a systemic pattern allows side-to-side comparisons.
- Maximize sounds by:
  - Having the client take deep breaths with an open mouth each time you move the stethoscope.
  - Placing the diaphragm stethoscope directly on the skin to prevent muffling or distortion of sounds.
  - Facilitating breathing by medicating for pain, giving clear directions, and assisting the client to a sitting position.

HEALTH HISTORY: REVIEW OF SYSTEMS

QUESTIONS TO ASK

- Do you have any chronic lung conditions such as asthma or emphysema? Do you take any medications for your respiratory problems?
- Have you ever had pneumonia? If so, when?
- Do you get coughs and colds frequently?
- Do you have environmental allergies?
- Do you ever have shortness of breath or difficulty breathing with activity?
- Do you have a cough now? Do you cough up sputum? If so, what does it look like?
- Do you currently or have you ever smoked? If you no longer smoke, when did you quit? How long did you smoke? If you do currently smoke, when did you start and how much do you smoke? Are you interested in quitting?
- Are you exposed to secondhand smoke?
- Are you exposed to environmental pollutants in your work area or residence?
- Has anyone in your family had lung cancer or tuberculosis? Have you had any exposure to tuberculosis?
- Do you receive an influenza vaccine every year?
- Have you received a pneumonia vaccine?
- Have you had a TB test?

INSPECTION

SHAPE: The anteroposterior diameter is one third to one half of the transverse diameter.

SYMMETRY: The chest is symmetric with no deformities of the ribs, sternum, scapula, or vertebrae, and equal movements during respiration.

ICS: No excessive retractions.

RESPIRATORY EFFORT
- Rate and pattern: 12 to 20/min and regular
- Character of breathing (diaphragmatic, abdominal, thoracic)
- Use of accessory muscles
- Chest wall expansion
- Depth of respirations: unlabored, quiet breathing

COUGH: If productive, note the color and consistency of sputum.

TRACHEA: Midline.

PALPATION

- Surface characteristics include tenderness, lesions, lumps, and deformities. Tenderness is an unexpected finding. Avoid deep palpation if the client reports pain or tenderness.
- Chest excursion or expansion of the posterior thorax: With thumbs aligned parallel along the spine at the level of the tenth rib, and the hands flattened around the client's back, instruct the client to take a deep breath. Move your thumbs outward approximately 5 cm (2 in) when the client takes a deep inspiration.

Vocal (tactile) fremitus

- Palpate the chest wall using the palms of both hands, comparing side to side from top to bottom.
- Ask the client to say "99" each time you move your hands.

EXPECTED FINDINGS: Vibration is symmetric and more pronounced at the top, near the level of the tracheal bifurcation.

PERCUSSION

- Compare sounds from side to side.
- Percussion of the thorax elicits resonance.

UNEXPECTED FINDINGS AND SIGNIFICANCE
- **Dullness:** In fluid or solid tissue, this can indicate pneumonia or a tumor.
- **Hyperresonance:** In the presence of air, this can indicate pneumothorax or emphysema.

AUSCULTATION

EXPECTED SOUNDS

Bronchial: Loud, high-pitched, hollow quality, expiration longer than inspiration over the trachea

Bronchovesicular: Medium pitch, blowing sounds and intensity with equal inspiration and expiration times over the larger airways

Vesicular: Soft, low-pitched, breezy sounds, inspiration three times longer than expiration over most of the peripheral areas of the lungs

UNEXPECTED OR ADVENTITIOUS SOUNDS

Crackles or rales: Fine to coarse bubbly sounds (not cleared with coughing) as air passes through fluid or re-expands collapsed small airways

Wheezes: High-pitched whistling, musical sounds as air passes through narrowed or obstructed airways, usually louder on expiration

Rhonchi: Coarse, loud, low-pitched rumbling sounds during either inspiration or expiration resulting from fluid or mucus, can clear with coughing

Pleural friction rub: Dry, grating, or rubbing sound as the inflamed visceral and parietal pleura rub against each other during inspiration or expiration

Absence of breath sounds: From collapsed or surgically removed lobes

Heart

This examination includes measuring heart rate and blood pressure, examining the jugular veins, and auscultating heart sounds.

EQUIPMENT
- Stethoscope
- Blood pressure cuff
- Wristwatch or clock that allows for counting seconds
- Two rulers

Cardiac cycle and heart sounds

- Closure of the mitral and tricuspid valves signals the beginning of ventricular systole (contraction) and produces the **S1 sound** (lub). Place the diaphragm of the stethoscope at the apex.
- Closure of the aortic and pulmonic valves signals the beginning of ventricular diastole (relaxation) and produces the **S2 sound** (dub). Place the diaphragm of the stethoscope at the aortic area.
- An **S3 sound** (ventricular gallop) indicates rapid ventricular filling and can be an expected finding in children and young adults. Use the bell of the stethoscope.
- An **S4 sound** reflects a strong atrial contraction and can be an expected finding in older and athletic adults and children. Use the bell of the stethoscope. Ⓒ
- **Dysrhythmias** occur when the heart fails to beat at regular successive intervals.
- **Gallops** are extra heart sounds. Use the bell of the stethoscope.
  - **Ventricular gallop** occurs after S2, sounds like "Ken-tuck'-y"
  - **Atrial gallop** occurs before S1, sounds like "Ten'-es-see"
- **Murmurs** are audible when blood volume in the heart increased or its flow is impeded or altered. Use the bell of the stethoscope to hear the characteristic blowing or swishing sound. Can be asymptomatic or a finding of heart disease.
  - **Systolic murmurs** occur just after S1.
  - **Diastolic murmurs** occur just after S2.
- **Thrills** are a palpable vibration that can accompany murmurs or cardiac malformation.
- **Bruits** are blowing or swishing sounds that indicate obstructed peripheral blood flow. Use the bell of the stethoscope.

Auscultatory sites for the heart

Aortic: Just right of the sternum at the second ICS

Pulmonic: Just left of the sternum at the second ICS

Erb's point: Just left of the sternum at the third ICS

Tricuspid: Just left of the sternum at the fourth ICS

Apical/mitral: Left midclavicular line at the fifth ICS

HEALTH HISTORY: REVIEW OF SYSTEMS

QUESTIONS TO ASK
- Do you have any problems with your heart? Do you take any medications for your heart?
- Have you had any history of heart trouble, preexisting diabetes, lung disease, obesity, or hypertension?
- Do you have high blood pressure or high cholesterol?
- Do your feet and ankles ever swell?
- Do you cough frequently?
- Do you have chest pain? When? How long does it last? How often does it occur? Describe the pain. Do you also feel it in your arms, neck, or jaw?
- What are you doing before the pain begins?
- Do you have any other symptoms with the pain (nausea, shortness of breath, sweating, dizziness)?
- What have you tried to relieve the pain? Does it work?
- Describe your energy level. Are you frequently tired? Do you have unusual fatigue?
- Do you have fainting spells or dizziness? If so, how often? When was the last time?
- What is your stress level?
- Do currently or have a history of smoking, drinking alcohol, using caffeine, using prescriptive or recreational drugs?
- Describe your exercise habits.
- Describe your dietary pattern and intake.
- Are you familiar with the risk factors for heart disease?
- Does anyone in your family have health problems related to the heart?

INSPECTION AND PALPATION

VITAL SIGNS: Pulse and blood pressure reflect cardiovascular status.

Peripheral vascular system

Inspect jugular veins with the client in bed with the head of the bed at a 30° to 45° angle to assess for right-sided heart failure.

APPEARANCE: no neck vein distention

JUGULAR VENOUS PRESSURE (JVP): Measure at less than 2.5 cm (1 in) above the sternal angle using the following technique:
- Place one ruler vertically at the sternal angle.
- Locate the pulsation in the external jugular vein and place the straight edge of another ruler parallel to the floor at the level of the pulsation.
- Line up the two rulers as a T square, keeping the horizontal ruler at the level of pulsation.
- Measure JVP at the level where the horizontal ruler intersects the vertical ruler.
- Bilateral pressures greater than 2.5 cm (1 in) are considered elevated, and a finding of right-sided heart failure. One-sided pressure elevation indicates obstruction.
  - Examine one carotid artery at a time. If you occlude both arteries simultaneously during palpation, the client loses consciousness as a result of inadequate circulation to the brain.

Heart

APICAL PULSE OR POINT OF MAXIMAL IMPULSE (PMI)

- Can be visible just medial to the left midclavicular line at the fourth or fifth ICS. With female clients, displace the breast tissue.
- Palpate where you visualized it. Otherwise, try to palpate the location to feel the pulsations.

HEAVES (OR LIFTS) are unexpected, visible elevations of the chest wall that indicate heart failure, and are often along the left sternal border or at the PMI.

THRILLS: Use the palm of the hand to feel for vibration similar to that of a purring kitten. This is an unexpected finding.

AUSCULTATION

Heart

- Positioning the client in three different ways allows for optimal assessment of heart sounds, as some positions amplify extra or abnormal sounds.
  - Sitting, leaning forward
  - Lying supine
  - Turned toward the left side (best position for auscultating extra heart sounds or murmurs)
- Use both the diaphragm and the bell of the stethoscope in a systematic manner to listen at all of the auscultatory sites.
- To measure the heart rate, listen and count for 1 min. Determine if the rhythm is regular. If a dysrhythmia exists, check for a pulse deficit (radial pulse slower than apical pulse). Report a difference in pulse rates to the provider immediately.

Peripheral vascular system

LOCATIONS TO ASSESS FOR BRUITS

- **Carotid arteries:** Over the carotid pulses
- **Abdominal aorta:** Just below the xiphoid process
- **Renal arteries:** Midclavicular lines above the umbilicus on the abdomen
- **Iliac arteries:** Midclavicular lines below the umbilicus on the abdomen
- **Femoral arteries:** Over the femoral pulses

Abdomen

- This examination includes observing the shape of the abdomen, palpating for masses, and auscultating for vascular sounds.
- Use the techniques of inspection, auscultation, percussion, and palpation. Note that this changes the usual order of assessment techniques. Auscultate just after inspection, because percussion and palpation can alter bowel sounds.
- EQUIPMENT
  - Stethoscope
  - Tape measure or ruler
  - Marking pen
- Ask the client to urinate before the abdominal examination. Have the client lie supine with arms at sides and knees slightly bent.
- Imagine vertical and horizontal lines through the umbilicus to divide the abdomen into four quadrants with the xiphoid process as the upper boundary and the symphysis pubis as the lower boundary.
  - Right upper quadrant
  - Left upper quadrant
  - Right lower quadrant
  - Left lower quadrant

HEALTH HISTORY: REVIEW OF SYSTEMS

QUESTIONS TO ASK

- Do you ever have nausea, vomiting, or cramping?
- Have you had any change in your appetite? Do you have any food intolerances? Any recent weight changes?
- Do you have any difficulty with swallowing, belching or gas?
- Have you had any vomit containing blood?
- Do you have any problems with your bowels? Do you get diarrhea? Constipation? When was your last bowel movement? Do you often use laxatives or enemas?
- Have you had any black or tarry stools?
- Do you take aspirin or ibuprofen? If so, how often?
- Do you ever have heartburn? When? How often?
- Have you had any low abdominal or back pain? Any tenderness in these areas?
- Have you had any abdominal surgery, injuries, or diagnostic tests in this area?
- Has anyone in your family had colon cancer?
- For clients over 50: Do you have routine colonoscopies?
- Are you aware of the warning signs of colon cancer?
- Do you drink alcohol? If so, how much?
- What do you eat and drink on a typical day?
- Do you have any dietary restrictions or special practices?
- Do you have any health problems related to the stomach or bowels? Do you take any medications for these problems? Do you have any family history of these conditions?

INSPECTION

- Note any guarding or splinting of the abdomen.
- Inspect the umbilicus for position, shape, color, inflammation, discharge, and masses.

ASSESS THE SKIN FOR

- **Lesions:** Bruising, rashes, or other primary lesions
- **Scars:** Location and length
- **Silver striae or stretch marks** (expected findings)
- **Dilated veins:** An unexpected finding possibly reflecting cirrhosis or inferior vena cava obstruction
- **Jaundice, cyanosis, or ascites:** Possibly reflecting cirrhosis

SHAPE OR CONTOUR

- **Flat:** In a horizontal line from the xiphoid process to the symphysis pubis
- **Convex:** Rounded
- **Concave:** A sunken appearance
- **Distended:** A large protrusion of the abdomen due to fat, fluid, or flatus
  - **Fat:** The client has rolls of fat tissue along her sides, and the skin does not look taut.
  - **Fluid:** The flanks also protrude, and when the client turns onto her side, the protrusion moves to the dependent side.
  - **Flatus:** The protrusion is mainly midline, and there is no change in the flanks.
  - **Hernias:** Protrusions through the abdominal muscle wall are visible, especially when the client raises her head.

MOVEMENT OF THE ABDOMINAL WALL

- **Peristalsis:** Wavelike movements visible in thin adults or in clients who have intestinal obstructions.
- **Pulsations:** Regular beats of movement midline above the umbilicus are expected findings in thin adults, but a pulsating mass is unexpected.

29.1 Abdominal assessment

right upper quadrant | left upper quadrant
right lower quadrant | left lower quadrant

AUSCULTATION

Bowel sounds result from the movement of air and fluid in the intestines. The most appropriate time to auscultate bowel sounds is in between meals.

- TECHNIQUE: Listen with the diaphragm of the stethoscope in all four quadrants.
- EXPECTED SOUNDS: High-pitched clicks and gurgles 5 to 35 times/min. To make the determination of absent bowel sounds, you must hear no sounds after listening for a full 5 min.
- UNEXPECTED SOUNDS: Loud, growling sounds (borborygmi) are hyperactive sounds and indicate increased gastrointestinal motility. Possible causes include diarrhea, anxiety, bowel inflammation, and reactions to some foods.

Friction rubs result from the rubbing together of inflamed layers of the peritoneum.

- Listen with the diaphragm over the liver and spleen.
- Ask the client to take a deep breath while you listen for any grating sounds (like sandpaper rubbing together).

PERCUSSION

- Expect to hear tympany over most of the abdomen. A lower-pitch tympany over the gastric bubble in the left upper quadrant is common.
- Expect dullness over the liver or a distended bladder.
- The liver span is a measurement of liver size at the right midclavicular line.
  - Establish the lower border of the liver by percussing upward from below the umbilicus at the right midclavicular line until tympany turns to dullness.
  - Make a mark.
  - Establish the upper border by percussing downward, starting at the right midclavicular line over the lung until resonance turns to dullness.
  - Make a mark.
  - Measure the distance between the two marks for the size of the liver span.
  - The expected finding is 6 to 12 cm (2.4 to 4.7 in).
- Assess for kidney tenderness by fist percussion over the costovertebral angles at the scapular lines on the back. The expected finding is no tenderness.

PALPATION

Palpate tender areas last.

Light

- Use the finger pads on one hand to palpate to a depth of 1.3 cm (0.5 in) in each quadrant.
- Expect softness, no nodules, and no guarding.
- The bladder is palpable if full; otherwise, it is nonpalpable.

Deep

TWO-HANDED APPROACH: The top hand depresses the bottom hand 2.5 to 7.5 cm (1 to 3 in) in depth. The bottom hand assesses for organ enlargement or masses.

EXPECTED FINDINGS: The stool can be palpable in the descending colon.

Rebound tenderness (Blumberg's sign)

An indication of irritation or inflammation somewhere in the abdominal cavity. Use the following technique in all four quadrants.

- Apply firm pressure for 4 seconds with the hand at a 90° angle and with the fingers extended.
- After releasing the pressure, observe the client's response to see if releasing the pressure caused pain.
- Ask about pain and tenderness.
- Never palpate an abdominal mass, tender organs, or surgical incisions deeply.

For all systems in this chapter

EXPECTED CHANGES WITH AGING

Breasts

- With menopause, glandular tissue atrophies. Adipose tissue replaces it, making it feel softer and more pendulous. The atrophied ducts can feel like thin strands.
- Nipples no longer have erectile ability and can invert.

Lungs

- Chest shape changes so that the AP diameter becomes similar to the transverse diameter (barrel chest), resulting in decreased vital capacity.
- Chest excursion or expansion diminishes.
- Cough reflex diminishes.
- Cilia ineffectively removes dust and irritants from the airways.
- Alveoli dwindle, airway resistance increases, and the risk of pulmonary infection increases.
- Kyphosis, an increased curvature of the thoracic spine due to osteoporosis and weakened cartilage, results in vertebral collapse and impairment of respiratory effort.

Cardiovascular system

- Systolic hypertension (widened pulse pressure) is a common finding with atherosclerosis.
- The PMI becomes more difficult to palpate because the AP diameter of the chest widens.
- Coronary blood vessel walls thicken and become more rigid with a narrowed lumen.
- Cardiac output decreases and strength of contraction leads to poor activity tolerance.
- Heart valves stiffen due to calcification.
- The left ventricle thickens.
- Pulmonary vascular tension increases.
- Systolic blood pressure rises.
- Peripheral circulation diminishes.

Abdomen

- Weaker abdominal muscles declining in tone and more adipose tissue result in a rounder, more protruding abdomen.
- Peritoneal inflammation is more difficult to detect due to less pain, guarding, fever, and rebound tenderness.
- Saliva, gastric secretions, and pancreatic enzymes decrease.
- Esophageal peristalsis and small-intestine motility decrease.

SAMPLE DOCUMENTATION

Breasts conical, symmetric in size, and without masses or lesions. Nipples and areolae darker pigmented and symmetric. Everted nipples without discharge. No palpable axillary or clavicular lymph nodes. No pain or tenderness.

Respiratory rate 16/min and regular. Respirations easy and unlabored. Thorax has a greater transverse than AP diameter. No chest wall deformities. Trachea midline. Movement symmetric with 5 cm of expansion. Equal tactile fremitus. Resonant sounds throughout. Vesicular sounds primarily over the bases bilaterally. No adventitious sounds. No cough, shortness of breath, difficulty breathing.

Heart rhythm and rate regular at 72/min. Blood pressure 118/76 mm Hg. No thrills or heaves. PMI approximately 1 cm at the fifth ICS left midclavicular line. S1 louder at the apex than S2. S2 loudest in the pulmonary area on inspiration. No extra heart sounds, murmurs, or bruits. JVP 2 cm bilaterally. No chest pain or discomfort.

Abdomen flat with active bowel sounds every 10 to 20 seconds in all four quadrants. No bruits or friction rubs. Abdomen soft, nontender, and without masses or enlargement of spleen or liver. Liver span 8 cm. No rebound or costovertebral tenderness. Bladder not palpable. No pain or discomfort in abdominal region.

Application Exercises

1. A nurse in a provider's office is preparing to perform a breast examination for an older adult client who is postmenopausal. Which of the following findings should the nurse expect? (Select all that apply.)

   A. Smaller nipples

   B. Less adipose tissue

   C. Nipple discharge

   D. More pendulous

   E. Nipple inversion

2. A nurse in a provider's office is preparing to auscultate and percuss a client's thorax as part of a comprehensive physical examination. Which of the following findings should the nurse expect? (Select all that apply.)

   A. Rhonchi

   B. Crackles

   C. Resonance

   D. Tactile fremitus

   E. Bronchovesicular sounds

3. During an abdominal examination, a nurse in a provider's office determines that a client has abdominal distention. The protrusion is at midline, the skin over the area is taut, and the nurse notes no involvement of the flanks. Which of the following possible causes of distention should the nurse suspect?

   A. Fat

   B. Fluid

   C. Flatus

   D. Hernias

4. During a cardiovascular examination, a nurse in a provider's office places the diaphragm of the stethoscope on the left midclavicular line at the fifth intercostal space. Which of the following heart sounds is the nurse attempting to auscultate? (Select all that apply.)

   A. Ventricular gallop

   B. Closure of the mitral valve

   C. Closure of the pulmonic valve

   D. Closure of the tricuspid valve

   E. Murmur

5. A nurse in a provider's office is preparing to auscultate and percuss a client's abdomen as part of a comprehensive physical examination. Which of the following findings should the nurse expect? (Select all that apply.)

   A. Tympany

   B. High-pitched clicks

   C. Borborygmi

   D. Friction rubs

   E. Bruits

PRACTICE Active Learning Scenario

A nurse is teaching a group of newly licensed nurses about identifying chest landmarks to help them find the optimal locations for auscultation of the thorax. Use the ATI Active Learning Template: Basic Concept to complete this item.

UNDERLYING PRINCIPLES: List the seven key chest landmarks, along with their location on the thorax.

Application Exercises Key

1. A. **CORRECT:** In older adulthood, the nipples become smaller and flatter.

   B. Older adults have more adipose tissue and less glandular tissue in their breasts.

   C. Older adults have no nipple discharge, unless there is some underlying pathophysiology.

   D. **CORRECT:** In older adulthood, breasts become softer and more pendulous.

   E. **CORRECT:** Nipple inversion is common among older adults, due to fibrotic changes and shrinkage.

   Ⓝ *NCLEX® Connection: Physiological Adaptation, Pathophysiology*

2. A. Rhonchi are coarse sounds that result from fluid or mucus in the airways.

   B. Crackles are fine to coarse popping sounds that result from air passing through fluid or re-expanding collapsed small airways.

   C. **CORRECT:** Resonance is the expected percussion sound over the thorax. It is a hollow sound that indicates air inside the lungs.

   D. Tactile fremitus is an expected vibration the nurse can expect to feel or palpate as the client vocalizes. Speech creates sound waves, the vibrations of which travel from the vocal cords through the lungs and to the chest wall.

   E. **CORRECT:** Bronchovesicular sounds are expected breath sounds of medium pitch and intensity and of equal inspiration and expiration time. The nurse can expect to hear them over the larger airways.

   Ⓝ *NCLEX® Connection: Physiological Adaptation, Pathophysiology*

3. A. With fat, there are rolls of adipose tissue along the sides, and the skin does not look taut.

   B. With fluid, the flanks also protrude, and when the client turns onto one side, the protrusion moves to the dependent side.

   C. **CORRECT:** With flatus, the protrusion is mainly midline, and there is no change in the flanks.

   D. With hernias, protrusions through the abdominal muscle wall are visible, especially when the client raises her head.

   Ⓝ *NCLEX® Connection: Physiological Adaptation, Pathophysiology*

4. A. To auscultate a ventricular gallop (an S3 sound), the nurse places the bell of the stethoscope at each of the auscultatory sites.

   B. **CORRECT:** To auscultate the closure of the mitral valve, the nurse places the diaphragm of the stethoscope over the apex, or apical/mitral site, which is on the left midclavicular line at the fifth intercostal space.

   C. To auscultate the closure of the pulmonic valve, the nurse places the diaphragm of the stethoscope over the aortic area, which is just to the right of the sternum at the second intercostal space.

   D. **CORRECT:** To auscultate the closure of the tricuspid valve, the nurse places the diaphragm of the stethoscope over the apex, or apical/mitral site, which is on the left midclavicular line at the fifth intercostal space.

   E. To auscultate a murmur, the nurse places the bell of the stethoscope at various auscultatory sites.

   Ⓝ *NCLEX® Connection: Physiological Adaptation, Pathophysiology*

5. A. **CORRECT:** Tympany is the expected drumlike percussion sound over the abdomen. It indicates air in the stomach.

   B. **CORRECT:** Typical bowel sounds are high-pitched clicks and gurgles occurring about 35 times/min.

   C. Borborygmi are unexpected loud, growling sounds that indicate increased gastrointestinal motility. Possible causes include diarrhea, anxiety, bowel inflammation, and reactions to some foods.

   D. Friction rubs result from the rubbing together of inflamed layers of the peritoneum and are unexpected findings.

   E. Bruits indicate narrowed blood vessels and are unexpected findings.

   Ⓝ *NCLEX® Connection: Physiological Adaptation, Pathophysiology*

PRACTICE Answer

Using the ATI Active Learning Template: Basic Concept

UNDERLYING PRINCIPLES
- Midsternal line: through the center of the sternum
- Midclavicular line: through the midpoint of the clavicle
- Anterior axillary line: through the anterior axillary folds
- Midaxillary line: through the apex of the axillae
- Posterior axillary line: through the posterior axillary fold
- Right and left scapular lines: through the inferior angle of the scapula
- Vertebral line: along the center of the spine

Ⓝ *NCLEX® Connection: Health Promotion and Maintenance, Techniques of Physical Assessment*

UNIT 2 HEALTH PROMOTION
SECTION: HEALTH ASSESSMENT/DATA COLLECTION

CHAPTER 30 *Integumentary and Peripheral Vascular Systems*

Assess the integumentary (skin, hair, scalp, and nails) and peripheral vascular systems at the same time.

First, examine the upper extremities while the client is sitting or recumbent. Then remove stockings/socks, and drape the client to expose the entire lower extremity at once. Make side-to-side comparisons to evaluate for variations of symmetry. Examine lesions individually. Use the Braden scale or a similar assessment tool to predict pressure-ulcer risk. Inspect and palpate simultaneously. Q̲EBP

Equipment includes adequate lighting, gloves for palpating open or draining lesions, a flexible ruler or tape measure to measure the size and depth of lesions in centimeters, and a gown or drape to cover the client.

HEALTH HISTORY: REVIEW OF SYSTEMS

QUESTIONS TO ASK
- Have you noticed any change in your skin color? If so, is the change widespread or just in one area?
- Do you have a rash? Where? Does it itch? How long have you had it? What have you used to treat the rash?
- Is your skin excessively dry or oily? Does this change with the seasons? Do you use anything to treat it?
- Have you developed any new moles or lesions? Have any of the moles or lesions changed in any way (color, borders, size)?
- How often are you out in the sun? Do you use sunscreen or wear protective clothing and a hat?
- Do you have any swelling? If in your legs, is it in both legs? Does the swelling cause pain? What do you do to relieve the swelling? Does it occur at any particular time of day?

INSPECTION AND PALPATION

Hair, skin, and nails

- Assess the color of the hair, nails, and skin for uniformity. Hair color can vary due to dyes or from aging changes. Typically, skin color varies from ivory to ruddy to deep brown. Color changes are more difficult to notice in dark-skinned clients.
  - **Pallor:** loss of color
    - LOCATION: face, conjunctivae, nail beds, palms, lips, buccal mucosa
    - INDICATION: Anemia, shock, or lack of blood flow
  - **Cyanosis:** bluish
    - LOCATION: nail beds, lips, mouth mucosa, skin, palms
    - INDICATION: Hypoxia or impaired venous return
  - **Jaundice:** yellow to orange
    - LOCATION: skin, sclera, mucous membranes
    - INDICATION: Liver dysfunction, red blood–cell destruction
  - **Erythema:** redness
    - LOCATION: face, skin, trauma and pressure sore areas
    - INDICATION: Inflammation, localized vasodilation, substance use, sun exposure, rash, elevated body temperature
- Note cleanliness of the hair, skin, and nails, as well as any odors.
- Expect firm nail bases and nail angles to be approximately 160°. Note the curvature of the nail plate in relationship to the tissue just before the cuticle.
  - Clubbing, an angle of the nail greater than 160°, can result from chronic low oxygen saturation related to heart and lung disease (emphysema, chronic bronchitis). (The angle of the nail and base can eventually exceed 180°.)
- Expect pink, symmetric nail beds. Capillary refill assesses circulation to the periphery. Assess capillary refill by applying firm pressure to the nail bed to blanch it. Quick release of the pressure should result in a brisk return of color (within 3 seconds).
- Expect even hair distribution patterns and symmetric hair loss, as with male pattern baldness. Note any infestations of the hair or skin. Alopecia can result from endocrine disorders and poor nutrition.
- Expect skin color of the extremities to be symmetric and similar to the rest of the body.
  - Brown pigmentation changes with venous insufficiency.
  - Shiny and translucent skin without hair on the toes and foot indicates arterial insufficiency.
- Palpate the temperature of the skin with the dorsal part of the hand and assess for symmetry of temperature, and expect warmth. Note changes reflecting circulation impairment or environmental temperature. Slightly cooler temperatures of the hands or feet are acceptable.
- Expect smooth, soft, even skin. Hair can be smooth, coarse, or fine. Thicker skin of the palms and soles of the feet is an expected finding.

- Assess skin turgor by lifting and releasing a fold of skin on the forearm or sternum to verify that it returns quickly into place. Tenting is a delay in the skin returning to its usual place. Poor turgor indicates dehydration or aging, increasing the risk for skin breakdown.
- Moisture in the axillae is an expected finding. Otherwise, the skin should be dry. Note diaphoresis, oiliness, or excessive dryness with flaking or scaling.

Peripheral arteries

- Palpate the peripheral pulses for strength (amplitude) and equality (symmetry).
  - **Strength (amplitude):** The same from beat to beat
  - Grade strength as
    - 0 = Absent, unable to palpate
    - 1+ = Diminished, weaker than expected
    - 2+ = Brisk, expected
    - 3+ = Increased
    - 4+ = Full volume, bounding
  - **Equality:** Symmetric in quality and quantity from the right side of the body to the left
- With the exception of the carotid arteries, palpate pulse sites bilaterally to make comparisons.
  - **Carotid pulse:** On either side of the trachea, just medial to the sternocleidomastoid muscle on the neck
  - **Radial pulse:** On the radial (or thumb) side of each wrist
  - **Brachial pulse:** In the antecubital fossa above the elbow
  - **Femoral pulse:** Midway between the symphysis pubis and the anterosuperior iliac spine
  - **Popliteal pulse:** Behind the knee, deep in the popliteal fossa, just lateral to midline
  - **Dorsalis pedis pulse:** On the top of the foot, along a line with the groove between the first toe and the extensor tendons of the great toe
  - **Posterior tibial pulse:** Behind and below the medial malleolus of the ankles
- Inspect peripheral veins for varicosities, redness, and swelling.

Edema

Edema is an accumulation of fluid in the tissues most often from direct trauma or impaired venous return. The presence of edema causes swelling with the skin appearing shiny and tight.

- Assess the swelling for discoloration, location, and tenderness. In the extremities, measure the circumference of the swollen body area and compare both sides.
- Evaluate pitting by compressing the skin for at least 5 seconds over a bony prominence (behind the medial malleolus, the dorsum of foot, or over the shin) and then assess. The depth of pitting reflects the degree of edema.
  - 1+ = Trace, 2 mm, rapid skin response
  - 2+ = Mild, 4 mm, 10- to 15-second skin response
  - 3+ = Moderate, 6 mm, prolonged skin response
  - 4+ = Severe, 8 mm, prolonged skin response

Lesions

Examine skin lesions for size, color, shape, consistency, elevation, location, distribution, configuration, tenderness, fluid, and drainage. Measure the height, width, and depth of lesions. Observe a lesion for any odor, exudate, the amount and consistency of the exudate and document.

Primary lesions arise from healthy skin tissue. Common examples include the following.
- **Macule**
  - Nonpalpable, skin color change, smaller than 1 cm
  - EXAMPLES: Freckle, petechiae
- **Papule**
  - Palpable, circumscribed, solid elevation of skin, smaller than 1 cm
  - EXAMPLE: Elevated nevus
- **Nodule**
  - Palpable, circumscribed, deep, firm, 1 to 2 cm
  - EXAMPLE: Wart
- **Vesicle**
  - Serous fluid-filled, smaller than 1 cm
  - EXAMPLES: Blister, herpes simplex, varicella
- **Pustule**
  - Pus-filled, varies in size
  - EXAMPLE: Acne
- **Tumor**
  - Solid mass, deep, larger than 1 to 2 cm
  - EXAMPLE: Epithelioma
- **Wheal**
  - Palpable, irregular borders, edematous
  - EXAMPLE: Insect bite
- **Atrophy**
  - Thinning of skin with loss of normal skin furrow. Skin is shiny and translucent
  - EXAMPLE: Arterial insufficiency

Secondary lesions result from a change in a primary lesion. Common examples include the following.
- **Erosion**
  - Lost epidermis, moist surface, no bleeding
  - EXAMPLE: Ruptured vesicle
- **Crust**
  - Dried blood, serum, or pus
  - EXAMPLE: Scab
- **Scale**
  - Flakes of skin that exfoliate
  - EXAMPLES: Dandruff, psoriasis, eczema
- **Fissure**
  - Linear crack
  - EXAMPLE: Tinea pedis
- **Ulcer**
  - Loss of epidermis and dermis with possible bleeding, scarring
  - EXAMPLES: Venous stasis ulcer, pressure ulcer

Common examples of **skin lesions in various age groups** include the following.

- CHILDREN
  - Diaper dermatitis
  - Intertrigo
  - Impetigo
  - Atopic dermatitis (eczema)
- ADULTS
  - Primary contact dermatitis
  - Tinea pedis (ringworm of the foot)
  - Psoriasis
  - Labial herpes simplex (cold sores)
- OLDER ADULTS Ⓒ
  - Lentigines (liver spots)
  - Seborrheic keratosis
  - Acrochordons (skin tags)
  - Sebaceous hyperplasia

Vascular lesions result from aging changes or blood-vessel damage in or near the skin. Common examples include the following.

- **Spider angioma:** Red center with radiating red legs, up to 2 cm, possibly raised
- **Cherry angioma:** Red, 1 to 3 cm, round, possibly raised
- **Spider vein:** Bluish, spider-shaped or linear, up to several inches in size
- **Petechiae/purpura:** Deep reddish purple, flat, petechiae 1 to 3 mm, purpura larger than 3 mm
- **Ecchymosis:** Purple fading to green or yellow over time, variable in size, flat
- **Hematoma:** Raised ecchymosis

EXPECTED CHANGES WITH AGING

Integumentary system

- Skin thin and translucent, dry, flaky, tears easily, loss of elasticity and wrinkling
- Thinning of hair
- Slow growth of nails with thickening
- Decline in glandular structure and function (less oil, moisture, sweat)
- Uneven pigmentation
- Slow wound healing
- Little subcutaneous tissue over bony prominences

Peripheral vascular system

- Thicker, more rigid peripheral blood vessel walls with a narrowed lumen leading to poor peripheral circulation
- Higher systolic blood pressure

SAMPLE DOCUMENTATION

Skin pink, warm, and dry. Turgor brisk, skin elastic. Rough, thickened skin over heels, elbows, and knees; otherwise, smooth. A 0.5 cm brown papule on right forearm and a 2.5 cm scar on left knee. Scalp dry with slight dandruff. Hair brown, clean, smooth, straight, evenly distributed on the head. Axillary and pubic hair evenly distributed with no infestations. Nails short and firm with no clubbing. Capillary refill < 3 seconds. No edema. Pulses palpable, 2+, and equal bilaterally.

Application Exercises

1. A nurse in a provider's office is preparing to assess a client's skin as part of a comprehensive physical examination. Which of the following findings should the nurse expect? (Select all that apply.)

   A. Capillary refill less than 3 seconds
   B. 1+ pitting edema in both feet
   C. Pale nail beds in both hands
   D. Thick skin on the soles of the feet
   E. Numerous light brown macules on the face

2. A nurse is assessing an older adult client who has significant tenting of the skin over his forearm. Which of the following factors should the nurse consider as a cause for this finding? (Select all that apply.)

   A. Thin, parchment-like skin
   B. Loss of adipose tissue
   C. Dehydration
   D. Diminished skin elasticity
   E. Excessive wrinkling

3. A nurse is assessing postoperative circulation of the lower extremities for a client who had knee surgery. The nurse should include which of the following? (Select all that apply.)

   A. Range of motion
   B. Skin color
   C. Edema
   D. Skin lesions
   E. Skin temperature

4. A nurse is performing skin assessments on a group of clients. Which of the following lesions should the nurse identify as vesicles? (Select all that apply.)

   A. Acne
   B. Warts
   C. Psoriasis
   D. Herpes simplex
   E. Varicella

5. A nurse is performing an integumentary assessment for a group of clients. Which of the following findings should the nurse recognize as requiring immediate intervention?

   A. Pallor
   B. Cyanosis
   C. Jaundice
   D. Erythema

Application Exercises Key

1. A. **CORRECT:** The nurse should expect capillary refill in less than 3 seconds as an expected finding.

   B. The nurse should not expect pitting edema, which can reflect excess fluid that has accumulated in body tissues.

   C. The nurse should not expect pallor in the nail beds, which can reflect anemia or impaired circulation.

   D. **CORRECT:** The nurse should expect thicker skin on the palms of the hands and the soles of the client's feet.

   E. **CORRECT:** The nurse should expect light brown macules on the face, such as freckles, .

   Ⓝ *NCLEX® Connection: Physiological Adaptation, Pathophysiology*

2. A. The older adult client as aging occurs will have skin that becomes thin and translucent and is not a factor for tenting of the skin.

   B. **CORRECT:** Tenting is a delay in the skin returning to its normal place after pinching. Tenting is a manifestation of aging skin and loss of subcutaneous tissue that provides recoil in younger skin.

   C. **CORRECT:** Tenting is a delay in the skin returning to its normal place after pinching. Dehydration can cause the skin to tent, which can easily develop in the older adult client.

   D. **CORRECT:** Tenting is a delay in the skin returning to its normal place after pinching. Tenting in the older adult client is a manifestation of aging skin and loss of elasticity.

   E. The older adult client who has aging skin does become wrinkled, but is not a factor for tenting of the skin

   Ⓝ *NCLEX® Connection: Physiological Adaptation, Pathophysiology*

3. A. Determining range of motion helps the nurse evaluate joint function, not circulation.

   B. **CORRECT:** The nurse should assess the peripheral vascular system to verify adequate circulation to the client's legs, which includes skin color. Pallor and cyanosis reflect inadequate circulation.

   C. **CORRECT:** The nurse should assess the peripheral vascular system to verify adequate circulation to the client's legs, which includes edema. Edema reflects inadequate venous circulation.

   D. Inspecting for skin lesions is part of an integumentary assessment, but it does not evaluate circulation. Some skin lesions do reflect inadequate circulation, but they would not have developed in the immediate postoperative period.

   E. **CORRECT:** The nurse should assess the peripheral vascular system to verify adequate circulation to the client's legs, which includes skin temperature. Coolness of the extremity compared with the nonoperative extremity indicates inadequate circulation.

   Ⓝ *NCLEX® Connection: Physiological Adaptation, Illness Management*

4. A. Acne lesions are pustules, not vesicles.

   B. Warts are nodules, not vesicles.

   C. Psoriasis lesions are scales, not vesicles.

   D. **CORRECT:** Herpes simplex lesions are vesicles, which are circumscribed fluid-filled skin elevations. Eczema and impetigo also cause vesicles to appear on the skin.

   E. **CORRECT:** Varicella (chickenpox) lesions are vesicles, which are circumscribed fluid-filled skin elevations. Eczema and impetigo also cause vesicles to appear on the skin.

   Ⓝ *NCLEX® Connection: Physiological Adaptation, Pathophysiology*

5. A. The nurse should report pallor, which can indicate anemia or circulation difficulties. However, another assessment finding is the priority.

   B. **CORRECT:** The priority finding when using the airway, breathing, circulation (ABC) approach to care is cyanosis, which an indication of hypoxia (inadequate oxygenation). Therefore, the nurse should immediately report this finding to the provider.

   C. The nurse should report jaundice, which can indicate liver dysfunction or red blood cell destruction. However, another assessment finding is the priority.

   D. The nurse should report erythema, which can indicate inflammation. However, another assessment finding is the priority.

   Ⓝ *NCLEX® Connection: Physiological Adaptation, Illness Management*

PRACTICE Active Learning Scenario

A nurse is reviewing the questions to ask when interviewing clients as part of an integumentary and peripheral vascular assessment. Use the ATI Active Learning Template: Basic Concept to complete this item.

NURSING INTERVENTIONS: Identify at least five questions to ask prior to beginning the inspection and palpation portions of the assessment.

PRACTICE Answer

Using the ATI Active Learning Template: Basic Concept

NURSING INTERVENTIONS

- Have you noticed any changes in your skin color? If so, is the change widespread or just in one area?
- Do you have a rash? Where? Does it itch? How long have you had it? What have you used to treat the rash?
- Is your skin excessively dry or oily? Does this change with the seasons? Do you use anything to treat it?
- Have you developed any new moles or lesions? Have any of the moles or lesions changed in any way (color, borders, size)?
- How often are you out in the sun? Do you use sunscreen or wear protective clothing and a hat?
- Do you have any swelling? If in your legs, is it in both legs? Does the swelling cause pain? What do you do to relieve the swelling? Does it occur at any particular time of day?

Ⓝ *NCLEX® Connection: Reduction of Risk Potential, System Specific Assessments*

CHAPTER 31 *Musculoskeletal and Neurosensory Systems*

This examination includes muscles, joints, range of motion, mental status, cranial nerves, and motor and sensory function.

Musculoskeletal system

- Examination of the musculoskeletal system includes assessing both its structure and function.
- Assessment involves examining each joint, muscle, and the surrounding tissues bilaterally and comparing findings for symmetry.
- Use the techniques of inspection and palpation to assess the musculoskeletal system.

EQUIPMENT
- Tape measure
- Drape or cover for privacy

ASSESS
- **Gait:** Manner or style of walking
- **Alignment:** Position of the joints, tendons, muscles, and ligaments while sitting, standing and lying
- **Symmetry, muscle mass**
- **Muscle tone:** Normal state of balanced muscle tension allowing one to maintain positions such as sitting or standing
- **Range of motion (ROM):** Maximum amount of movement of a joint – sagittal (left or right), transverse (side to side) and frontal (front to back).
- **Any involuntary movements**
- **Indications of inflammation:** Redness, swelling, warmth, tenderness, loss of function
- **Gross deformities**

EXPECTED RANGE OF MOTION OF JOINT MOVEMENT
- **Flexion:** Movement that decreases the angle between two adjacent bones
- **Extension:** Movement that increases the angle between two adjacent bones
- **Hyperextension:** Movement of a body part beyond its normal extended position
- **Supination:** Movement of a body part so the ventral (front) surface faces up
- **Pronation:** Movement of a body part so the ventral (front) surface faces down
- **Abduction:** Movement of an extremity away from the midline of the body
- **Adduction:** Movement of an extremity toward the midline of the body
- **Dorsiflexion:** Flexing the foot and toes upward
- **Plantar flexion:** Bending the foot and toes downward
- **Eversion:** Turning a body part away from midline
- **Inversion:** Turning a body part toward the midline
- **External rotation:** Rotating a joint outward
- **Internal rotation:** Rotating a joint inward

HEALTH HISTORY: REVIEW OF SYSTEMS

QUESTIONS TO ASK
- Do you have any pain in your joints or muscles?
- Do you have any stiffness, weakness, or twitching?
- Have you fallen recently?
- Are you able to care for yourself?
- Do you have any physical problems that limit your activities?
- Do you exercise or participate in sports on a regular basis?
- For postmenopausal women: What was your maximum height? Do you take calcium supplements?

INSPECTION

SYMMETRY: Observe and compare both sides of the body for symmetry.

HEIGHT: Measure for comparison over time. Gradual height loss is a common finding as a person ages. Ⓖ

POSTURE: Observe when the client is unaware. Expected finding: client standing with head erect with both shoulders and hips at equal heights bilaterally.

SPINE: Inspect from the side. Note the following curvatures:

Expected curvatures (posteriorly)
- Concave cervical spine
- Convex thoracic spine
- Concave lumbar spine
- Convex sacral spine

UNEXPECTED FINDINGS
- Kyphosis: exaggerated curvature of the thoracic spine (common among older adults) Ⓖ
- Lordosis: exaggerated curvature of the lumbar spine (common during the toddler years and pregnancy)
- Scoliosis: exaggerated lateral curvature

INSPECTION AND PALPATION

Expect equal range of motion (ROM) in the joints bilaterally.
- Assess passive ROM by moving the client's joints through his full range of movements. Do not move a joint past the point of pain or resistance. Qs
- Assess active ROM by having the client repeat the movements the nurse demonstrates.
- Assess joints for warmth, inflammation, edema, stiffness, crepitus, deformities, tenderness, limitations, and instability. Assess the following joints.
  - Temporomandibular joint
  - Shoulders
  - Elbows
  - Wrists and hands
  - Spine (scoliosis)
  - Hips
  - Knees
  - Ankles, feet

Muscles should be firm, symmetric, and have equal strength bilaterally. The dominant side is usually slightly larger; less than a 1 cm difference is not significant.
- Size variations
  - **Hypertrophy:** Enlargement of muscle due to strengthening
  - **Atrophy:** Decrease in muscle size due to disuse; feels soft and boggy
- During ROM, assess tone: slight resistance of the muscles during relaxation.
- Assess the strength of muscle groups by asking the client to push or pull against resistance. Expected finding: strength equal, or slightly stronger, on the dominant side of the body.
- Assess for muscle tremors.

Inspect and palpate the spine from the back for any lateral deviations or scoliosis.
- Instruct the client to bend at the waist with the arms reaching for the toes.
- Inspect and palpate down the spine using the thumb and forefinger.
- Inspect and palpate the spine again with the client standing.
- Expected finding: No tenderness, with spinal vertebrae that are midline.

Neurosensory system

- A neurological screening examination can evaluate the major indicators of neurological function and assist with recognition of areas of dysfunction.
- Integrate the neurological system with other assessments.

EXAMINATION COMPONENTS
- Mental status examination to test cerebral function
- Assessment of cranial nerves
- Motor function to test cerebellar function
- Sensory function
- Reflexes

EQUIPMENT
- Snellen and Rosenbaum eye charts
- Aromatic substances
- Tongue blades
- Penlight
- Sugar and salt
- Tuning fork
- Reflex hammer
- Cotton balls
- Two test tubes containing water (one cold, one warm)
- Pencil
- Paper clips
- Key

HEALTH HISTORY: REVIEW OF SYSTEMS

QUESTIONS TO ASK
- Do you have any dizziness or headaches?
- Do you ever have seizures? If so, what triggers them?
- Have you ever had a head injury or any loss of consciousness?
- Have you noticed any change in your vision, speech, ability to think clearly, loss of memory, or change in memory or behavior?
- Do you have any weakness, numbness, tremors, or tingling? If so, where?

INSPECTION

Mental status

- Describe levels of consciousness and observed behavior with the following terms.
  - **Alert:** The client is responsive and able to open his eyes and answer questions spontaneously and appropriately.
  - **Lethargic:** The client is able to open his eyes and respond but is drowsy and falls asleep readily.
  - **Obtunded:** The client responds to light shaking but can be confused and slow to respond.
  - **Stuporous:** The client requires painful stimuli (pinching a tendon or rubbing the sternum) to achieve a brief response. The client might not be able to respond verbally.
  - **Comatose:** There is no response to repeated painful stimuli. Abnormal posturing in clients who are comatose:
    - **Decorticate rigidity:** Flexion and internal rotation of upper extremity joints and legs
    - **Decerebrate rigidity:** Neck and elbow extension, with the wrists and fingers flexed
- Assess appearance by observing hygiene, grooming, and clothing choice. EXPECTED FINDINGS: client is clean and dressed appropriately for the environment or situation.
- Assess mood by inspecting mannerisms and actions during interactions. EXPECTED FINDINGS: client makes eye contact, and emotions correspond to the conversation and situation.

- Assess cognitive and intellectual processes:
  - Assess memory, both recent and remote.
    - Recent: Ask the client to repeat a series of numbers or a list of objects.
    - Remote: Ask the client to state his birth date or mother's maiden name (verifiable).
  - **Level of knowledge:** Ask the client what he knows about his current hospitalization or illness.
  - **Ability for calculation:** Ask the client to count backward from 100 in serials of 7.
  - **Abstract thinking:** Ask the client the interpretation of a cliché such as, "A bird in the hand is worth two in the bush." This demonstrates a higher level of thought processes.
  - **Insight:** Perform an objective assessment of the client's perception of illness.
  - **Judgment:** Ask the client about the solution to a specific dilemma. ("What would you do if you locked your keys in your car?")
  - **Thought process:** Note processing differences, such as a rapid change of topic (flight of ideas) and use of nonsense words ("hipsnippity").
  - **Thought content:** Note the presence of delusions, hallucinations, and other ideas the client presents during the interview.
- Expect speech and language rate and features, such as quality, quantity, and volume, to be articulate and responses meaningful and appropriate.

31.1 Cranial nerve functions

EARS, NOSE, MOUTH, AND THROAT	EYES	HEAD AND NECK	NEURO-LOGICAL		
✓				I (Olfactory)	SENSORY: smell
	✓			II (Optic)	SENSORY: visual acuity, visual fields
	✓			III (Oculomotor), IV (Trochlear), and VI (Abducens)	MOTOR: PERRLA, six cardinal positions of gaze
		✓		V (Trigeminal)	SENSORY: light touch sensation to the face (forehead, cheek, jaw) MOTOR: jaw opening, clenching, chewing
		✓		VII (Facial)	SENSORY: taste (salt/sweet) on anterior two thirds of the tongue MOTOR: facial movements
✓				VIII (Auditory)	SENSORY: hearing and balance
✓			✓	IX (Glossopharyngeal)	SENSORY: taste (sour/bitter) on posterior third of the tongue MOTOR: swallowing, speech sounds, gag reflex
✓				X (Vagus)	SENSORY: gag reflex MOTOR: swallowing, speech sounds
		✓		XI (Spinal accessory)	MOTOR: turning head, shrugging shoulders
✓				XII (Hypoglossal)	MOTOR: tongue movement

STANDARDIZED SCREENING TOOLS

- Use the Mini-Mental State Examination to assess cognitive status objectively. The tool evaluates:
  - Orientation to time and place
  - Attention and calculation of counting backward by sevens
  - Registration and recalling of objects
  - Language, including naming of objects, following of commands, and ability to write
  - Reading
- Use the Glasgow Coma Scale to obtain a baseline assessment of the client's level of consciousness and for ongoing assessment. Q EBP
  - This assessment looks at eye, verbal, and motor response, and assigns a number value based on the client's response.
  - The highest value possible is 15, indicating full consciousness.

Motor function

- Assess coordination by asking the client to extend his arms and rapidly touch his finger to his nose, alternating hands, and then doing it with his eyes closed. EXPECTED FINDINGS include smooth, coordinated movements.
- Assess gait when the client is unaware of the assessment. EXPECTED FINDING: Gait is steady, smooth, and coordinated.
- Assess balance using the following tests.
  - **Romberg test:** Ask the client to stand with his feet together, his arms at his sides, and his eyes closed. EXPECTED FINDING: The client stands with minimal swaying for at least 5 seconds.
  - **Heel-to-toe walk:** Ask the client to place the heel of one foot in front of the toes of the other foot as he walks in a straight line. EXPECTED FINDING: The client walks in a straight line without losing his balance.
- Muscle strength: Assess the strength of muscle groups by asking the client to push or pull against resistance. EXPECTED FINDING: Strength is equal or slightly stronger on the dominant side of the body.

Sensory function

Perform tests on all four extremities with the client's eyes closed.

- Assess pain sensation by alternating sharp and dull objects on the skin and asking the client to report what he feels.
- Assess temperature by using two test tubes containing water (one warm and one cold), and ask the client to identify which he feels.
- Assess light touch by asking the client to report when and where he feels a cotton ball touching his skin.
- Assess vibration by having the client report when and where he feels the handle of the vibrating tuning fork on his skin.

- Assess position by repositioning the client's appendages and asking him to report whether each is positioned up or down.
- Assess discrimination by using one of the following.
  - **Two-point discrimination:** Use open paper clips to determine the smallest distance between the two points at which the client can still feel the two points on his skin and not just one. Compare bilaterally. Minimal distance varies with the body part.
  - **Stereognosis:** Place a familiar object (key, cotton ball) in the client's hand, and ask him to identify it.
  - **Graphesthesia:** Trace a number on the client's palm with the blunt end of a pencil and ask him to identify it.

Deep-tendon reflexes (DTRs)

Using a reflex hammer, assess DTRs bilaterally and compare results for symmetry.

Biceps
- Flex arm 45°.
- Place the thumb on the tendon in antecubital fossa.
- Strike the thumb with a reflex hammer.
- EXPECTED RESPONSE: Flexion of the elbow

Brachioradialis
- Rest a forearm on the examiner's forearm with the wrist slightly pronated.
- Strike the tendon 2.5 to 5 cm above the wrist.
- EXPECTED RESPONSE: Pronation of the forearm and flexion of the elbow

Triceps
- Support the upper arm with the forearm hanging at a 90° angle.
- Strike the tendon above the elbow.
- EXPECTED RESPONSE: Extension of the elbow

Patellar
- With the upper leg supported and the lower leg dangling freely, strike the tendon below the knee.
- EXPECTED RESPONSE: Extension of the lower leg

Achilles
- Flex the knee, dorsiflex the foot, and strike the tendon above the heel.
- EXPECTED RESPONSE: Plantar flexion of the foot

Grade DTR responses as
- 4+ = Very brisk with clonus
- 3+ = More brisk than average
- 2+ = Expected
- 1+ = Diminished
- 0 = No response

EXPECTED CHANGES WITH AGING

Musculoskeletal system

- Reduced muscle mass
- Declines in speed, strength, resistance to fatigue, reaction time, coordination
- Osteoporosis (fragility of bones, loss of bone mass and height)
- Greater risk of fractures and vertebral compression
- Degenerative alterations in joints
- Limited range of motion
- Flexed elbows, hips, and knees
- Thinning intervertebral discs, kyphosis (with height loss), wider stance altering posture

Neurological system

- Some short–term memory decline
- Diminished/slowed reflex and motor responses, impulse transmission, and reaction times
- Altered vibration, position, hearing, vision, smell, and deep pain and temperature sensation
- Slower fine finger movement
- Decline in mental function probably related to less cognitive stimulation and solitude
- Fewer brain cells, smaller brain volume, deteriorating nerve cells, fewer neurotransmitters
- With infection, delirium more common than fever
- Greater risk of depression
- Impaired balance
- Decreased touch sensation

SAMPLE DOCUMENTATION

Full range of motion without pain in all joints and spine. No joint deformities, warmth, or swelling. Posture erect. Spine midline with expected cervical, thoracic, and lumbar curvatures. No scoliosis. Muscle strength equal and strong bilaterally.

Application Exercises

1. A nurse in a provider's office is preparing to assess a young adult male client's musculoskeletal system as part of a comprehensive physical examination. Which of the following findings should the nurse expect? (Select all that apply.)

   A. Concave thoracic spine posteriorly

   B. Exaggerated lumbar curvature

   C. Concave lumbar spine posteriorly

   D. Exaggerated thoracic curvature

   E. Muscles slightly larger on his dominant side

2. A nurse is assessing a client's neurosensory system. To evaluate stereognosis, the nurse should ask the client to close his eyes and identify which of the following items?

   A. A word she whispers 30 cm from his ear

   B. A number she traces on the palm of his hand

   C. The vibration of a tuning fork she places on his foot

   D. A familiar object she places in his hand

3. A nurse is caring for a client who reports pain with internal rotation of her right shoulder. This discomfort can affect the client's ability to perform which of the following activities?

   A. Mopping her floors

   B. Brushing the back of her hair

   C. Fastening her bra behind her back

   D. Reaching into a cabinet above her sink

4. A nurse is performing a neurosensory examination for a client. Which of the following assessments should the nurse perform to test the client's balance? (Select all that apply.)

   A. Romberg test

   B. Heel-to-toe walk

   C. Snellen test

   D. Spinal accessory function

   E. Rosenbaum test

5. A nurse is collecting data from an older adult client as part of a neurosensory examination. Which of the following findings should the nurse expect as changes associated with aging? (Select all that apply.)

   A. Slower light touch sensation

   B. Some vision and hearing decline

   C. Slower fine finger movement

   D. Some short-term memory decline

   E. Decreased risk of depression

Application Exercises Key

1. A. The nurse should expect the client to have a convex thoracic spine posteriorly.

   B. Although lordosis (an exaggerated lumbar curvature) is common among toddlers and pregnant women, the nurse should not expect this finding in a young adult male client.

   C. **CORRECT:** The nurse should expect the client to have a concave lumbar spine posteriorly.

   D. Although kyphosis (an exaggerated lumbar curvature) is common among older adults, the nurse should not expect this finding in a young adult client.

   E. **CORRECT:** The nurse should expect the client to have muscle size equal on both sides or slightly larger on the dominant side.

   Ⓝ *NCLEX® Connection: Physiological Adaptation, Pathophysiology*

2. A. Identifying a whispered word confirms that cranial nerve VIII is intact.

   B. Identifying a tracing on the palm confirms the client's sense of graphesthesia, which is the ability to use only the sensation of touch to recognize writing on the skin.

   C. Identifying the vibration of a tuning fork confirms the client's vibratory sense.

   D. **CORRECT:** Identifying a familiar object in the hand confirms the client's sense of stereognosis, which is tactile recognition.

   Ⓝ *NCLEX® Connection: Reduction of Risk Potential, System Specific Assessments*

3. A. The client who is mopping the floor requires flexion and extension of the shoulder.

   B. The client who is brushing the back of the hair requires external rotation of the shoulder.

   C. **CORRECT:** The client who is fastening a bra from behind requires internal rotation of the shoulder, so this activity will elicit pain.

   D. The client who is reaching for something up high requires external rotation of the shoulder.

   Ⓝ *NCLEX® Connection: Reduction of Risk Potential, System Specific Assessments*

4. A. **CORRECT:** For the Romberg test, the client stands with his eyes closed, arms at his side, and feet together. The nurse verifies balance if the client can stand with minimal swaying for at least 5 seconds.

   B. **CORRECT:** For the heel-to-toe walk, the client places the heel of one foot in front of the toes of the other foot as he walks in a straight line. The nurse verifies balance if the client can walk in a straight line without losing his balance.

   C. A Snellen eye chart tests visual acuity, not balance.

   D. Testing spinal accessory function verifies that cranial nerve XI is intact by asking the client to shrug his shoulders and turn his head against resistance.

   E. A Rosenbaum eye chart tests visual acuity, not balance.

   Ⓝ *NCLEX® Connection: Reduction of Risk Potential, Diagnostic Tests*

5. A. **CORRECT:** Touch sensation decreases for the client who is aging.

   B. **CORRECT:** Losses in vision, hearing, taste, and smell decline for the client who is aging.

   C. **CORRECT:** Fine finger movement slows, along with some reflex and motor responses for the client who is aging.

   D. **CORRECT:** Minimal decline in short-term memory is an expected finding for the client who is aging.

   E. The risk for depression typically increases for the client who is aging.

   Ⓝ *NCLEX® Connection: Health Promotion and Maintenance, Developmental Stages and Transitions*

PRACTICE Active Learning Scenario

A nurse is reviewing the expected range of motion of joint movement with a group of nursing students. What information should the nurse include in the review? Use the ATI Active Learning Template: Basic Concept to complete this item.

RELATED CONTENT: List the 13 common types of motion along with the actions that demonstrate them.

PRACTICE Answer

Using the ATI Active Learning Template: Basic Concept

RELATED CONTENT

- Flexion: a movement that decreases the angle between two adjacent bones
- Extension: a movement that increases the angle between two adjacent bones
- Hyperextension: movement of a body part beyond its normal extended position
- Supination: movement of a body part so the ventral (or front) surface faces up
- Pronation: movement of a body part so the ventral surface (or front) faces down
- Abduction: the movement of an extremity away from the midline of the body
- Adduction: the movement of an extremity toward the midline of the body
- Dorsiflexion: flexing the foot and toes upward
- Plantar flexion: bending the foot and toes downward
- Eversion: turning the body part away from midline
- Inversion: turning the body part toward the midline
- External rotation: rotating a joint outward
- Internal rotating: rotating a joint inward

Ⓝ *NCLEX® Connection: Physiological Adaptation, Pathophysiology*

When reviewing the following chapters, keep in mind the relevant topics and tasks of the NCLEX outline, in particular:

Client Needs: Psychosocial Integrity

COPING MECHANISMS: Assess client in coping with life changes and provide support.

CULTURAL AWARENESS/CULTURAL INFLUENCES ON HEALTH: Incorporate client cultural practice and beliefs when planning and providing care.

GRIEF AND LOSS: Assist the client in coping with suffering, grief, loss, dying, and bereavement.

END OF LIFE CARE: Identify end of life needs of the client.

RELIGIOUS AND SPIRITUAL INFLUENCES ON HEALTH: Identify the emotional problems of client or client needs that are related to religious/spiritual beliefs.

THERAPEUTIC COMMUNICATION
Allow time to communicate with the client.

Use therapeutic communication techniques to provide client support.

CHAPTER 32

CHAPTER 32 *Therapeutic Communication*

Communication is a complex process of sending, receiving, and comprehending messages between two or more people. It is a dynamic and ongoing process that creates a unique experience for the participants. When communication breaks down, the result can be workplace errors and the loss of professional credibility.

Communicating effectively is a skill that nurses must develop. Nurses use communication when providing care to demonstrate caring, establish therapeutic relationships, obtain and deliver information, and assist with changing behavior.

Therapeutic communication is foundational to the nurse-client relationship. Effective communication is key to ensuring clients' safety. Qs

BASIC COMMUNICATION

LEVELS OF BASIC COMMUNICATION

Intrapersonal communication: Communication within an individual. It is each person's "self-talk," the internal discussion when thinking but not outwardly verbalizing thoughts. It helps nurses assess clients and situations and think critically about them before communicating verbally.

Interpersonal communication: Communication between two people. This form of communication is the most common in nursing and requires an exchange of information with another individual. However, messages the receiver perceives can differ from what the sender intended.

Public communication: Communication within groups of people. Using this type of communication, many nurses teach, give community presentations, or write about nursing or health care topics and issues.

Transpersonal communication: Communication that addresses spiritual needs and provides interventions to meet these needs, such as prayer and meditation.

Small group communication: Communication within a group of people, often working toward a mutual goal, such as in committees, research teams, and support groups.

FUNCTIONAL COMPONENTS

Referent: The incentive or motivation for communication between two people

Sender: The person who initiates and transmits the message

Receiver: The person to whom the sender aims the message and who interprets the sender's message

Message: The verbal and nonverbal information the sender expresses and intends for the receiver

Channel: The method of transmitting and receiving a message (sight, hearing, touch, facial expression, body language)

Environment: The emotional and physical climate in which the communication takes place

Feedback: Can be verbal, nonverbal, positive, negative
- The message the receiver returns to the sender that indicates the receipt of the message
- An essential component of ongoing communication

Interpersonal variables: Factors that influence communication between the sender and the receiver, such as educational and developmental levels

METHODS OF COMMUNICATION

Verbal communication

Vocabulary
- These are the words that communicate a message the sender writes or speaks.
- Limited vocabulary or speaking another language can make it difficult for nurses to communicate with clients. Using medical or nursing jargon can decrease clients' understanding. Children and adolescents tend to use words differently than adults.

Credibility
- Trustworthiness and reliability of the individual. Nurses must be knowledgeable, consistent, honest, confident, and dependable.
- Lack of credibility creates a sense of uncertainty for clients.

Denotative and connotative meaning
- When communicating, participants must share meanings.
- Words that have multiple meanings can cause miscommunication if people interpret them differently.

Clarity and brevity
- The shortest, simplest communication is usually most effective.
- Long and complex communication can be difficult to understand.

Timing and relevance

- Knowing when to communicate makes the receiver more attentive to the message.
- When clients are uncomfortable or distracted, it can be difficult to convey the message.

Pacing

- The rate of speech can communicate a meaning the speaker did not intend.
- Speaking rapidly can suggest not having time for the clients.

Intonation

- The tone of voice can communicate a variety of feelings.
- Nurses communicate feelings such as acceptance, judgment, and dislike through their tone of voice.

Nonverbal communication

Nurses should be aware of how they communicate nonverbally and should determine the meaning of clients' nonverbal communication as well. Culture also affects interpretation. Attention to the following in both the communicator and the receiver is necessary. Q**PCC**

Appearance, posture, gait: Physical characteristics can convey professionalism. Body language and posture can demonstrate comfort and ease in the situation. The first impression is very important.

Facial expressions, eye contact, gestures: Facial expressions can reveal feelings that clients can easily misinterpret. Eye contact typically conveys interest and respect but varies with culture and situation. Gestures can enhance verbal communication or create their own messages.

Sounds: Crying or moaning can have multiple meanings, especially when other nonverbal communication accompanies it.

Territoriality, personal space: Lack of awareness of territoriality (right to space) and personal space (the area around an individual) can make clients perceive a threat and react defensively.

Electronic communication

Some facilities permit nurses to communicate with clients via email. An email encryption system is essential for assuring confidentiality. These facilities must also have guidelines that address when and how to use email and what information nurses may convey. Many clients welcome the use of technology in this way; for all clients, nurses must have their permission to communicate electronically and must respect their preferences. Email communication becomes part of the clients' medical record.

THERAPEUTIC COMMUNICATION

Therapeutic communication is the purposeful use of communication to build and maintain helping relationships with clients, families, and significant others.

- Nurses use interactive, purposeful communication skills to
  - Elicit and attend to clients' thoughts, feelings, concerns, and needs.
  - Express empathy and genuine concern for clients' and families' issues.
  - Obtain information and give feedback about clients' status.
  - Intervene to promote functional behavior and effective interpersonal relationships.
  - Evaluate clients' progress toward desired goals and outcomes.
- Children and older adults often require specific, age-appropriate techniques to enhance communication.
- Use of the nursing process depends on therapeutic communication among the nurse, client, family, significant other, and the interprofessional health care team. Q**TC**

CHARACTERISTICS

- Client-centered: Not social or reciprocal
- Purposeful, planned, and goal-directed

ESSENTIAL COMPONENTS Q**PCC**

Time: Plan for and allow adequate time to communicate with others.

Attentive behavior or active listening: Use this as a means of conveying interest, trust, and acceptance.

Caring attitude: Show concern and facilitate an emotional connection and support among nurses and clients, families, and significant others.

Honesty: Be open, direct, truthful, and sincere.

Trust: Demonstrate to clients, families, and significant others that they can rely on nurses without doubt, question, or judgment.

Empathy: Convey an objective awareness and understanding of the feelings, emotions, and behavior of clients, families, and significant others, including trying to envision what it must be like to be in their position.

Nonjudgmental attitude: A display of acceptance of clients, families, and significant others encourages open, honest communication.

NURSING PROCESS

ASSESSMENT/DATA COLLECTION

- Determine verbal and nonverbal communication needs for client-centered care.
  - Clients who have hearing, vision, or cognitive losses, are unresponsive, are aphasic, or do not speak the same language as the staff.
- Consider physical status.
- Consider the developmental level, and alter communication accordingly.
  - CHILDREN
    - Use simple, straightforward language.
    - Be aware of nonverbal messages because children are especially sensitive to nonverbal communication.
    - Enhance communication by being at the child's eye level.
    - Incorporate play in interactions.
  - OLDER ADULT CLIENTS
    - Recognize that many older adults require amplification of sound.
    - Make sure assistive devices such as glasses and hearing aids are available for clients who need them.
    - Minimize distractions, and face clients when speaking.
    - Speak in short and simple sentences.
    - Allow plenty of time for clients to respond.
    - Ask for input from caregivers or family to determine the extent of any communication deficits and how best to communicate. **Qpcc**
- Identify any cultural considerations that affect communication.
  - Provide an interpreter.
  - Address the client directly when the interpreter is present.
  - Provide educational materials and instructions in the client's language.

PLANNING

- Minimize distractions.
- Provide privacy.
- Identify mutually agreed-upon outcomes.
- Set priorities according to the clients' needs.
- Collaborate with other health care professionals when necessary.
- Plan adequate time for interventions.

IMPLEMENTATION

- Establish a trusting nurse–client relationship. Clients feel more at ease during the implementation phase when nurses establish a helping relationship.
- Provide empathetic responses and explanations by using observations, giving information, conveying hope, and using humor.
- Manipulate the environment to decrease distractions.

EFFECTIVE SKILLS AND TECHNIQUES

Silence: This allows time for meaningful reflection.

Presenting reality: This helps the client distinguish what is real from what is not and to dispel delusions, hallucinations, and faulty beliefs.

Active listening: This helps the nurse hear, observe, and understand what the client communicates and provide feedback.

Asking questions: This is a way to seek additional information.

Open-ended questions: This facilitates spontaneous responses and interactive discussion. It encourages the client to explore feelings and thoughts and avoids yes or no answers

Clarifying techniques: This helps the nurse determine whether the message the client received was accurate:
- **Restating:** Uses the client's exact words
- **Reflecting:** Directs the focus back to the client for him to examine his feelings
- **Paraphrasing:** Restates the client's feelings and thoughts for him to confirm what he has communicated
- **Exploring:** Allows the nurse to gather more information about important topics the client mentioned

Offering general leads, broad opening statements: This encourages the client to start and to continue talking.

Showing acceptance and recognition: This acknowledges the nurse's interest and nonjudgmental attitude.

Focusing: This helps the client concentrate on what is important.

Giving information: This provides factual details that the client might need for decision-making.

Summarizing: This emphasizes important points and reviews what the nurse and the client have discussed.

Offering self: This demonstrates a willingness to spend time with the client. The nurse may share limited personal information, but the focus should return to the client as soon as possible. Relevant self-disclosure by the nurse helps the client see that others share his experience and understand.

Touch: If appropriate, touch can communicate caring and provide comfort.

BARRIERS TO EFFECTIVE COMMUNICATION

- Asking irrelevant personal questions
- Offering personal opinions
- Stereotyping
- Giving advice
- Giving false reassurance
- Minimizing feelings
- Changing the topic
- Asking "why" questions or asking for explanations
- Challenging
- Offering value judgments
- Asking questions excessively (probing)
- Responding approvingly or disapprovingly (refusing)
- Being defensive
- Testing
- Judging
- Offering sympathy
- Arguing

COMMUNICATION AMONG HEALTH PROFESSIONALS

Nurses must communicate clearly, respectfully, and professionally with all staff members. Qᴛᴄ

Faulty communication among the members of the health care team can have a negative effect on the work environment and on clients' outcomes.

- **Incivility:** Rude dialogue or actions (sarcasm, eye rolling)
- **Bullying:** Repeated words or acts of intimidation
- **Lateral violence:** Abusive words or actions of peers (gossiping, exclusion of information, threats of harm, actual harm)

Application Exercises

1. A nurse is caring for a client who states, "I have to check with my wife and see if she thinks I am ready to go home." The nurse replies, "How do you feel about going home today?" Which clarifying technique is the nurse using to enhance communication with the client?

   A. Pacing

   B. Reflecting

   C. Paraphrasing

   D. Restating

2. Which of the following actions should the nurse take when using the communication technique of active listening? (Select all that apply.)

   A. Use an open posture.

   B. Write down what the client says to avoid forgetting details.

   C. Establish and maintain eye contact.

   D. Nod in agreement with the client throughout the conversation.

   E. Respond positively when giving feedback.

3. A nurse is caring for a client who is concerned about his impending discharge to home with a new colostomy because he is an avid swimmer. Which of the following statements should the nurse make? (Select all that apply.)

   A. "You will do great! You just have to get used it."

   B. "Why are you worried about going home?"

   C. "Your daily routines will be different when you get home."

   D. "Tell me about your support system you'll have after you leave the hospital."

   E. "Let me tell you about a friend of mine with a colostomy who also enjoys swimming."

4. Which of the following strategies should a nurse use to establish a helping relationship with a client?

   A. Make sure the communication is equally reciprocal between the nurse and the client.

   B. Encourage the client to communicate his thoughts and feelings.

   C. Give the nurse-client communication no time limits.

   D. Allow communication to occur spontaneously throughout the nurse-client relationship.

5. A nurse is caring for a school-age child who is sitting in a chair. To facilitate effective communication, which of the following actions should the nurse take?

   A. Touch the child's arm.

   B. Sit at eye level with the child.

   C. Stand facing the child.

   D. Stand with a relaxed posture.

PRACTICE Active Learning Scenario

A nurse manager is reviewing nonverbal communication with staff members. Use the ATI Active Learning Template: Basic Concept to complete this item.

RELATED CONTENT: List at least four examples of nonverbal communication.

UNDERLYING PRINCIPLES: Explain their effect on the communication.

Application Exercises Key

1. A. Pacing is a characteristic of verbal communication, not a clarifying technique.

    B. **CORRECT:** Reflecting directs the focus of the conversation back to the client so that he can further explore his own feelings.

    C. Paraphrasing restates the client's feelings for him to confirm what he has communicated. In this scenario, the client did not verbalize his feelings to the nurse.

    D. Restating uses the client's exact words. In this scenario, the nurse did not restate what the client stated.

    Ⓝ *NCLEX® Connection: Psychosocial Integrity, Therapeutic Communication*

2. A. **CORRECT:** Having an open posture, facing the client, and leaning forward are ways the nurse can demonstrate active listening.

    B. Writing down everything the client says can interfere with the nurse's ability to convey full attention and interest.

    C. **CORRECT:** Establishing and maintaining eye contact are ways the nurse can demonstrate active listening.

    D. If the nurse nods in agreement throughout the conversation, the client could interpret that as agreement with what the client is saying when instead the nurse meant to convey attending to and understanding what he is saying.

    E. **CORRECT:** Responding positively when giving feedback is a way the nurse can demonstrate active listening.

    Ⓝ *NCLEX® Connection: Psychosocial Integrity, Therapeutic Communication*

3. A. Giving false reassurance and minimizing the client's feelings are both barriers to effective communication.

    B. Although this might appear to help the client discuss his feelings, asking a "why" question is a barrier to effective communication.

    C. **CORRECT:** Presenting reality is an effective communication technique that can help the client focus on what will really happen after the changes the surgery has made.

    D. **CORRECT:** Asking open-ended questions and offering general leads and broad opening statements are effective communication techniques that encourage the client to express feelings through dialogue and offer additional information.

    E. **CORRECT:** Offering self is an effective communication technique that can convey understanding and share another's experience with the client. However, the nurse should return the focus to the client as soon as she communicates the relevant point.

    Ⓝ *NCLEX® Connection: Psychosocial Integrity, Therapeutic Communication*

4. A. The communication should not be reciprocal but client-focused.

    B. **CORRECT:** Therapeutic communication facilitates a helping relationship that maximizes the client's ability to express his thoughts and feelings openly.

    C. The nurse should limit therapeutic communication to the boundaries of the therapeutic relationship, including time.

    D. The nurse should plan therapeutic communication.

    Ⓝ *NCLEX® Connection: Psychosocial Integrity, Therapeutic Communication*

5. A. Touching can intimidate the child and block communication.

    B. **CORRECT:** The nurse should be at the same eye level as the child to facilitate communication.

    C. Standing can appear domineering and intimidating.

    D. Standing can appear domineering and intimidating, even with a relaxed posture.

    Ⓝ *NCLEX® Connection: Psychosocial Integrity, Therapeutic Communication*

PRACTICE Answer

Using ATI Active Learning Template: Basic Concept

RELATED CONTENT
- Appearance, posture, gait
- Facial expressions, eye contact, gestures
- Sounds
- Territoriality, personal space

UNDERLYING PRINCIPLES
- Appearance, posture, gait: Physical characteristics convey professionalism and can demonstrate comfort and ease in the situation.
- Facial expressions: Facial expressions can reveal feelings that clients could misinterpret.
- Eye contact: Eye contact conveys interest and respect but varies with culture and situation.
- Gestures: Gestures can enhance verbal communication or create their own messages.
- Sounds: Crying or moaning can have multiple meanings when clients also convey other nonverbal communication
- Territoriality, personal space: Lack of awareness of territoriality (right to space) and personal space (the area around an individual) can make clients perceive a threat and react defensively.

Ⓝ *NCLEX® Connection: Psychosocial Integrity, Therapeutic Communication*

CHAPTER 33 *Coping*

Coping describes how an individual deals with problems, such as illness and stress. Factors involved in coping and adaptation include the client's family dynamics, adherence to treatment regimens, and the role an individual can play in important relationships.

Stress, coping, adaptation, and adherence

Stress

- Stress describes changes in an individual's state of balance in response to stressors, the internal and external forces that disrupt that state of balance. Any stressor, whether it is perceived as "good" or "bad," produces a similar biological response in the body.
- Stress can be situational (adjusting to a chronic disease or a stressful job change).
- Stress can be developmental (varying with life stage). Adult stressors can include losing parents, having a baby, and getting married.
- Stress can be caused by sociocultural factors, including substance use, lack of education, and prolonged poverty.
- Research has shown that stress not only impairs and weakens the immune system but has been identified as a causal factor in numerous health conditions.

Coping

- Coping describes how an individual deals with problems and issues.
- Factors influencing an individual's ability to cope include the number, duration, and intensity of stressors; the individual's past experiences; the current support system; and available resources (financial).
- Coping strategies are unique to an individual and can vary greatly with each stressor.
- Caregiver burden results from the accumulated stress that family members experience after caring for a loved one over a period of time. Some responses include fatigue, difficulty sleeping, and illness (increased blood pressure, mental illness).
- Ego defense mechanisms: assist a person during a stressful situation or crisis by regulating emotional distress.

Adaptation

Coping behavior that describes how an individual handles demands imposed by the environment.

General adaptation syndrome (GAS)
Also known as "stress syndrome." Hans Selye developed a theory of adaptation that describes the stress reaction in three stages.
- **Alarm reaction:** Body functions are heightened to respond to stressors. Hormones (epinephrine, norepinephrine, cortisone) are released, which cause elevated blood pressure and heart rate, heightened mental alertness, increased secretion of epinephrine and norepinephrine, and increased blood flow to muscles.
- **Resistance stage:** Body functions normalize while responding to the stressor. The body attempts to cope with the stressor and return to homeostasis. Stabilization of BP, heart rate and hormones will occur.
- **Exhaustion stage:** Body functions are no longer able to maintain a response to the stressor and the client cannot adapt. The end of this stage results in recovery or death.

Adherence

- The commitment and ability of the client and family to follow a given treatment regimen.
- Commitment to the regimen increases adherence.
- Complicated regimen interferes with adherence.
- Involvement of the client and significant support people in the planning stage increases adherence.
- Adverse effects of medications diminish adherence.
- Coping mechanisms, such as denial, can cause non-adherence.
- Available resources increase adherence.

ASSESSMENT/DATA COLLECTION

- Ask the client questions related to Qpcc
  - Current stress, perception of stressors, and ability to cope
  - Support systems
  - Adherence to healthy behaviors and/or the treatment regimen
  - Sleep patterns
  - Altered elimination patterns, changes in appetite, and weight loss or gain
- Observe the client's appearance and eye contact, verbal, motor and cognitive status during the assessment.
- Measure vital signs.
- Observe for irritability, anxiety, and tension.
- Thoroughly assess each client to ensure client centered clinical decisions required for safe nursing care.

PATIENT-CENTERED CARE

NURSING CARE

Stress

- Encourage health promotion strategies, including regular exercise, optimal nutrition, and adequate sleep and rest.
- Assist with time management, and determine priority tasks.
- Encourage appropriate relaxation techniques, including breathing exercises, massage, imagery, yoga, and meditation.
- Listen attentively, and take the time to understand the client's perspective.
- Control the environment to reduce the number of external stressors, including noise and breaks in the continuity of care.
- Identify available support systems.
- Use effective communication techniques to foster the expression of feelings.

Coping

- Be empathetic in communication, and encourage the client to verbalize feelings.
- Identify the client's and family's strengths and abilities.
- Encourage client's autonomy with decision-making.
- Discuss the client's and family's abilities to deal with the current situation.
- Encourage the client to describe coping skills used effectively in the past.
- Identify available community resources, and refer the client for counseling if needed.

Adherence

- Put instructions in writing.
- Allow the client to give input into the treatment regimen.
- Simplify treatment regimens as much as possible.
- Follow up with the client to address any questions or problems.

Family systems and family dynamics

- Family is defined by the client, and it consists of the individual structures and roles. It is typically two or more people whose relationships create a bond and influence their mutual development, support, goals, and resources.
- Consider five realms of processes involved in family function during a family assessment: interactive, developmental, coping, integrity, health.
- Assessment of a family can focus on family as a context, a client, or a system.
- Families and clients are not mutually exclusive; family-centered care creates a holistic approach to nursing care.
- Family dynamics are constantly evolving due to the processes of family life and developmental stages of the family members.

CURRENT TRENDS

FASTEST-GROWING POPULATION: Those older than 65 years, leading to caregiver issues

DECLINING ECONOMIC STATUS OF FAMILIES (increased unemployment)

FAMILY VIOLENCE and its endless cycle **Qs**

ANY ACUTE OR CHRONIC ILLNESS THE DISRUPTS THE FAMILY UNIT (can include end-of-life care issues)

HOMELESSNESS: Lack of stable environment, financial issues, inadequate access to health care (fastest-growing homeless population is families with children). The homeless population is increasing due to lack of affordable housing.

ATTRIBUTES OF FAMILIES

- Structure dictates the family's ability to cope.
  - Rigid structure is dictatorial and strict.
  - Open structure includes few or no boundaries, consistent behavior, or consequences.
  - Either structure can provide positive or negative outcomes.
- Function describes the course of action the family uses to reach its goals, including members' communication skills, problem-solving abilities, and available resources.

ASSESSMENT/DATA COLLECTION

- Assess all clients within the context of the family.
- Assess a family by looking at its structure and function.
- Identify who is a family member, what role each family member plays, and the dynamic interactions within the family.
- Listen attentively, and use the therapeutic communication techniques of reflection and restatement to clarify the family's concerns.
- Cultural variables: all of which can differ between and within generations
  - Perception of events
  - Rites and rituals
  - Health beliefs

PATIENT-CENTERED CARE

NURSING CARE

- Identify and adapt family strengths to perceived stressor(s).
  - Communication
  - Adaptability
  - Nurturing
  - Crisis as a growth element
  - Parenting skills
  - Resiliency
- Set realistic goals with the family.
- Provide information about support networks and community resources. Q<small>TC</small>
  - Child and adult day care
  - Caregiver support groups
- Promote family unity.
- Ensure safety for families at risk for violence.
- Encourage conflict resolution.
- Minimize family process disruption effects.
- Remove barriers to health promotion.
- Increase family members' abilities to participate.
- Perform interventions that the family cannot perform.
- Evaluate goals within the context of the family by checking back to ensure that goals were realistic and achievable.

Situational role changes

- A role is the function a person adopts within their life. Seldom is it limited to one role, but rather is multidimensional and is often relative to the role of others.
  - Grandparent
  - Parent
  - Dependent child
  - Employee/employer
  - Committee member
  - Community activist
- Stress affects roles in many ways.
- The presence of stressors delays a client's return to health in the same way that the presence of a foreign body or infection delays the healing of a wound.
- Illness causes role stress by creating a situation in which roles can change simply due to the effect and progression of the illness.
- Nurses must be aware of a client's roles in life, as well as how the situation of illness might change these roles, either temporarily or permanently.
- A basic assumption is that a client can either advance or regress in the face of a situational role change.

TYPES OF ROLE PROBLEMS

Role conflict: This develops when a person must assume opposing roles with incompatible expectations. Role conflicts can be interpersonal (when parents expect adolescents to participate in sports and perform household tasks) or inter-role (when a mother wants to stay at home with her infant, but family finances require her to work).

Sick role: Expectations of others and society regarding how one should behave when sick (caring for self while sick and continuing to provide childcare to grandchildren).

Role ambiguity: Uncertainty about what is expected when assuming a role; creates confusion.

Role strain: The frustration and anxiety that occurs when a person feels inadequate for assuming a role (caring for a parent dementia).

Role overload: More responsibility and roles than are manageable; very common (assuming the role of student, employee, and parent).

SITUATIONAL ROLE CHANGES

- Caused by situations other than physical growth and development (marriage, job changes, divorce)
- Can disrupt one or more of the client's roles in life (with illness or hospitalization)
- With resolution, can contribute to healing in the physical, mental, and spiritual realms

TEMPORARY ROLE CHANGES: The client will resume the role when illness resolves.

PERMANENT ROLE CHANGES: Illness has altered the level of the client's health to a point that previous roles are no longer available.

ASSESSMENT/DATA COLLECTION

- Identify the client's roles as perceived as owning and by significant others.
- Validate any discrepancies.
- Identify the effect that the loss or addition of a role is having on the client (grieving the loss of a role).
- Identify who will now take on the client's role while the client cannot and make referrals as appropriate.

PATIENT-CENTERED CARE

NURSING CARE Q℀

- Provide short-term care to provide relief for the family caregiver.
- Provide encouragement during times of stress.
- Seek congruence among perceived roles.
- Prepare the client for the anticipated situational crisis.
- Anticipate role conflict or overload on the client's part.
- Help the client improve relationships by supplementing specific role behaviors.
- Explore which roles the client can relinquish.
- Help the client improve personal judgment of self-worth given the current situational role change.
- Counsel the client about roles that are permanently altered.
- Refer the client to community services for outpatient adaptation to lost or new roles.
- Refer the client to social services for assistance in some roles.
- Evaluate the client after acceptance of the role change(s) to assess adaptation.

Application Exercises

1. A nurse is caring for a client whose partner passed away 4 months ago and who has been recently diagnosed with diabetes mellitus. He is tearful and states, "How could you possibly understand what I am going through?" Which of the following responses should the nurse make?

   A. "It takes time to get over the loss of a loved one."

   B. "You are right. I cannot really understand. Perhaps you'd like to tell me more about what you're feeling."

   C. "Why don't you try something to take your mind off your troubles, like watching a funny movie."

   D. "I might not share your exact situation, but I do know what people go through when they deal with a loss."

2. A nurse is caring for a client awaiting transport to the surgical suite for a coronary artery bypass graft. Just as the transport team arrives, the nurse takes the client's vital signs and notes an elevation in blood pressure and heart rate. The nurse should recognize this response as which part of the general adaptation syndrome (GAS)?

   A. Exhaustion stage

   B. Resistance stage

   C. Alarm reaction

   D. Recovery reaction

3. A nurse is caring for a client who has left-sided hemiplegia resulting from a cerebrovascular accident. The client works as a carpenter and is now experiencing a situational role change based on physical limitations. The client is the primary wage earner in the family. Which of the following describes the client's role problem?

   A. Role conflict

   B. Role overload

   C. Role ambiguity

   D. Role strain

4. A nurse is caring for a client who has a new diagnosis of type 2 diabetes mellitus. Which of the following nursing interventions for stress, coping, and adherence to the treatment plan should the nurse initiate at this time? (Select all that apply.)

   A. Suggest coping skills for the client to use in this situation.

   B. Allow the client to provide input in the treatment plan.

   C. Assist the client with time management, and address the client's priorities.

   D. Provide extensive instructions on the client's treatment regimen.

   E. Encourage the client in the expression of feelings and concerns.

5. A nurse is caring for a family who is experiencing a crisis. Which of the following approaches should the nurse use when working with a family using an open structure for coping with crisis?

   A. Prescribing tasks unilaterally

   B. Delegating care to one member

   C. Speaking to the primary client privately

   D. Convening a family meeting

PRACTICE Active Learning Scenario

A nurse manager is reviewing coping factors with the members of her team. Use the ATI Active Learning Template: Basic Concept to complete this item.

RELATED CONTENT: List at least four factors that influence an individual's ability to cope.

NURSING INTERVENTIONS: List three interventions the nurse can take to assist the client in coping with a stressful event or situation.

Application Exercises Key

1. A. Telling the client it will take more time to heal belittles the client's feelings and gives false reassurance.

   B. **CORRECT:** By stating that she is not in his situation, the nurse is using the therapeutic communication technique of validation, whereby she shows sensitivity to the meaning behind his behavior. She is also creating a supportive and nonjudgmental environment, and inviting him to express his frustrations.

   C. Telling the client to try a distraction dismisses the client's feelings and gives common advice instead of expert advice.

   D. Saying she knows what clients feel is presumptive and inappropriate.

   (N) *NCLEX® Connection: Psychosocial Integrity, Therapeutic Communication*

2. A. Although the exhaustion stage is a component of GAS, body functions are no longer able to respond to the stressor in this stage.

   B. Although the resistance stage is a component of GAS, body functions normalize in an attempt to cope with the stressor in this stage.

   C. **CORRECT:** As a component of GAS, body functions, such as blood pressure and heart rate, are heightened in order to respond to the stressor in the alarm stage.

   D. Although not technically a component of GAS, recovery reaction is an alternative to the exhaustion stage, but it would not account for an elevation in blood pressure and heart rate.

   (N) *NCLEX® Connection: Reduction of Risk Potential, Changes/Abnormalities in Vital Signs*

3. A. **CORRECT:** The client is experiencing role conflict because his career is extremely physical, and he can no longer perform his job duties. However, the client is the primary wage earner in the family.

   B. Although the client can feel overloaded and overwhelmed, role overload occurs when the client is trying to juggle too many roles.

   C. The client is not experiencing role ambiguity because his job duties and his physical limitations are quite clear.

   D. The client is not experiencing role strain. That occurs when one feels inadequate for assuming a role.

   (N) *NCLEX® Connection: Psychosocial Integrity, Coping Mechanisms*

4. A. Although it can seem helpful to suggest specific coping skills for the client, it is best to allow the client to discuss coping skills that have worked in the past.

   B. **CORRECT:** Allowing the client to contribute to the treatment plan allows for greater adherence to the plan.

   C. **CORRECT:** Helping the client to prioritize is an intervention that can reduce levels of stress for the client because many times time management is extremely difficult in times of stress.

   D. Although it is necessary to provide complete information on treatment plans, simplifying treatment regimens as much as possible allows for greater adherence to the treatment plan.

   E. **CORRECT:** By using effective communication techniques, encouraging the client to verbalize feelings is an intervention for stress, coping, and adherence that allows the client to reduce stress, validate emotions, and start planning for valid concerns.

   (N) *NCLEX® Connection: Psychosocial Integrity, Coping Mechanisms*

5. A. Prescribing tasks is too rigid for acceptance by a family with an open structure.

   B. Delegating care is too rigid for acceptance by a family with an open structure.

   C. Speaking to the primary client privately excludes the family.

   D. **CORRECT:** An open structure is loose, and convening a family meeting would give all family members input and an opportunity to express their feelings.

   (N) *NCLEX® Connection: Psychosocial Integrity, Coping Mechanisms*

PRACTICE Answer

Using ATI Active Learning Template: Basic Concept

RELATED CONTENT
- Number of stressors
- Duration of the stressors
- Intensity of the stressors
- Individual's past experiences
- Current support system
- Available resources (financial)

NURSING INTERVENTIONS
- Be empathetic in communication, and encourage the client to verbalize feelings.
- Identify the client's and family's strengths and abilities.
- Discuss the client's and family's abilities to deal with the current situation.
- Encourage the client to describe coping skills used effectively in the past.
- Identify available community resources, and refer the client for counseling if needed.

(N) *NCLEX® Connection: Psychosocial Integrity, Coping Mechanisms*

Self-Concept and Sexuality

Self-concept is the way individuals feel and view themselves. This involves conscious and unconscious thoughts, attitudes, beliefs, and perceptions. Body image, a component of self-concept, refers to the way individuals perceive their appearance, size, and body structure/function.

Sexuality and sexual orientation are integrated into individuals' personalities as well as their general health. Sexuality encompasses their sense of maleness and/or femaleness and their physical and emotional connections with others.

Individuals' sexuality and sexual health are influenced by self-concept, body image, gender identity, and sexual orientation.

Nurses should assess their own comfort levels with issues related to sexuality because clients usually can sense any discomfort nurses have about these issues. Skills that nurses use in dealing with clients' sexuality issues are a knowledge of sexual growth and development, and an understanding of how health problems and treatments affect sexuality.

Self-concept

- Self-concept is subjective and includes self-identity, body image, role performance, and self-esteem.
  - Individuals who have high self-esteem are better equipped to cope successfully with life's stressors.
  - Stressors that affect self-concept include unrealistic expectations, surgery, chronic illness, and changes in role performance.
- Individuals who have positive self-concepts tend to feel good about themselves.
- Individuals who have positive self-esteem feel capable and competent.
- Individuals' self-concepts can be adversely affected by physical, spiritual, emotional, sexual, familial, and sociocultural stressors.

Body image

- Body image changes with growth and development. During adolescence, hormonal changes include the development of secondary sex characteristics that influence body image. Among older adults, changes in mobility, thinning and graying of hair, and decreased visual and hearing acuity are just a few factors that affect body image. Ⓒ
- Stressors that affect body image include loss of body parts due to an amputation, mastectomy, or hysterectomy; loss of body function due to arthritis, spinal cord injury, or stroke; and an unattainable body ideal.
- External influences (media, others' perceptions and responses, cultural standards) can affect body image.
- Clients who have a negative body image perception tend to be at risk for suicidal ideations.

Sexuality

- Sexuality and sexual health are vital components of general health and part of a nursing assessment.
- Sexual health occurs when relationships are safe, enjoyable, and respected.
- Aspects of sexual health include knowledge of sexual behavior, understanding of expected growth and development, and access to appropriate health care resources for preventing and treating problems related to sexual health.
- Sexuality is affected by developmental stage. For example, during adolescence, primary and secondary sex characteristics develop, menarche occurs, relationships involving sexual activity can develop, and masturbation is common.
- Sexuality is influenced by culture. Various cultures view premarital sex, homosexuality, and polygamy differently.
- Sexuality affects health status. Certain conditions can alter sexual expression. For example, the presence of a sexually transmitted infection can cause fear of transmission to a partner, leading to a decrease in sexual desire.
- Some prescription medications affect sexual functioning. Diuretics decrease vaginal lubrication, cause erectile dysfunction, and reduce sexual desire. Erectile dysfunction can also be caused by antidepressant medications.
- Use the PLISSIT assessment tool for sexuality
  - **P: Permission** (obtain permission to discuss this with client)
  - **LI: Limited information** (related to sexual health patterns)
  - **SS: Specific suggestions** (based upon assessment data make appropriate suggestions)
  - **IT: Intensive therapy** (more referral if needed)

ASSESSMENT/DATA COLLECTION

- Posture
- Appearance
- Demeanor
- Eye contact
- Grooming
- Unusual behavior

EXPECTED FINDINGS
- Cultural background
- Quality of relationships
- Feelings related to recent body image changes, self-concept, and issues of sexuality
- Coping mechanisms used in the past
- Evaluation of self-worth

PATIENT-CENTERED CARE

Self-concept

- How one values oneself
- Suggest a healthier lifestyle (exercise, diet, stress management).
- Encourage the client to verbalize fears or anxieties.
- Use therapeutic communication skills to assist the client with self-awareness.
- Encourage the use of effective coping skills.
- Reinforce successes and strengths.

Body image

- Establish a therapeutic relationship with the client. A caring and nonjudgmental manner puts the client at ease and fosters meaningful communication.
- Ensure privacy and confidentiality. Let the client know that sensitive issues are safe to discuss.
- A person's perception about their appearance
- Identify individuals who can be at risk for body image disturbances.
- Acknowledge anger, depression, and denial as feelings to be expected when adjusting to body changes.
- Encourage the client to participate in the plan of care.
- Arrange for a visit from a volunteer who has experienced a similar body image change.

Sexuality

- Allow the client to discuss issues and concerns related to sexuality.
- Be straightforward with questions in relaxed manner. ("Are you, or have you been, concerned about sexual functioning since your surgery?")
- Ask client to describe factors that influence sexual desire.
- Health promotion: Determine the client's current knowledge base regarding sexuality, and provide education as needed based upon developmental level such as: contraception, sexually transmitted infections prevention, and immunizations.
- Acute care: Increase awareness by introducing or clarifying information and referring the client for counseling if necessary.
- Inform the client of available resources and support groups.
- Never assume that sexual function is not a concern.
- Discuss alternative means of sexual expression if the client experiences a change in body functioning or structure (hugging, cuddling).

Application Exercises

1. A nurse in an ambulatory care clinic is caring for a client who had a mastectomy 6 months ago. The client tells the nurse that she has not had much desire for sexual relations since her surgery, stating, "My body is so different now." Which of the following responses should the nurse make?

   A. "Really, you look just fine to me. There's no need to feel undesirable."

   B. "I'm interested in finding out more about how your body feels to you."

   C. "Consider an afternoon at a spa. A facial will make you feel more attractive."

   D. "It's still too soon to expect to feel normal. Give it a little more time."

2. A nurse is caring for a group of clients on a medical-surgical unit. Which of the following clients are at risk for body image disturbances? (Select all that apply.)

   A. 30-year-old male client following laparoscopic appendectomy

   B. 45-year-old female client following mastectomy

   C. 20-year-old female client following left above-the-knee amputation

   D. 65-year-old male client following cardiac catheterization

   E. 55-year-old male client following stroke with right-sided hemiplegia

3. A nurse is caring for a client who is 3 days postoperative following a below-the-knee amputation as a result of a motor vehicle crash. Which of the following client statements indicates to the nurse that the client has a distorted body image?

   A. "I'll be able to function exactly as I did before the accident."

   B. "I just can't stop crying."

   C. "I am so mad at that guy who hit us. I wish he lost a leg."

   D. "I don't even want to look at my leg. You can check the dressing."

4. A nurse is caring for a client who is recovering from a myocardial infarction and a cardiac catheterization. The client states, "I am concerned that things might be a little, you know, 'different' with my wife when I get home." Which of the following statements should the nurse make?

   A. "Sounds like something you should discuss with her when you get home."

   B. "It sounds like you are concerned about sexual functioning. Let's discuss your concerns."

   C. "Oh, I wouldn't be too concerned. Things will be fine as soon as we get you home."

   D. "Just make sure you take your medication as directed, and you should be fine."

5. A nurse is teaching a group of clients how to care for their colostomies. Which of the following statements should alert the nurse that one of the clients is having an issue with self-concept?

   A. "I was having difficulty with attaching the appliance at first, but my wife was able to help."

   B. "I'll never be able to care for this at home. Can't you just send a nurse to the house?"

   C. "I met a neighbor who also has a colostomy, and he taught me a few things."

   D. "It may take me a while to get the hang of this. I have to admit, I am pretty nervous."

PRACTICE Active Learning Scenario

A nurse manager is reviewing self-concept assessment findings with her staff. Use the ATI Active Learning Template: System Disorder to complete this item.

EXPECTED FINDINGS: List at least six.

Application Exercises Key

1. A. Telling the client she looks fine is using the nontherapeutic communication technique of giving an opinion. Assuming she feels undesirable is using the nontherapeutic communication technique of interpreting.

   B. **CORRECT:** Showing interest in the client is applying the therapeutic communication technique of offering self. Asking more about how the client feels is applying the therapeutic communication technique of encouraging a description of perception.

   C. Suggesting a facial is using the nontherapeutic communication technique of giving advice.

   D. Telling her it is too soon to feel normal and to give it more time is belittling the client's feelings and giving false reassurance.

   Ⓝ *NCLEX® Connection: Psychosocial Integrity, Coping Mechanisms*

2. A. Based on the concept of body image, an appendectomy would not place a client at high risk for a body image disturbance.

   B. **CORRECT:** Having a mastectomy involves a change in the physical appearance of a woman and can lead to body image disturbances related to femininity and sexuality.

   C. **CORRECT:** Having an above-the-knee amputation involves a change in physical appearance and can lead to body image disturbances related to function, health, and strength.

   D. Depending on the client's prognosis postcatheterization, the client can experience some limitations. However, in general, a cardiac catheterization would not place a client at high risk for a body image disturbance.

   E. **CORRECT:** Having right-sided hemiplegia involves a change in physical appearance and can lead to body image disturbances related to function, health, and strength.

   Ⓝ *NCLEX® Connection: Psychosocial Integrity, Coping Mechanisms*

3. A. Denial is a normal and expected reaction when adjusting to body changes.

   B. Depression and sadness are normal and expected reactions when adjusting to body changes.

   C. Anger is a normal and expected reaction when adjusting to body changes.

   D. **CORRECT:** Refusing to look at the leg or the dressing indicates that the client is having difficulty acknowledging the fact that the leg has been amputated. This would imply a distorted body image.

   Ⓝ *NCLEX® Connection: Psychosocial Integrity, Coping Mechanisms*

4. A. The nurse should allow the client to discuss issues and concerns related to sexuality and not dismiss his concerns.

   B. **CORRECT:** The nurse is acknowledging and allowing the client to discuss his concerns regarding sexual functioning.

   C. False reassurance should not be used. The client has valid concerns. The nurse also is dismissing the client's feelings.

   D. The nurse is not allowing the client to express his feelings and is displaying false reassurance, which should not be used because the client has valid concerns.

   Ⓝ *NCLEX® Connection: Psychosocial Integrity, Coping Mechanisms*

5. A. Although the client was having difficulty at first, the client expressed how he was able to use his resources, resulting in a positive outcome, and does not show signs of self-concept issues.

   B. **CORRECT:** This client is displaying a lack of interest in learning how to care for the colostomy and dependence on others to care for him. The nurse should suspect issues with self-concept with this client.

   C. This client is displaying a positive self-concept by reaching out and using his resources to learn additional information regarding the colostomy.

   D. Expression of feelings is a sign of positive self-concept even if the client admits being nervous or hesitant regarding caring for the colostomy on his own.

   Ⓝ *NCLEX® Connection: Psychosocial Integrity, Coping Mechanisms*

PRACTICE Answer

Using the ATI Active Learning Template: System Disorder

EXPECTED FINDINGS

- Cultural background
- Quality of relationships
- Feelings related to recent body image changes, self-concept, and issues of sexuality
- Coping mechanisms used in the past
- Expectations
- Posture
- Appearance
- Demeanor
- Eye contact
- Grooming
- Unusual behavior

Ⓝ *NCLEX® Connection: Psychosocial Integrity, Coping Mechanisms*

UNIT 3   PSYCHOSOCIAL INTEGRITY

CHAPTER 35 *Cultural and Spiritual Nursing Care*

Clients vary widely in their cultural and spiritual backgrounds and belief systems. Nurses must examine their own beliefs before providing optimal cultural and spiritual care to their clients.

CULTURE

Culture is a collection of learned, adaptive, and socially and intergenerationally transmitted behaviors, values, beliefs, and customs that form the context from which a group interprets the human experience. Culture includes language, communication style, traditions, religions, art, music, dress, health beliefs, and health practices. These components can be shared by members of an ethnic, racial, social, or religious group.

- Ethnicity (the shared identity, bond, or kinship people feel with their country of birth or place of ancestral origin) affects culture.
- Culture influences health beliefs; health practices; and manifestations of, responses to, and treatment of illness or injury. Culture evolves over time and is shared by members of a group who have similar needs and life experiences.
- Many cultures consider the mind–body–spirit to be a single entity. Therefore, no distinction is made between physical and mental illness.
- The predominant culture in the U.S. is anglicized or English-based, with a general cultural tendency to do the following.
  - Express positive and negative feelings freely.
  - Prefer direct eye contact when communicating.
  - Address people in a casual manner.
  - Prefer a strong handshake as a way of greeting.
- Although everyone within a culture shares cultural values, diversity exists, forming subcultures based on age, gender, sexual orientation, marital status, family structure, income, education level, religious views, and life experiences.

EVOLUTION OF CULTURE

Culture evolves as the following.
- **Knowledge**
- **Values**
  - Values guide decision-making and behavior. For example, if health promotion and maintenance are valued, monthly breast self-examinations are done.
  - Values develop unconsciously during childhood.
- **Beliefs**
- **Morals and law**
- **Customs and habits**

CULTURALLY RESPONSIVE NURSING CARE

- Culturally responsive nursing care involves the delivery of care that transcends cultural boundaries and considers a client's culture as it affects health, illness, and lifestyle. Communication, dietary preferences, and dress are influenced by culture.
- Within the context of culturally responsive nursing care is terminology that describes how nurses approach clients' culture. Qpcc
  - **Culturally sensitive** means that nurses are knowledgeable about the cultures prevalent in their area of practice.
  - **Culturally appropriate** means that nurses apply their knowledge of a client's culture to their care delivery.
  - **Culturally competent** means that nurses understand and address the entire cultural context of each client within the realm of the care they deliver.
  - **Culturally responsive** nursing care improves communication, fosters mutual respect, promotes sensitive and effective care, and increases adherence with the treatment plan as clients' and families' needs are met. Culturally responsive nursing care should encourage client decision-making by introducing self-empowerment strategies.
  - **Cultural imposition** is a key prerequisite to the delivery of culturally responsive nursing care is the nurses' understanding and awareness of their own culture and any cultural biases that might affect care delivery.
- Nurses should accommodate each client's cultural beliefs and values whenever possible, unless they are in direct conflict with essential health practices. The goal is to provide culturally competent care.

BARRIERS TO CULTURALLY RESPONSIVE NURSING CARE

- Language, communication, and perception of time differences
- Culturally inappropriate tests and tools that lead to misdiagnosis
- Ethnic variations in drug metabolism related to genetics
- Ethnocentrism is the belief that one's culture is superior to others. Ethnocentric ideas interfere with the provision of cultural nursing care.

SPIRITUALITY

Spirituality can play an important role in clients' abilities to achieve balance in life, maintain health, seek health care, and deal with illness and injury. Hope, faith, and transcendence are integral components of spirituality.

- Spiritual distress is a challenge to belief systems or spiritual well-being. It often arises as a result of catastrophic events. The client can display hopelessness and decreased interactions with others.
- When faced with health care issues such as acute, chronic, or life-limiting illness, clients often find ways to cope through the use of spiritual practices. Clients who begin to question their belief systems and are unable to find support from those belief systems can experience spiritual distress.
- Nursing interventions are directed at identification, restoration, and/or reconnection of clients and families to spiritual strength. Qᴘᴄᴄ

Spirituality implies connectedness.
  - **Intrapersonal:** within one's self
  - **Interpersonal:** with others and the environment
  - **Transpersonal:** with an unseen higher power

Faith is a belief in something or a relationship with a higher power. Faith can be defined by a culture or a religion.

Hope is a concept that includes anticipation and optimism and provides comfort during times of crisis.

Religion is a system of beliefs practiced outwardly to express one's spirituality.

SPIRITUAL RITUALS AND OBSERVANCES

Buddhism

BIRTH RITUALS AND HEALTH CARE DECISIONS
- Can refuse care on holy days.
- Can refuse analgesics or strong sedatives.

DIETARY RITUALS
- Some are vegetarians.
- Can avoid alcohol and tobacco.
- Clients might fast on holy days.

DEATH RITUALS
- Clients can request a priest to deliver last rites.
- Chanting is common.
- Brain death is not considered as a requirement for death.

Christianity

BIRTH RITUALS AND HEALTH CARE DECISIONS: Some baptize infants at birth.

DIETARY RITUALS
- Some avoid alcohol, tobacco, and caffeine.
- Might fast during Lent.
- Some wish to receive the Holy Communion.

DEATH RITUALS: Some give last rites.

Hinduism

BIRTH RITUALS AND HEALTH CARE DECISIONS
- Those practicing Hinduism do not prolong life.
- Personal hygiene and cleanliness are valued.

DIETARY RITUALS: Some are vegetarians.

DEATH RITUALS
- Clients might want to lie on the floor while dying.
- A thread is placed around the neck/wrist.
- The family pours water into the mouth.
- The family bathes the body.
- Clients might want to be cremated.

Islam

BIRTH RITUALS AND HEALTH CARE DECISIONS
- Women must be cared for by female providers, especially during childbirth.
- Women often must wear head and/or body covering when in the presence of males who are not immediate family.
- Have strict rules regarding hand washing.
- Must pray five times a day facing Mecca.

DIETARY RITUALS
- Clients avoid alcohol and pork.
- Clients can fast during Ramadan.

DEATH RITUALS
- Dying clients confess their sins.
- The body faces Mecca.
- The body is washed and enveloped in a white cloth.
- A prayer is said.

Jehovah's Witnesses

BIRTH RITUALS AND HEALTH CARE DECISIONS: Might not accept blood transfusions, even in life-threatening situations.

DIETARY RITUALS: Clients avoid foods having or prepared with blood.

DEATH RITUALS: Clients can choose burial or cremation.

Judaism

BIRTH RITUALS AND HEALTH CARE DECISIONS: On the eighth day after birth, males are circumcised.

DIETARY RITUALS: Some practice a kosher diet.

DEATH RITUALS
- Someone stays with the body.
- A burial society prepares the body.

Mormonism

BIRTH RITUALS AND HEALTH CARE DECISIONS: Children are baptized at age 8 by immersion.

DIETARY RITUALS: Clients avoid alcohol, tobacco, and caffeine.

DEATH RITUALS
- Last rites include wearing temple clothes for burial.
- Burial is preferred.

ASSESSMENT/DATA COLLECTION

To meet a client's cultural needs, a nurse must first perform a cultural assessment to identify those needs. Qᴘᴄᴄ

Cultural background and acculturation

Example: The client was born in Central America and has been a resident of New York for 2 years.

Health and wellness beliefs/practices

Example: The client relies on folk medicine to treat or prevent illness.

Family patterns

Example: The client is from a patriarchal culture where the oldest male family member makes decisions for all family members.

Verbal and nonverbal communication

Example: Within the client's culture, it is disrespectful to make direct eye contact.

Space and time orientation

Example: Within the client's culture, little importance is placed on how past behavior affects future health.

Nutritional patterns

Example: The client believes that some foods have healing properties.

Meaning of pain

Example: Within the client's culture, pain is viewed as a punishment for misbehavior or sin.

Death rituals

Example: Within the client's culture, suicide is acceptable.

Care of ill family members

Example: The client expects the entire family to remain at the client's bedside during an illness.

Perform the cultural assessment in a language that is common to both nurse and client, or use a facility-approved medical interpreter. Inform the interpreter of questions that might be asked.

4 C'S CULTURAL ASSESSMENT

Nurses may use the 4 C's of Culture by Slavin, Galanti, and Kuo (2012).
- What do you **call** the problem you are having now?
- How do you **cope** with the problem?
- What are your **concerns** regarding the problem?
- What do you think **caused** the problem?

OTHER QUESTIONS
- When did the problem start?
- What does the illness do to you? How does it work?
- What makes it better or worse?
- How severe is the illness?
- What treatments have you tried? How do you think it should be treated?
- What are the chief problems the illness has caused you?
- What do you fear most about the illness?

NONVERBAL BEHAVIOR

- Assess the client's gestures, vocal tones, and inflections.
- Culturally competent nurses must understand how nonverbal behaviors vary among cultures. Qᴘᴄᴄ

Tone of voice

ASIAN: Many use a soft tone of voice to convey respect.

ITALIAN AND MIDDLE EASTERN: Many use a loud tone of voice.

Eye contact

AMERICAN: Use direct eye contact. Lack of direct eye contact implies deception or embarrassment.

MIDDLE EASTERN: Usually avoid making direct eye contact with nonrelated members of the opposite gender. Direct eye contact can be seen as rude, hostile, or sexually aggressive.

ASIAN: Can believe that direct eye contact is disrespectful.

NATIVE AMERICAN: Can believe that direct eye contact leads to soul loss or soul theft.

Touch

AMERICAN: Can use touch during conversations between intimate partners or family members.

ITALIAN AND LATIN AMERICAN: Can view frequent touch as a sign of concern, interest, and warmth.

NATIVE AMERICANS: View touch as a form of aggression.

Use of space

ANGLO-AMERICAN/NORTH EUROPEANS (ENGLISH, SWISS, SCANDINAVIAN, GERMAN): Tend to keep their distance during communication except in intimate or family relationships.

ITALIAN, FRENCH, SPANISH, RUSSIAN, LATIN AMERICAN, MIDDLE EASTERN: Prefer closer personal contact and less distance between individuals during communication.

METHODS FOR ASSESSING CULTURE

Observation: Study the client and his environment for examples of cultural relevance.

Interview
- Establish a therapeutic relationship with the client. This can be hindered by misinterpretations of communication. Nurses should develop transcultural communication skills. Qᴘᴄᴄ
- Use focused, open-ended, nonjudgmental questions.
- Paraphrasing the client's communication will decrease misinterpretations.

Participation

- Become involved in culturally related activities outside of the health care setting.
- Maintain awareness of population demographics (review census data).
  - Number of members in a practice area
  - Average educational and economic levels
  - Typical occupations
  - Commonly practiced religious spiritual beliefs
  - Prevalence of illnesses/health issues
  - Most commonly held health, wellness, illness, and death beliefs
  - Social organization

SPIRITUAL ASSESSMENT

- A spiritual assessment includes several components.
  - **Primary:** self-reflection (nurses) on personal beliefs and spirituality
  - **Initial:** identifying the client's religion, if any
  - **Focused:** ongoing, as nurses identify the clients at risk for spiritual distress
- Spirituality is a highly subjective area requiring the development of rapport and trust among the client, family, and provider.

ASSESSMENT OF THE CLIENT

- Faith/beliefs
- Perception of life and self-responsibility
- Satisfaction with life
- Culture
- Fellowship and the client's perceived place in the community
- Rituals and practices
- Incorporation of spirituality within profession or workplace
- Client expectations for health care in relation to spirituality (traditional vs. alternative paths, such as shamans, priests, prayer)

PATIENT-CENTERED CARE

Death rituals

Death rituals vary among cultures. Facilitate practices and offer appropriate spiritual care whenever possible.

Pain

- Recognize that how clients react to, display, and relieve pain varies by culture.
- Use an alternative to the pain scale (0 to 10) because it might not appropriately reflect pain for all cultures.
- Explore religious beliefs that influence the meaning of pain.

Nutrition

- Provide food choices and preparation consistent with cultural beliefs.
- When possible, allow the client's family/caregiver to bring in food (as long as it meets the client's dietary restrictions), and allow clients to consume foods that they view as a treatment for illness.
- Communicate ethnicity-related food intolerances/allergies to the dietary staff.

Communication

- Improve nurse-client communication when cultural variations exist by establishing rapport with client and family.
- Use facility-approved interpreters when the communication barrier is significant enough to affect the exchange of information between the nurse and the client.
- Use nonverbal communication with caution because it can have a different meaning for the client than for the nurse.
- Apologize if cultural traditions or beliefs are violated.

Family patterns and gender roles

Communicate with and include the person who has the authority to make decisions in the family.

Culture and life transitions

Assist families as they mark rituals (rites of passage) that symbolize cultural values. Common events expressed with cultural rituals are puberty, pregnancy, childbirth, dying, and death.

Repatterning

Changing one's lifestyle for a new and beneficial one
- Accommodate clients' cultural beliefs and values as much as possible.
- Attempt to repattern that belief to one that is compatible with health promotion, when a cultural value or behavior hinders a client's health and wellness.
- Plan and implement appropriate interventions, with knowledge of cultural differences and respect for the client and family.

Using an interpreter

The Joint Commission requires that an interpreter be available in health care facilities in the client's language (2010).
- Use only a facility-approved medical interpreter. Do not use the client's family or friends, or a nondesignated employee to interpret. Qrc
- Inform the interpreter about the reason for and the type of questions that will be asked, the expected response (brief or detailed), and with whom to converse.
- Interpreters must recognize their role without being biased of the client's response.
- Allow time for the interpreter and the family to be introduced and become acquainted before starting the interview.
- Refrain from making comments about the family to the interpreter because the family might understand some of the discussion.
- Ask one question at a time.
- Direct the questions to the client, not to the interpreter.
- Use lay terminology if possible, knowing that some words might not have an equivalent word in the client's language.
- Do not interrupt the interpreter, the client, or the family as they talk.
- Do not try to interpret answers.
- Following the interview, ask the interpreter for any additional thoughts about the interview and the client's and family's responses, both verbal and nonverbal.

Addressing spirituality

- Identify the client's perception of the existence of a higher power.
- Facilitate growth in the client's abilities to connect with a higher power.
- Look for environmental, behavioral, or verbal cues to assess a client's spirituality, such as a Bible at bedside, praying at bedtime, or talking about God.
- Assist the client to feel connected or reconnected to a higher power.
  - Allow time and/or resources for the practice of religious rituals.
  - Provide privacy for prayer, meditation, or the reading of religious materials.
- Use your facility's pastoral care department if appropriate.
- Facilitate development of a positive outcome in a particular situation.
- Provide stability for the person experiencing a dysfunctional spiritual mood.

- Establish a caring presence in being with the client and family rather than merely performing tasks for them.
- Support all healing relationships.
  - Using a holistic approach to care: seeing the large picture for the client
  - Using client-identified spiritual resources and needs
- Be aware of diet therapies included in spiritual beliefs.
- Support religious rituals.
  - Icons
  - Statues
  - Prayer rugs
  - Devotional readings
  - Music
- Support restorative care.
  - Prayer
  - Meditation
  - Grief work
- Evaluation of care is ongoing and continuous, with a need for flexibility as the client and family process the current crisis through their spiritual identity.

Application Exercises

1. A nurse is using an interpreter to communicate with a client. Which of the following actions should the nurse use when communicating with a client and his family? (Select all that apply.)
   A. Talk to the interpreter about the family while the family is in the room.
   B. Ask the family one question at a time.
   C. Look at the interpreter when asking the family questions.
   D. Use lay terms if possible.
   E. Do not interrupt the interpreter and the family as they talk.

2. A nurse is caring for a client who shares the nurse's religious background. Which of the following information should the nurse anticipate?
   A. Members of the same religion share similar feelings about their religion.
   B. A shared religious background generates mutual regard for one another.
   C. The same religious beliefs can influence individuals differently.
   D. The nurse and client should discuss the differences and commonalities in their beliefs.

3. A nurse is caring for a client who is crying while reading from his devotional book. Which of the following interventions should the nurse take?
   A. Contact the hospital's spiritual services.
   B. Ask him what is making him cry.
   C. Provide quiet times for these moments.
   D. Turn on the television for a distraction.

4. A nurse is planning care for a client who is a devout Muslim and is 3 days postoperative following a hip arthroplasty. The client is scheduled for two physical therapy sessions today. Which of the following statements by the nurse indicates culturally appropriate care to the client?
   A. "I will make sure the menu includes kosher options."
   B. "I will discuss the daily schedule with the client to make sure the client will have time for prayer."
   C. "I will make sure to use direct eye contact when speaking with this client."
   D. "I will make sure daily communion is available for this client."

5. A nurse is caring for a client who is a Jehovah's Witness and is scheduled for surgery as a result of a motor vehicle crash. The surgeon tells the client that a blood transfusion is essential. The client tells the nurse that based on his religious values and mandates, he cannot receive a blood transfusion. Which of the following responses should the nurse make?
   A. "I believe in this case you should really make an exception and accept the blood transfusion."
   B. "I know your family would approve of your decision to have a blood transfusion."
   C. "Why does your religion mandate that you cannot receive any blood transfusions?"
   D. "Let's discuss the necessity for a blood transfusion with your religious and spiritual leaders and come to a reasonable solution."

Application Exercises Key

1. A. Talking to the interpreter about the family while the family is in the room would hinder communication between the family and the nurse/interpreter.

   B. **CORRECT:** Asking the family one question at a time will promote effective communication between the family and the nurse/interpreter.

   C. Looking at the interpreter instead of the family while the family is in the room would hinder communication between the family and the nurse/interpreter.

   D. **CORRECT:** Using lay terms will promote effective communication between the family and the nurse/interpreter.

   E. **CORRECT:** Not interrupting will promote effective communication between the family and the nurse/interpreter.

   Ⓝ *NCLEX® Connection: Psychosocial Integrity, Cultural Awareness/Cultural Influences on Health*

2. A. It would be stereotyping to assume that all members of a specific religion had the same beliefs. Feelings and ideas about religion and spiritual matters can be quite diverse, even within a specific culture.

   B. Mutual regard does not necessarily follow a shared religious background.

   C. **CORRECT:** Members of any particular religion should be assessed for individual feelings and ideas.

   D. Due to boundary issues, the nurse's beliefs are not part of a therapeutic client relationship. It is the client's beliefs that are important.

   Ⓝ *NCLEX® Connection: Psychosocial Integrity, Religious Influences on Health*

3. A. Contacting the hospital's spiritual services presumes there is a problem.

   B. Asking the client about the crying could be interpreted as discounting or being disrespectful of the client's beliefs.

   C. **CORRECT:** Providing privacy and time for the reading of religious materials supports the client's spiritual health.

   D. Providing a distraction could be interpreted as discounting or being disrespectful of the client's beliefs.

   Ⓝ *NCLEX® Connection: Psychosocial Integrity, Religious Influences on Health*

4. A. Clients of the Jewish culture, not Islam, require their food to be kosher.

   B. **CORRECT:** Devout Muslims pray five times per day. Without proper awareness and planning, the client can refuse necessary treatments, such as physical therapy, if adequate prayer times are not planned for and incorporated into the client's day.

   C. American culture appreciates direct eye contact. In Middle Eastern cultures, direct eye contact can be perceived as rude, hostile, or sexually aggressive.

   D. Daily communion is a ritual to consider for a Catholic client, not for a Muslim client.

   Ⓝ *NCLEX® Connection: Psychosocial Integrity, Cultural Awareness/Cultural Influences on Health*

5. A. The nurse should not impose her opinion onto the client and ask him to go against his religious beliefs.

   B. The nurse should not make an assumption on behalf of the client's family.

   C. Asking a "why" question can appear judgmental or accusatory.

   D. **CORRECT:** Involving the client's religious and spiritual leaders is a culturally responsive action at this point. Alternative forms of blood products can be discussed, and a plan reasonable to all can be reached.

   Ⓝ *NCLEX® Connection: Psychosocial Integrity, Cultural Awareness/Cultural Influences on Health*

PRACTICE Active Learning Scenario

A nurse educator is conducting a class on culturally responsive nursing care. Use the ATI Active Learning Template: Basic Concept to complete this item.

RELATED CONTENT: List five examples of subculture categories than can exist within a culture.

PRACTICE Answer

Using the ATI Active Learning Template: Basic Concept

RELATED CONTENT

Although everyone within a culture shares cultural values, diversity exists. Forming subcultures is based on the following.

- Age
- Gender
- Sexual orientation
- Marital status
- Family structure
- Income
- Education level
- Religious views
- Life experiences

Ⓝ *NCLEX® Connection: Psychosocial Integrity, Cultural Awareness/Cultural Influences on Health*

UNIT 3   PSYCHOSOCIAL INTEGRITY

CHAPTER 36 *Grief, Loss, and Palliative Care*

Clients experience loss in many aspects of their lives. Grief is the inner emotional response to loss and is exhibited through thoughts, feelings, and behaviors. Bereavement includes both grief and mourning (the outward display of loss) as the individual deals with the death of a significant individual in their life.

Palliative or end-of-life care is an important aspect of nursing care and attempts to meet the client's physical, spiritual, emotional, and psychosocial needs. End-of-life issues include decision-making in a highly stressful time during which the nurse must consider the desires of the client and the family. Decisions are shared with other health care personnel for a smooth transition during this time of stress, grief, and bereavement.

ADVANCE DIRECTIVES

Advance directives: Legal documents that direct end-of-life issues
- **Living will:** Directive documents for medical treatment per the client's wishes
- **Health care proxy** (also known as durable power of attorney for health care): A document that appoints someone to make medical decisions when the client is no longer able to do so on his own behalf

TYPES OF LOSS

Necessary loss: A loss related to a change that is part of the cycle of life that is anticipated but still can be intensely felt. This type of loss can be replaced by something different or better.

Actual loss: Any loss of a valued person, item, or status, such as loss of a job that can be recognized by others

Perceived loss: Any loss defined by the client that is not obvious or verifiable to others

Maturational or developmental loss: Any loss normally expected due to the developmental processing of life. These losses are associated with normal life transitions and help to develop coping skills (e.g., child leaving home for college).

Situational loss: Any unanticipated loss caused by an external event (e.g., family loses home during tornado)

Anticipatory loss: Experienced before the loss happens

THEORIES OF GRIEF

KÜBLER-ROSS MODEL Q𝐄𝐁𝐏

Denial: The client has difficulty believing a terminal diagnosis or loss.

Anger: The client lashes out at other people or things.

Bargaining: The client negotiates for more time or a cure.

Depression: The client is overwhelmingly saddened by the inability to change the situation.

Acceptance: The client acknowledges what is happening and plans for the future by moving forward.

> Stages might not be experienced in order, and the length of each stage varies from person to person.

FACTORS INFLUENCING LOSS, GRIEF, AND COPING ABILITY

- Individual's current stage of development
- Gender
- Interpersonal relationships and social support networks
- Type and significance of the loss
- Culture and ethnicity
- Spiritual and religious beliefs and practices
- Prior experience with loss
- Socioeconomic status

FACTORS THAT CAN INCREASE AN INDIVIDUAL'S RISK FOR DYSFUNCTIONAL GRIEVING
- Being exceptionally dependent upon the deceased
- A person dying unexpectedly at a young age, through violence or in a socially unacceptable manner
- Inadequate coping skills or lack of social supports
- Lack of hope or preexisting mental health issues, such as depression or substance use disorder

ASSESSMENT/DATA COLLECTION

MANIFESTATIONS OF GRIEF REACTIONS

Normal grief

- This grief is considered uncomplicated.
- Emotions can be negative, such as anger, resentment, withdrawal, hopelessness, and guilt but should change to acceptance with time.
- Some acceptance should be evident by 6 months after the loss.
- Somatic complaints can include chest pain, palpitations, headaches, nausea, changes in sleep patterns, and fatigue.

Anticipatory grief

- This grief implies the "letting go" of an object or person before the loss, as in a terminal illness.
- Individuals have the opportunity to start the grieving process before the actual loss.

Complicated grief

- **Unresolved or chronic grief** is a type of complicated grief.
- This grief involves difficult progression through the expected stages of grief.
- Usually, the work of grief is prolonged. The manifestations of grief are more severe, and they can result in depression or exacerbate a preexisting disorder.
- The client can develop suicidal ideation, intense feelings of guilt, and lowered self-esteem.
- Somatic complaints persist for an extended period of time.

Disenfranchised grief

This grief entails an experienced loss that cannot be publicly shared or is not socially acceptable, such as suicide and abortion.

NURSING INTERVENTIONS

FACILITATE MOURNING Qpcc

- Grant time for the grieving process.
- Identify expected grieving behaviors, such as crying, somatic manifestations, and anxiety.
- Use therapeutic communication related to the client's stage of grief. Name the emotion the client is feeling. For example, the nurse can say, "You sound as though you are angry. Anger is a normal feeling for someone who has lost a loved one. Tell me about how you are feeling."
- Use active listening, open-ended questions, paraphrasing, clarifying, and/or summarizing, while using therapeutic communication.
- Use silence and personal presence to facilitate mourning.
- Avoid communication that inhibits the open expression of feelings, such as offering false reassurance, giving advice, changing the subject, and taking the focus away from the grieving individual.
- Assist the grieving individual to accept the reality of the loss.
- Support efforts to "move on" in the face of the loss.
- Encourage the building of new relationships.
- Provide continuing support. Encourage the support of family and friends.
- Assess for evidence of ineffective coping, such as a client refusing to leave the home months after his partner died.
- Share information about mourning and grieving with the client, who might not realize that feelings, such as anger toward the deceased, are expected.
- Encourage attendance at bereavement or grief support groups. Provide information about available community resources.
- Initiate referrals for individual psychotherapy for clients who have difficulty resolving grief.
- Ask the client whether contacting a spiritual advisor would be acceptable, or encourage the client to do so.
- Participate in debriefing provided by professional grief and mental health counselors.

Palliative care

- The nurse serves as an advocate for the client's sense of dignity and self-esteem by providing palliative care at the end of life.
- Goal is to learn to live fully with an incurable condition.
- Palliative care improves the quality of life of clients and their families facing end-of-life issues.
- Palliative care is appropriate for any client who has a chronic or curable illness, regardless of the stage of the disease process. Assessment of the client's family is very important as well.
- Palliative care interventions focus on the relief of physical manifestations (such as pain) as well as addressing spiritual, emotional, and psychosocial aspects of the client's life.
- Palliative care can be provided by an interprofessional team of physicians, nurses, social workers, physical therapists, massage therapists, occupational therapists, music/art therapists, touch/energy therapists, and chaplains. Qtc
- Hospice care is a comprehensive care delivery system, that can be performed in a variety of settings, and can be implemented when a client is not expected to live longer than 6 months. Further medical care aimed toward a cure is stopped, and the focus becomes enhancing quality of life and supporting the client toward a peaceful and dignified death.

ASSESSMENT/DATA COLLECTION

- Determine the client's sources of strength and hope.
- Identify the desires and expectations of the client and family for end-of-life care.

CHARACTERISTICS OF DISCOMFORT
- Pain
- Anxiety
- Restlessness
- Dyspnea
- Nausea or vomiting
- Dehydration
- Diarrhea or constipation
- Urinary incontinence
- Inability to perform ADLs

MANIFESTATIONS OF APPROACHING DEATH
- Decreased level of consciousness
- Muscle relaxation of the face
- Labored breathing (dyspnea, apnea, Cheyne-Stokes respirations), "death rattle"
- Hearing is not diminished
- Touch diminished, but client is able to feel the pressure of touch
- Mucus collecting in large airways
- Incontinence of bowel and/or bladder
- Mottling (cyanosis) occurring with poor circulation
- Pupils no longer reactive to light
- Pulse slow and weak and blood pressure dropping
- Cool extremities
- Perspiration
- Decreased urine output
- Inability to swallow

NURSING INTERVENTIONS

- Promote continuity of care and communication by limiting assigned staff changes.
- Assist the client and family to set priorities for end-of-life care.

PHYSICAL CARE

- Give priority to controlling findings.
- Administer medications (such as morphine) that manage pain, air hunger, and anxiety.
- Perform ongoing assessment to determine the effectiveness of treatment and the need for modifications of the treatment plan, such as lower or higher doses of medications.
- Manage adverse effects of medications.
- Reposition the client to maintain airway patency and comfort.
- Maintain the integrity of skin and mucous membranes.
- Provide caring touch (holding the client's hand).
- Provide an environment that promotes dignity and self-esteem.
  - Remove products of elimination as soon as possible to maintain a clean and odor-free environment.
  - Offer comfortable clothing.
  - Provide careful grooming for hair, nails, and skin.
  - Encourage family members to bring in comforting possessions to make the client feel at home.
- If appropriate, encourage the use of relaxation techniques, such as guided imagery and music.
- Promote decision-making in food selection, activities, and health care to give the client as much control as possible.
- Encourage the client to perform ADLs as able and willing to do so.

PSYCHOSOCIAL CARE Qpcc

- Use an interprofessional approach.
- Provide care and foster support to the client and family.
- Use volunteers when appropriate to provide nonmedical care.
- Use therapeutic communication to develop and maintain and facilitate communication between the client, family, and the provider.
- Facilitate the understanding of information regarding disease progression and treatment choices.
- Facilitate communication between the client, the family, and the provider.
- Encourage the client to participate in religious practices that bring comfort and strength, if appropriate.
- Assist the client in clarifying personal values in order to facilitate effective decision-making.
- Encourage the client to use coping mechanisms that have worked in the past.
- Be sensitive to comments made in the presence of clients who are unconscious because hearing is the last sensation lost.

PREVENTION OF ABANDONMENT AND ISOLATION

- Prevent the fear of dying alone.
- Make your presence known by answering call lights in a timely manner and making frequent contact.
- Keep the client informed of procedure and assessment times.
- Allow family members to stay overnight.
- Determine where the client is most comfortable, such as in a room close to the nurses' station.

SUPPORT FOR THE GRIEVING FAMILY

- Suggest that family members plan visits to promote the client's rest.
- Ensure that the family receives appropriate information as the treatment plan changes.
- Provide privacy so family members have the opportunity to communicate and express feelings among themselves without including the client.
- Determine family members' desire to provide physical care while maintaining awareness of possible caregiver fatigue. Provide instruction as necessary.
- Educate the family about physical changes to expect as the client moves closer to death.
- Allow families to express feelings

Postmortem care

- Nurses are responsible for following federal and state laws regarding requests for organ or tissue donation, obtaining permission for autopsy, ensuring the certification and appropriate documentation of the death, and providing postmortem (after-death) care.
- After postmortem care is completed, the client's family becomes the nurse's primary focus. Qᴘᴄᴄ

NURSING INTERVENTIONS

CARE OF THE BODY

- Provide care with respect and compassion while attending to the desires of the client and family per their cultural, religious, and social practices. Check the client's religion and make attempts to comply.
- Recognize that the provider certifies death by pronouncing the time and documenting therapies used, and actions taken prior to the death.

PREPARING THE BODY FOR VIEWING

- Maintain privacy.
- Remove all tubes (unless organs are to be donated or this is a medical examiner's case).
- Remove all personal belongings to be given to the family.
- Cleanse and align the body supine with a pillow under the head, arms with palms of hand down outside the sheet and blanket, dentures in place, and eyes closed.
- Apply fresh linens with absorbent pads on bed and a gown.
- Brush/comb the client's hair. Replace any hairpieces.
- Remove excess supplies, equipment, and soiled linens from the room.
- Dim the lights and minimize noise to provide a calm environment.

VIEWING CONSIDERATIONS

- Ask the family whether they would like to visit with the body, honoring any decision.
- Clarify where the client's personal belongings should go: with the body or to a designated person.
- Adhere to the same procedures when the client is an infant, with the following exceptions.
  - Swaddle the infant's body in a clean blanket.
  - Transport the infant in the nurse's arms or in an infant carrier based on facility protocol.
  - Offer mementos of the infant (identification bracelets, footprints, the cord clamp, a lock of hair, photos).

POSTVIEWING

- Apply identification tags according to facility policy.
- Complete documentation.
- Remain aware of visitor and staff sensibilities during transport.

ORGAN/TISSUE DONATION

- Recognize that requests for tissue and organ donations must be made by specifically trained personnel.
- Provide support and education to family members as decisions are being made. Use private areas for any family discussions concerning donation.
- Be sensitive to cultural and religious influences.
- Maintain ventilatory and cardiovascular support for vital organ retrieval.

AUTOPSY CONSIDERATIONS

- The provider typically approaches the family about performing an autopsy.
- The nurse's role is to answer the family members' questions and support their choices.
- Autopsies can be conducted to advance scientific knowledge regarding disease processes, which can lead to the development of new therapies.
- The law can require an autopsy to be performed if the death is due to homicide, suicide, or accidental death, or if death occurs within 24 hr of hospital admission.
- Most facilities require that all tubes remain in place for an autopsy.
- Documentation and completion of forms following federal and state laws typically includes the following.
  - Who pronounced the death and at what time
  - Consideration of and preparation for organ donation
  - Description of any tubes or lines left in or on the body
  - Disposition of personal articles
  - Who was notified, and any decisions made
  - Location of identification tags
  - Time the body left the facility and the destination

CARE OF NURSES WHO ARE GRIEVING

- Caring long-term for clients can create personal attachments for nurses.
- Nurses can use coping strategies.
  - Going to the client's funeral
  - Communicating in writing to the family
  - Attending debriefing sessions with colleagues
  - Using stress management techniques
  - Talking with a professional counselor

Application Exercises

1. A nurse is caring for a client who has terminal lung cancer. The nurse observes the client's family assisting with all ADLs. Which of the following rationales for self-care should the nurse communicate to the family?

   A. Allowing the client to function independently will strengthen her muscles and promote healing.

   B. The client needs to be given privacy at times for self-reflecting and organizing her life.

   C. The client's sense of loss can be lessened through retaining control of certain areas of her life.

   D. Performing ADLs is required prior to discharge from an acute care facility.

2. A nurse is caring for a client who has stage IV lung cancer and is 3 days postoperative following a wedge resection. The client states, "I told myself that I would go through with the surgery and quit smoking, if I could just live long enough to attend my daughter's wedding." Based on Kübler-Ross' model, which stage of grief is the client experiencing?

   A. Anger

   B. Denial

   C. Bargaining

   D. Acceptance

3. A nurse is consoling the partner of a client who just expired after a long battle with liver cancer. The partner is displaying grief and states, "I hate him for leaving me." Which of the following statements by the nurse successfully facilitate mourning for the grieving partner? (Select all that apply.)

   A. "Would you like me to contact the chaplain to come speak with you?"

   B. "You will feel better soon. You have been expecting this for a while now."

   C. "Let's talk about your children and how they are going to react."

   D. "You know, it is quite normal to feel anger toward your husband at this time."

   E. "Tell me more about how you are feeling."

4. A nurse is caring for a client who has a terminal illness. Death is expected within 24 hr. The client's family is at the bedside and asks the nurse about anticipated findings at this time. Which of the following findings should the nurse include in the discussion?

   A. Regular breathing patterns

   B. Warm extremities

   C. Increased urine output

   D. Decreased muscle tone

5. A nurse is assisting a newly licensed nurse with postmortem care of a client. The family wishes to view the body. Which of the following statements by the newly licensed nurse indicate an understanding of the procedure? (Select all that apply.)

   A. "I will remove the dentures from the body."

   B. "I will make sure the body is lying completely flat."

   C. "I will apply fresh linens and place a clean gown on the body."

   D. "I will remove all equipment from the bedside."

   E. "I will dim the lights in the room."

PRACTICE Active Learning Scenario

A nurse educator is teaching a module on palliative care to a group of newly licensed nurses. Use the ATI Active Learning Template: Basic Concept to complete this item.

NURSING INTERVENTIONS: List five physical care interventions and five psychological care interventions appropriate for the care of a client who is dying.

Application Exercises Key

1. A. Strengthening of muscles is not a priority of palliative care.

    B. Privacy for periods of self-reflection can be achieved at times apart from performance of ADLs.

    C. **CORRECT:** Allowing the client as much control as possible maintains dignity and self-esteem.

    D. Performance of ADLs is not a criterion for discharge from an acute care facility.

    Ⓝ *NCLEX® Connection: Psychosocial Integrity, End of Life Care*

2. A. This client statement does not display anger.

    B. The client is not denying the severity of the diagnosis and prognosis.

    C. **CORRECT:** The client is displaying bargaining by attempting to negotiate more time to live to see his daughter get married.

    D. Although the client might have accepted his diagnosis and prognosis, this client statement does not convey coming to terms with the situation.

    Ⓝ *NCLEX® Connection: Psychosocial Integrity, End of Life Care*

3. A. **CORRECT:** Asking the grieving individual whether she would like spiritual support at this time is an acceptable nursing intervention to facilitate mourning.

    B. The nurse should avoid giving false reassurance and offering assumptions while intervening to facilitate mourning.

    C. The nurse should avoid changing the subject and bringing the focus away from the grieving individual while intervening to facilitate mourning.

    D. **CORRECT:** The nurse should educate the grieving individual on the grieving process and expected emotions at this time.

    E. **CORRECT:** The nurse should encouraging the open communication of feelings by using therapeutic communication to facilitate mourning.

    Ⓝ *NCLEX® Connection: Psychosocial Integrity, Therapeutic Communication*

4. A. Labored breathing and irregular patterns are indicative of imminent death.

    B. Cool extremities would be indicative of imminent death.

    C. Decreased urine output would be indicative of imminent death.

    D. **CORRECT:** Muscle relaxation is an expected finding when a client is approaching death.

    Ⓝ *NCLEX® Connection: Psychosocial Integrity, End of Life Care*

5. A. The nurse should insert the client's dentures so that the face looks as natural as possible.

    B. The body should not be completely flat. One pillow is placed under the head and shoulders to prevent discoloration of the face.

    C. **CORRECT:** The body and the environment should be as clean as possible. This includes washing soiled areas of the body and applying fresh linens and a clean gown.

    D. **CORRECT:** The environment should be as clutter-free as possible. The nurse should remove all equipment and supplies from the bedside.

    E. **CORRECT:** Dimming the lights helps to provide a calm environment for the family.

    Ⓝ *NCLEX® Connection: Basic Care and Comfort, Personal Hygiene*

PRACTICE Answer

Using the ATI Active Learning Template: Basic Concept

NURSING INTERVENTIONS

Physical care

- Give priority to controlling findings.
- Administer medications that manage pain, air hunger, and anxiety.
- Perform ongoing assessment to determine the effectiveness of treatment and the need for modifications of the treatment plan, such as lower or higher doses of medications.
- Manage adverse effects of medications.
- Reposition the client to maintain airway patency and comfort.
- Maintain the integrity of skin and mucous membranes.
- Provide an environment that promotes dignity and self-esteem.
- Remove products of elimination as soon as possible to maintain a clean and odor-free environment.
- Offer comfortable clothing.
- Provide careful grooming for hair, nails, and skin.
- Encourage family members to bring in comforting possessions to make the client feel at home.
- If appropriate, encourage the use of relaxation techniques, such as guided imagery and music.
- Promote decision-making in food selection, activities, and health care to give the client as much control as possible.
- Encourage the client to perform ADLs as able and willing to do so.

Psychosocial care

- Use an interprofessional approach.
- Provide care to the client and family.
- Use volunteers when appropriate to provide nonmedical care.
- Use therapeutic communication to develop and maintain a nurse-client relationship.
- Facilitate the understanding of information regarding disease progression and treatment choices.
- Facilitate communication between the client, family, and provider.
- Encourage the client to participate in religious practices that bring comfort and strength, if appropriate.
- Assist the client in clarifying personal values in order to facilitate effective decision-making.
- Encourage the client to use coping mechanisms that have worked in the past.
- Be sensitive to comments made in the presence of clients who are unconscious because hearing is the last sensation lost.

Ⓝ *NCLEX® Connection: Basic Care and Comfort, Non-Pharmacological Comfort Interventions*

NCLEX® Connections

When reviewing the following chapters, keep in mind the relevant topics and tasks of the NCLEX outline, in particular:

Client Needs: Basic Care and Comfort

ASSISTIVE DEVICES
Assess the client's use of assistive devices.

Assist client to compensate for a physical or sensory impairment.

ELIMINATION: Provide skin care to clients who are incontinent.

MOBILITY/IMMOBILITY: Apply knowledge of nursing procedures and psychomotor skills when providing care to clients with immobility.

NON-PHARMACOLOGICAL COMFORT INTERVENTIONS
Recognize complementary therapies and identify potential contraindications.

Plan measures to provide comfort interventions to clients with anticipated or actual impaired comfort.

NUTRITION AND ORAL HYDRATION: Evaluate client intake and output and intervene as needed.

PERSONAL HYGIENE: Assess the client for personal hygiene habits/routine.

REST AND SLEEP: Schedule client care activities to promote adequate rest.

CHAPTER 37 *Hygiene*

Personal hygiene needs vary with clients' health status, social and cultural practices, and the daily routines they follow at home. For most clients, personal hygiene includes bathing, oral care, nail and foot care, perineal care, hair care, and shaving (especially for men).

Because personal hygiene has a profound effect on overall health, comfort, and well-being, it is an integral component of individualized nursing care plans. When clients become ill, have surgery, or are injured and are unable to manage their own personal hygiene needs, it becomes the nurse's responsibility to meet those needs.

Before beginning any personal care delivery, it is important to evaluate the client's ability to participate in personal hygiene. Encourage clients to participate in any way they can. Integrate assessment, range of motion exercises, and dressing changes while providing hygiene care.

HYGIENE CARE

Bathing

- Bathe clients to cleanse the body, stimulate circulation, provide relaxation, and enhance healing.
- Bathing clients is often delegated to the assistive personnel. However, the nurse is responsible for data collection and client care.
- Bathe clients whose health problems have exhausted them or limited their mobility.
  - Give a complete bath to clients who can tolerate it and whose hygiene needs warrant it.
  - Partial baths are useful when clients cannot tolerate a complete bath, need particular cleansing of odorous or uncomfortable areas, or can perform part of the bath independently.
  - Therapeutic baths are used to promote comfort and/or provide treatment, such as soothe itchy skin.

Oral hygiene

Proper oral hygiene helps decrease the risk of infection for clients living in long-term care facilities, especially from the transmission of pathogens that can cause pneumonia.

Foot care

- Foot care prevents skin breakdown, pain, and infection.
- Foot care is extremely important for clients who have diabetes mellitus, and a qualified professional must perform it. Qs

Perineal care

Perineal care helps maintain skin integrity, relieve discomfort, and prevent transmission of micro-organisms (catheter care).

CULTURAL AND SOCIAL PRACTICES

- Clients vary in their hygiene preferences and practices. These include bathing routines, oral care, grooming preferences, and health beliefs.
- Culture also plays an important role, because some cultures have unique hygiene practices. Be sure to be respectful and observant of each client's specific cultural needs.
- Consider the client's personal preference regarding hygiene practices.
- Socioeconomic status can affect clients' hygiene status. If a client is homeless, alter discharge instructions and follow-up care accordingly.
- Respect each client's dignity. Many clients are dealing with a loss of control when others must provide their hygiene care. Reassure clients and allow them to have as much control as possible. Qpcc

SAFETY Qs

- Before starting any care, understand how to complete each task to avoid injuring the client. This includes knowing the equipment and what the proper techniques are for each hygiene procedure.
- Never leave clients in a position where injury could occur during routine hygiene care. For example, avoid leaving a client who is at risk for aspiration alone with oral hygiene supplies.
- Adjust the bed to comfortable working height and lower the bed upon completion of the task.

CONSIDERATIONS FOR OLDER ADULTS Ⓒ

- Older adults' skin is drier, thinner, and will not tolerate as much bathing as younger adults' skin.
- Older adults have higher incidences of infection and periodontal disease due to the weakening of the periodontal membrane.
- Dentures must fit correctly, or they can cause digestive issues, pain, and discomfort. Dentures are a client's personal property. Never leave them on a meal tray or in a place where they could be damaged or lost.
- Dry mouth is common in older adults due to decreased saliva production and the use of certain medications (antihypertensives, diuretics, anti-inflammatory agents, antidepressants).
- Poor nutritional status is often due to dental problems, socioeconomic status, or a limited ability to prepare healthful foods.

ASSESSMENT/DATA COLLECTION

- Inspect the skin for color, hydration, texture, turgor, and any lesions or other impaired integrity.
- Check the condition of the gums and teeth for dryness or inflammation of the oral mucosa. Does the client report any pain?
- Assess the skin surfaces, including the feet and nails, and note the shape and size of each foot, any lesions, and areas of dryness or inflammation. Significant alterations can indicate neuropathy and/or vascular insufficiency. Are all pulses palpable and equal bilaterally?
- Identify hygiene preferences to understand how clients perform hygiene at home and what additional education and care to provide.
- Monitor for safety issues (altered positioning, decreased mobility) and the ability to participate in self-care. Alter the plan of care according to the client's capabilities.

PATIENT-CENTERED CARE

NURSING CONSIDERATIONS

Giving a bed bath

- Collect supplies, provide for privacy, and explain the procedure to the client.
- Apply gloves.
- Lock the wheels on the bed.
- Adjust the bed to a comfortable working position.
- Place a bath blanket over the client, and remove the client's gown.
- Obtain warm bath water.
- Wash the client's face first. Allow the client to perform this task if able.
- Perform the bath systematically by starting with the client's trunk and upper extremities and continuing to the client's lower extremities. Keep cleaned areas covered with a blanket or towel.
- Wash with long, firm strokes from distal to proximal. Use light strokes over lower extremities for clients who have a history of deep vein thrombosis. Qs
- Apply lotion and powder (if neither is contraindicated), and a clean gown.
- Change water if cool or as indicated, and use fresh water to perform perineal care.
- Document skin assessment, type of bath, and the client's response.

TO CHANGE LINENS ON AN OCCUPIED BED

- Adjust the bed to a comfortable working height.
- Don gloves.
- Roll the bottom linens up in the bottom sheet or mattress pad under the client who is turned on his side, facing the opposite direction. For safety purposes, adjust and lower side rails accordingly.
- Apply clean bottom linens to the bed (draw sheets are optional), and extend them to the middle of the bed with the remainder of the linen fan-folded underneath the client.
- Have the client roll over the linens and face the opposite direction, then remove the used linens (keep away from your uniform) and apply the clean linens. Make sure the linens are free from wrinkles.
- Apply the upper sheet and blanket.
- To remove the pillowcase, insert one hand into the opening, grab the pillow, and turn the pillowcase inside-out.
- Apply the clean pillowcase by grasping the center of the closed end, turning the case inside-out, fitting the pillow into the corner of the case, and pulling the case until it is right-side out over the pillow.

Foot care

- It is important to prevent any infection or pain that can interfere with gait. A qualified professional should perform foot care for clients who have diabetes mellitus, peripheral vascular disease, or immunosuppression to evaluate the feet and prevent injury.
- Instruct clients at risk for injury to do the following. Qs
  - Inspect the feet daily, paying specific attention to the area between the toes.
  - Use lukewarm water, and dry the feet thoroughly.
  - Apply moisturizer to the feet, but avoid applying it between the toes.
  - Avoid over-the-counter products that contain alcohol or other strong chemicals.
  - Wear clean cotton socks daily.
  - Check shoes for any objects, rough seams, or edges that can cause injury.
  - Cut the nails straight across, and use an emery board to file nail edges.
  - Avoid self-treating corns or calluses.
  - Wear comfortable shoes that do not restrict circulation.
  - Do not apply heat unless prescribed.
  - Contact the provider if any indications of infection or inflammation appear.

Perineal care

It is important to maintain skin integrity to relieve discomfort and prevent transmission of infection (catheter care).

PRINCIPLES OF PERINEAL CARE

- Provide privacy.
- Maintain a professional demeanor.
- Remove any fecal material from the skin.
- Cleanse the perineal area from front to back (perineum to rectum).
- Dry thoroughly.
- Retract the foreskin of male clients to wash the tip of the penis, clean from the meatus outward in a circular motion, then replace the foreskin.

Oral hygiene

- Check for aspiration risk, impaired swallowing, or decreased gag reflex. Qs
- Clients who have fragile oral mucosa require gentle brushing and flossing.
- Have suction apparatus ready at the bedside when providing oral hygiene to clients who are unconscious to help prevent aspiration. Do not place fingers into an unconscious client's mouth (the client could bite down on your fingers). Position the client on his side with his head turned toward you in either a semi-Fowler's position, or with the head of the bed flat. This will allow fluid and oral secretions to collect in the dependent side of the client's mouth and drain out. Qs
- Perform denture care for clients who are unable to do so themselves. Dentures are very fragile, so handle with care.
  - Remove the dentures with a gloved hand, pulling down and out at the front of the upper denture, and lifting up and out at the front of the lower denture.
  - Place the dentures in a denture cup, emesis basin, or on a washcloth in the sink.
  - Brush in a horizontal back and forth motion with a soft brush and denture cleaner.
  - Rinse dentures in tepid water.
  - Store the dentures in a denture cup. Label the cup with the client's name.
  - Place the dentures in the cup with water to keep them moist, or help the client reinsert the dentures.

Nail care

- Observe the size, shape, and condition of the nails and nail beds.
- Check for cracking, clubbing, and fungus.
- Before cutting any client's nails, check the facility's policy. Some require a prescription from the provider, while others allow only a podiatrist or other qualified professional to cut some or all clients' nails.
- Foot and nail care vary from the standard when caring for a client who has diabetes mellitus or peripheral vascular disease. Do not soak the feet due to the risk of infection, and do not cut the nails. Instead, file nails using a nail file. Do not apply lotion between the fingers or toes because the moisture can cause skin irritation and breakdown. QEBP

Hair care

- Caring for the hair and scalp is important for clients' appearance and sense of well-being, and is an essential component of personal hygiene. Take into consideration the client's cultural and personal preferences. **Q**_{pcc}
- Brush or comb the hair daily to remove tangles, massage the scalp, stimulate circulation to the scalp, and distribute natural oils along the shaft of the hair. Use a soft-bristled brush to prevent injury or trauma to the scalp and a wide-toothed comb or hair pick to comb through tightly curled hair.
- For clients who cannot shower but can sit in a chair and lean back, shampoo the hair at the sink. For clients on bed rest, use a plastic shampoo trough. Dry or no-rinse shampoos and shampoo caps are also options for clients on bed rest.
- Start shampooing the hair at the hairline and work toward the neck. To wash the hair on the back of the head, gently lift the head with one hand and shampoo with the other.
- Place a folded or rolled towel behind the neck to pad the edge of the sink. Then rinse, comb, and dry the hair.

Shaving

- Safety is important. Clients who are prone to bleeding, receiving anticoagulants, or have low platelet counts should use an electric razor. **Q**_s
- Soften the skin with warm water.
- Apply soap (bar soap not recommended) or shaving cream.
- Hold the skin taut.
- Move the razor over the skin in the direction of hair growth using long strokes on large areas of the face and short strokes around the chin and lips.
- Be sure to communicate with clients about personal shaving preferences.

Application Exercises

1. A nurse is performing mouth care for a client who is unconscious. Which of the following actions should the nurse take?

    A. Turn the client's head to the side.

    B. Place two fingers in the client's mouth to open.

    C. Brush the client's teeth once per day.

    D. Inject a mouth rinse into the center of the client's mouth.

2. A nurse is instructing a client who has diabetes mellitus about foot care. Which of the following guidelines should the nurse include? (Select all that apply.)

    A. Inspect the feet daily.

    B. Use moisturizing lotion on the feet.

    C. Wash the feet with warm water and let them air dry.

    D. Use over-the-counter products to treat abrasions.

    E. Wear cotton socks.

3. A nurse is planning care for a client who develops dyspnea and feels tired after completing her morning care. Which of the following actions should the nurse include in the client's plan of care?

    A. Schedule rest periods during morning care.

    B. Discontinue morning care for 2 days.

    C. Perform all care as quickly as possible.

    D. Ask a family member to come in to bathe the client.

4. A nurse is beginning a complete bed bath for a client. After removing the client's gown and placing a bath blanket over him, which of the following areas should the nurse wash first?

    A. Face

    B. Feet

    C. Chest

    D. Arms

5. A nurse is preparing to perform denture care for a client. Which of the following actions should the nurse plan to take?

    A. Pull down and out at the back of the upper denture to remove.

    B. Brush the dentures with a toothbrush and denture cleaner.

    C. Rinse the dentures with hot water after cleaning them.

    D. Place the dentures in a clean, dry storage container after cleaning them.

PRACTICE Active Learning Scenario

A nurse is about to perform perineal care for a client whose ability to assist with care is limited. Use the ATI Active Learning Template: Nursing Skill to complete this item.

DESCRIPTION OF SKILL: List the steps the nurse should take to perform this procedure.

1. A. **CORRECT:** The nurse should position the client's head on the side, unless contraindicated, to reduce the risk of aspiration.

    B. The nurse should not insert fingers into the client's mouth because the client might bite down on the fingers.

    C. The nurse should brush the client's teeth at least twice per day.

    D. The nurse should gently inject a mouth rinse into the side of the client's mouth to reduce the risk for aspiration.

    Ⓝ *NCLEX® Connection: Reduction of Risk Potential, Potential for Complications of Diagnostic Tests/Treatments/Procedures*

2. A. **CORRECT:** Clients who have diabetes mellitus are at increased risk for infection and diminished sensitivity in the feet, so they should inspect them daily.

    B. **CORRECT:** The client should use moisturizing lotions (but not between the toes) to help keep the skin smooth and supple.

    C. The client should wash the feet with lukewarm water and dry the feet thoroughly.

    D. Over-the-counter products often contain harmful chemicals that can cause skin impairment.

    E. **CORRECT:** The client should wear clean cotton socks each day.

    Ⓝ *NCLEX® Connection: Reduction of Risk Potential, Potential for Alterations in Body Systems*

3. A. **CORRECT:** Planning for rest periods during morning care will help prevent fatigue and continue to foster independence.

    B. Fatigue and dyspnea do not eliminate the need for morning care.

    C. Performing all of the client's care quickly might affect the client's self-esteem and reduce his independence.

    D. Having a family member bathe the client reduces his self-esteem and independence, and does not reduce the client's fatigue.

    Ⓝ *NCLEX® Connection: Basic Care and Comfort, Rest and Sleep*

4. A. **CORRECT:** The greatest risk to a client during bathing is the transmission of pathogens from one area of the body to another. The nurse should begin with the cleanest area of the body and proceed to the least clean area. The face is generally the cleanest area, and washing it first follows a systematic head-to-toe approach to client care.

    B. The client is at risk for infection from pathogens on the client's feet. Therefore, the nurse should wash another area first.

    C. The client is at risk for infection from pathogens on the client's chest. Therefore, the nurse should wash another area first.

    D. The client is at risk for infection from pathogens on the client's arms. Therefore, the nurse should wash another area first.

    Ⓝ *NCLEX® Connection: Safety and Infection Control, Standard Precautions/Transmission–Based Precautions/Surgical Asepsis*

5. A. The nurse remove the upper dentures with a gloved hand, pulling down and out at the front of the upper denture.

    B. **CORRECT:** Brushing the dentures thoroughly with a toothbrush and denture cleaner removes debris that accumulates on and between the teeth.

    C. Using hot water to rinse dentures can damage some denture materials. The nurse should use tepid water to rinse dentures.

    D. Dentures should be moist when not in use to prevent warping and to facilitate insertion. The nurse should store them in water in a denture cup with the client's identification on the cup.

    Ⓝ *NCLEX® Connection: Basic Care and Comfort, Assistive Devices*

PRACTICE Answer

Using the ATI Active Learning Template: Nursing Skill

DESCRIPTION OF SKILL
- Provide privacy.
- Maintain a professional demeanor.
- Remove any fecal material from the skin.
- Cleanse the perineal area from front to back.
- Dry skin thoroughly.
- Retract the foreskin of male clients to wash the tip of the penis, clean from the meatus outward in a circular motion, then replace the foreskin.

Ⓝ *NCLEX® Connection: Safety and Infection Control, Standard Precautions/Transmission–Based Precautions/Surgical Asepsis*

CHAPTER 38 Rest and Sleep

Adequate amounts of sleep and rest promote health. Too little sleep leads to inability to concentrate, poor judgment, moodiness, irritability, and increased risk for accidents.

Chronic sleep loss can increase risks of obesity, depression, hypertension, diabetes mellitus, heart attack, and stroke.

SLEEP CYCLE

The sleep cycle consists of four stages of **nonrapid eye movement (NREM) sleep** and a period of **rapid eye movement (REM) sleep**. Typically, after Stage 1 of NREM sleep, people cycle four to six times through the other stages of sleep per night. With each cycle, the length of time in REM sleep increases. NREM sleep accounts for 75% to 80% of sleep time.

Stage 1 NREM

- Very light sleep
- Only a few minutes long
- Vital signs and metabolism beginning to decrease
- Awakens easily
- Feels relaxed and drowsy

Stage 2 NREM

- Deeper sleep
- 10 to 20 min long
- Vital signs and metabolism continuing to slow
- Requires slightly more stimulation to awaken
- Increased relaxation

Stage 3 NREM

- Initial stages of deep sleep
- 15 to 30 min long
- Vital signs continuing to decrease but remain regular
- Difficult to awaken
- Relaxation with little movement

Stage 4 NREM

- Called delta sleep
- Deepest sleep
- 15 to 30 min long
- Vital signs low
- Very difficult to awaken
- Physiologic rest and restoration
- Enuresis, sleepwalking, sleeptalking possible
- Repair and renewal of tissue

REM

- Vivid dreaming
- About 90 min after falling asleep
- Longer with each sleep cycle
- Average length 20 min
- Varying vital signs
- Very difficult to awaken
- Cognitive restoration

SLEEP DURATION

Sleep averages vary with the developmental stage, with infants and toddlers averaging 9 to 15 hr/day. This declines gradually throughout childhood, with adolescents averaging 9 to 10 hr/day and adults 7 to 8 hr/day.

COMMON SLEEP DISORDERS

Insomnia

- The most common sleep disorder, this is the inability to get an adequate amount of sleep and to feel rested. It might mean difficulty falling asleep, difficulty staying asleep, awakening too early, or not getting refreshing sleep.
- **Acute insomnia** lasts a few days possibly due to personal or situational stressors.
- **Chronic insomnia** lasts a month or more.
- Some people have **intermittent insomnia**, sleeping well for a few days and then having insomnia for a few days.
- Women and older adults are more prone to insomnia.

Sleep apnea

- More than five breathing cessations lasting longer than 10 seconds per hour during sleep, resulting in decreased arterial oxygen saturation levels.
- Sleep apnea can be a single disorder or a mixture of the following
  - **Central:** Central nervous system dysfunction in the respiratory control center of the brain that fails to trigger breathing during sleep.
  - **Obstructive:** Structures in the mouth and throat relax during sleep and occlude the upper airway.

Narcolepsy

- Sudden attacks of sleep or excessive sleepiness during waking hours.
- It often happens at inappropriate times and increases the risk for injury.

ASSESSMENT/DATA COLLECTION

- Ask about sleep patterns, history, and any recent changes.
- Identify the usual sleep requirements.
- Ask about sleep problems (type, manifestations, timing, seriousness, related factors, aftereffects). Qpcc
- Use a linear or visual scale with "best sleep" on one end and "worst sleep" on the opposite end and ask for a sleep rating on a 0 to 10 scale.
- Check for common factors that interfere with sleep.

FACTORS THAT INTERFERE WITH SLEEP

Illness: Can require more sleep or disrupt sleep, such as nocturia.

Current life events: Traveling more, change in work hours.

Emotional stress or mental illness: Anxiety, fear, grief.

Diet: Caffeine consumption, heavy meals before bedtime.

Exercise: Promotes sleep if at least 2 hr before bedtime. Otherwise can disrupt sleep.

Fatigue: Exhausting or stressful work makes falling asleep difficult.

Sleep environment: Too light, the wrong temperature, or too noisy (children, pets, loud noise, snoring partner).

Medications: Some can induce sleep but interfere with restorative sleep. Others (bronchodilators, antihypertensives) cause insomnia.

NURSING CONSIDERATIONS

- Help clients establish and follow a bedtime routine.
- Limit waking clients during the night.
- Promote a quiet hospital environment.
- Help with personal hygiene needs or a back rub prior to sleep to increase comfort. Qpcc
- Consider continuous positive airway pressure (CPAP) devices for clients who have sleep apnea.
- Consult the provider about trying sleep-promoting over-the-counter products (melatonin, valerian, chamomile).
- As a last resort, suggest that the provider prescribe a pharmacological agent. Medications of choice for insomnia are benzodiazepine-like medications, which include the sedative-hypnotics zolpidem, eszopiclone, and zaleplon.

CLIENT EDUCATION

- Exercise regularly at least 2 hr before bedtime.
- Establish a bedtime routine and a regular sleep pattern.
- Arrange the sleep environment for comfort.
- Limit alcohol, caffeine, and nicotine at least 4 hr before bedtime.
- Limit fluids 2 to 4 hr before bedtime.
- Engage in muscle relaxation if anxious or stressed.

CLIENT EDUCATION FOR NARCOLEPSY Qs

- Exercise regularly.
- Eat small meals that are high in protein.
- Avoid activities that increase sleepiness (sitting too long, warm environments, drinking alcohol).
- Avoid activities that could cause injury should the client fall asleep (driving, heights).
- Take naps when drowsy or when narcoleptic events are likely.
- Take prescribed stimulants.

Application Exercises

1. A nurse in a provider's office is caring for a client who states that, for the past week, she has felt tired during the day and cannot sleep at night. Which of the following responses should the nurse ask when collecting data about the client's difficulty sleeping? (Select all that apply.)

   A. "Does your lack of sleep interfere with your ability to function during the day?"

   B. "Do you feel confused in the late afternoon?"

   C. "Do you drink coffee, tea, or other caffeinated drinks? If so, how many cups per day?"

   D. "Has anyone ever told you that you seem to stop breathing for a few seconds while you are asleep?"

   E. "Tell me about any personal stress you are experiencing."

2. A nurse is talking with a client about ways to help him sleep and rest. Which of the following recommendations should the nurse give to the client to promote sleep and rest? (Select all that apply.)

   A. Practice muscle relaxation techniques.

   B. Exercise each morning.

   C. Take an afternoon nap.

   D. Alter the sleep environment for comfort.

   E. Limit fluid intake at least 2 hr before bedtime.

3. A nurse is caring for an older adult client who has been following the facility's routine and bathing in the morning. However, at home, she always takes a warm bath just before bedtime. Now she is having difficulty sleeping at night. Which of the following actions should the nurse take first?

   A. Rub the client's back for 15 min before bedtime.

   B. Offer the client warm milk and crackers at 2100.

   C. Allow the client to take a bath in the evening.

   D. Ask the provider for a sleeping medication.

4. A nurse is preparing a presentation at a local community center about sleep hygiene. When explaining rapid eye movement (REM) sleep, which of the following characteristics should the nurse include? (Select all that apply.)

   A. REM sleep provides cognitive restoration.

   B. REM sleep lasts about 90 min.

   C. It is difficult to awaken a person in REM sleep.

   D. Sleepwalking occurs during REM sleep.

   E. Vivid dreams are common during REM sleep.

5. A nurse is instructing a client who has a new diagnosis of narcolepsy about measures that might help with self-management. Which of the following statements should the nurse identify as an indication that the client understands the instructions?

   A. "I'll add plenty of carbohydrates to my meals."

   B. "I'll take a short nap whenever I feel a little sleepy."

   C. "I'll make sure I stay warm when I am at my desk at work."

   D. "It's okay to drink alcohol as long as I limit it to one drink per day."

PRACTICE Active Learning Scenario

A nurse on a medical unit is collecting data from a client who reports a persistent inability to sleep. Use the ATI Active Learning Template: Basic Concept to complete this item.

UNDERLYING PRINCIPLES: List at least three common factors that might be interfering with the client's sleep.

NURSING INTERVENTIONS: List at least three strategies the nurse can implement to help the client sleep while in the hospital.

Application Exercises Key

1. A. **CORRECT:** Daytime sleepiness, which can interfere with functioning, is common during the day when people cannot sleep at night.

   B. Chronic sleep deprivation or lack of rapid eye movement sleep can cause confusion, but sleep difficulties for 1 week should not result in confusion.

   C. **CORRECT:** Caffeinated drinks act as a stimulant and can interfere with sleep.

   D. **CORRECT:** Periods of apnea warrant a prompt referral for diagnostic sleep studies.

   E. **CORRECT:** Emotional stress is the most common cause of short-term sleep problems.

   Ⓝ *NCLEX® Connection: Basic Care and Comfort, Rest and Sleep*

2. A. **CORRECT:** Relaxation techniques, especially muscle relaxation, can help promote sleep and rest.

   B. **CORRECT:** Following an exercise routine regularly, at least 2 hr prior to bedtime, can help promote rest and sleep.

   C. Napping during the day can keep some people from getting the sleep they need during their usual sleeping hours.

   D. **CORRECT:** For example, rather than trying to sleep with a restless pet at the foot of the bed, move the pet to another sleep area.

   E. **CORRECT:** Limiting fluids for a few hours before bedtime helps minimize getting up to urinate.

   Ⓝ *NCLEX® Connection: Basic Care and Comfort, Rest and Sleep*

3. A. Rubbing the client's back can help promote sleep, but there is another option the nurse should try first.

   B. Offering the client warm milk and crackers can help promote sleep, but there is another option the nurse should try first.

   C. **CORRECT:** When providing nursing care, the nurse should first use the least restrictive intervention. Of these options, allowing the client to follow her usual bedtime routine represents the least change, so it is the first intervention to try.

   D. Asking for a prescription for sleep medication can help, but there is another option the nurse should try first.

   Ⓝ *NCLEX® Connection: Basic Care and Comfort, Rest and Sleep*

4. A. **CORRECT:** Cognitive and brain tissue restoration occur during REM sleep.

   B. REM sleep lasts an average of 20 min. It typically begins about 90 min after falling asleep.

   C. **CORRECT:** In this stage, awakening is difficult. Awakening is relatively easy in stages 1 and 2 of non-REM sleep.

   D. Sleepwalking and sleeptalking tend to occur during stage 4 of non-REM sleep.

   E. **CORRECT:** Dreaming does occur in other stages, but it is less vivid and possibly less colorful.

   Ⓝ *NCLEX® Connection: Physiological Adaptation, Pathophysiology*

5. A. Clients who have narcolepsy should eat light, high-protein meals.

   B. **CORRECT:** Clients who have narcolepsy should take short naps to reduce feelings of drowsiness.

   C. Clients who have narcolepsy should avoid sitting for prolonged periods in warm environments.

   D. Clients who have narcolepsy should avoid ingesting any substance that could increase drowsiness, such as alcohol.

   Ⓝ *NCLEX® Connection: Basic Care and Comfort, Rest and Sleep*

PRACTICE Answer

Using the ATI Active Learning Template: Basic Concept

UNDERLYING PRINCIPLES

- Illness
- Current life events (travel, change in work hours)
- Emotional stress or mental illness (anxiety, fear)
- Caffeine consumption
- Heavy meals before bedtime
- Exercise within 2 hr of bedtime
- Sleep environment that is noisy, too light, or the wrong temperature
- Medications that cause insomnia

NURSING INTERVENTIONS

- Help clients establish and follow a bedtime routine.
- Limit waking clients during the night.
- Promote a quiet hospital environment.
- Assist with personal hygiene needs.
- Offer a back rub.
- Request a prescription for a sleep medication from the provider.

Ⓝ *NCLEX® Connection: Basic Care and Comfort, Rest and Sleep*

CHAPTER 39 *Nutrition and Oral Hydration*

Nutrients provide energy for cellular metabolism, tissue maintenance and repair, organ function, growth and development, and physical activity. Water, the most basic of all nutrients, is crucial for all body fluid and cellular functions.

The proper balance of nutrients and fluid along with consideration of energy intake and requirements is essential for ensuring adequate nutritional status. Early recognition and treatment of clients who are malnourished or at risk can have a positive influence on client outcomes.

A nutritional assessment helps identify areas to modify, either through adding or avoiding specific nutrients or by increasing or decreasing caloric intake.

When planning a nutritional or hydration intervention, it is important to consider beliefs and culture, the environment, and the presentation of the food, as well as any illnesses or allergies clients might have. Qpcc

BASIC NUTRIENTS THE BODY REQUIRES

Carbohydrates provide most of the body's energy and fiber. Each gram produces 4 kcal. They provide glucose, which burns completely and efficiently without end products to excrete. Sources include whole grain breads, baked potatoes, brown rice, and other plant foods.

Fats provide energy and vitamins. No more than 35% of caloric intake should be from fat. Each gram produces 9 kcal. Sources include olive oil, salmon, and egg yolks.

Proteins contribute to the growth, maintenance, and repair of body tissues. Each gram produces 4 kcal. Sources of complete protein include beef, whole milk, and poultry.

Vitamins are necessary for metabolism. The fat-soluble vitamins are A, D, E, and K. The water-soluble vitamins include C and B complex (eight vitamins). Qebp

Minerals complete essential biochemical reactions in the body (calcium, potassium, sodium, iron).

Water is critical for cell function and replaces fluids the body loses through perspiration, elimination, and respiration.

FACTORS AFFECTING NUTRITION AND METABOLISM

Religious and cultural practices guide food preparation and choices. Qpcc

Financial issues prevent some clients from buying foods that are high in protein, vitamins, and minerals.

Appetite decreases with illness, medications, pain, depression, and unpleasant environmental stimuli.

Negative experiences with certain foods or familiarity with foods clients like help determine preferences.

Environmental factors such as sedentary lifestyles, work schedules, and widespread access to less healthy foods contribute to obesity.

Disease and illness can affect the functional ability to prepare and eat food. Qs

Medications can alter taste and appetite and can interfere with the absorption of certain nutrients.

Age affects nutritional requirements.

AGE

Newborns and infants (birth to 1 year)
- High energy requirements
- Breast milk (ideally) or formula to provide
  - 108 kcal/kg of weight the first 6 months
  - 98 kcal/kg of weight the second 6 months
- Solid food starting at 4 to 6 months of age
- No cow's milk or honey for the first year

Toddlers (12 months to 3 years) and preschoolers (3 to 6 years)
- Toddlers and preschoolers need fewer calories per kg of weight than infants do.
- Toddlers and preschoolers need increased protein from sources other than milk.
- Calcium and phosphorus are important for bone health.
- Nutrient density is more important than quantity.

School-age children (6 to 12 years)
- School-age children need supervision to consume adequate protein and vitamins C and A.
- They tend to eat foods high in carbohydrates, fats, and salt.
- They grow at a slower and steadier rate, with a gradual decline in energy requirements.

Adolescents (12 to 20 years)
- Metabolic demands are high and require more energy.
- Protein, calcium, iron, iodine, folic acid, and vitamin B needs are high.
- One-fourth of dietary intake comes from snacks.
- Increased water consumption is important for active adolescents.
- Body image and appearance, fast foods, peer pressure, and fad diets influence adolescents' diet.

Young adults (20 to 35 years) and middle adults (35 to 65 years)
- There is a decreased need for most nutrients (except during pregnancy).
- Calcium and iron are essential minerals for women.
- Good oral health is important.

Older adults (over 65 years)
- A slower metabolic rate requires fewer calories.
- Thirst sensations diminish.
- Older adults need the same amount of most vitamins and minerals as younger adults.
- Calcium is important for both men and women.
- Many older adults require carbohydrates that provide fiber and bulk to enhance gastrointestinal function.

EATING DISORDERS

Anorexia nervosa
- Significantly low body weight for gender, age, developmental level, and physical health.
- Fear of being fat
- Self-perception of being fat
- Consistent restriction of food intake or repeated behavior that prevents weight gain

Bulimia nervosa: a cycle of binge eating followed by purging (vomiting, using diuretics or laxatives, exercise, fasting)
- Lack of control during binges
- Average at least one cycle of binge eating and purging per week for at least 3 months

Binge-eating disorder: repeated episodes of binge eating
- Feels a loss of control when binge eating, followed by an emotional response such as guilt, shame, or depression
- Does not use compensatory behaviors, such as purging
- Binge-eating episodes can range from 1 to more than 14 times per week
- Clients are often overweight or obese.

OBESITY

A BMI of 25 is the upper boundary of healthy weight (25 to 29.9 is considered overweight for an adult; 30 or greater is considered obese).

ASSESSMENT/DATA COLLECTION

Dietary history should include the following.
- Number of meals per day
- Fluid intake
- Food preferences, amounts
- Food preparation, purchasing practices, access
- History of indigestion, heartburn, gas
- Allergies
- Taste
- Chewing and swallowing
- Appetite
- Elimination patterns
- Medication use
- Activity levels
- Religious, cultural food preferences and restrictions
- Nutritional screening tools

CLINICAL MEASURES

- Height, weight to calculate BMI and ideal body weight

BMI = weight (kg) ÷ height (m²)
Step 1: Determine the client's weight in kg and height in m
Step 2: Multiply the client's height by itself to determine the m² value
Step 3: Divide the weight in kg by the height value from step 2. The result is the client's BMI.

- Skinfold measurements
- Laboratory values of cholesterol, triglycerides, hemoglobin, electrolytes, albumin, prealbumin, transferrin, lymphocyte count, nitrogen balance

INTAKE AND OUTPUT

- Record I&O.
- Monitor I&O for clients who have fluid or electrolyte imbalances.
- Weigh clients each day at the same time, after voiding, and while wearing the same type of clothes.
- If using bed scales, use the same amount of linen each day, and reset the scale to zero if possible.

EXPECTED FINDINGS OF POOR NUTRITION

- Nausea, vomiting, diarrhea, constipation
- Flaccid muscles
- Mental status changes
- Loss of appetite
- Change in bowel pattern
- Spleen, liver enlargement
- Dry, brittle hair and nails
- Loss of subcutaneous fat
- Dry, scaly skin
- Inflammation, bleeding of gums
- Poor dental health
- Dry, dull eyes
- Enlarged thyroid
- Prominent protrusions over bony areas
- Weakness, fatigue
- Change in weight
- Poor posture

NURSING INTERVENTIONS

- Assist in advancing the diet as prescribed.
- Instruct clients about the appropriate diet regimen.
- Provide interventions to promote appetite (good oral hygiene, favorite foods, minimal environmental odors).
- Educate clients about medications that can affect nutritional intake.
- Assist clients with feeding to promote optimal independence.
- Individualize menu plans according to clients' preferences. Qᴘᴄᴄ
- Assist with preventing aspiration. Qₛ
  - Position in Fowler's position or in a chair.
  - Support the upper back, neck, and head.
  - Have clients tuck their chin when swallowing to help propel food down the esophagus.
  - Avoid the use of a straw.
  - Observe for aspiration and pocketing of food in the cheeks or other areas of the mouth.
  - Observe for indications of dysphagia, such as coughing, choking, gagging, and drooling of food.
  - Keep clients in semi-Fowler's position for at least 1 hr after meals.
  - Provide oral hygiene after meals and snacks.

- Provide therapeutic diets.
  - **Clear liquid:** liquids that leave little residue (clear fruit juices, gelatin, broth)
  - **Full liquid:** clear liquids plus liquid dairy products, all juices, pureed vegetables
  - **Pureed:** clear and full liquids plus pureed meats, fruits, scrambled eggs
  - **Mechanical soft:** clear and full liquids plus diced or ground foods
  - **Soft/low-residue:** foods that are low in fiber and easy to digest
  - **High-fiber:** whole grains, raw and dried fruits
  - **Low sodium:** no added salt or 1 to 2 g sodium
  - **Low cholesterol:** no more than 300 mg/day of dietary cholesterol
  - **Diabetic:** balanced intake of protein, fats, and carbohydrates of about 1,800 calories
  - **Dysphagia:** pureed food and thickened liquids
  - **Regular:** no restrictions
- Administer and monitor enteral feedings via nasogastric, gastrostomy, or jejunostomy tubes.
- Administer and monitor parenteral nutrition to clients who are unable to use their gastrointestinal tract to acquire nutrients. Parenteral nutrients include lipids, electrolytes, minerals, vitamins, dextrose, and amino acids.
- Maintain fluid balance.
  - Administer IV fluids.
  - Restrict oral fluid intake (maintaining strict I&O).
    - Remove the water pitcher from the bedside.
    - Inform the dietary staff of the amount of fluid to serve with each meal tray. Qᴘᴄᴄ
    - Inform the staff of each shift of the amount of fluid clients may have in addition to what they receive with each meal tray.
    - Record all oral intake, and inform the family of the restriction.
  - Encourage oral intake of fluids.
    - Provide fresh drinking water.
    - Remind and encourage a consistent fluid intake.
    - Ask about beverage preferences.

Application Exercises

1. A nurse is caring for a client who is at high risk for aspiration. Which of the following actions should the nurse take?

   A. Give the client thin liquids.

   B. Instruct the client to tuck her chin when swallowing.

   C. Have the client use a straw.

   D. Encourage the client to lie down and rest after meals.

2. A nurse is preparing a presentation about basic nutrients for a group of high school athletes. She should explain that which of the following nutrients provides the body with the most energy?

   A. Fat

   B. Protein

   C. Glycogen

   D. Carbohydrates

3. A nurse is caring for a client who requires a low-residue diet. The nurse should expect to see which of the following foods on the client's meal tray?

   A. Cooked barley

   B. Pureed broccoli

   C. Vanilla custard

   D. Lentil soup

4. A nurse is caring for a client who weighs 80 kg (176 lb) and is 1.6 m (5 ft 3 in) tall. Calculate her body mass index (BMI) and determine whether this client's BMI indicates that she is of a healthy weight, overweight, or obese.

5. A nurse in a senior center is counseling a group of older adults about their nutritional needs and considerations. Which of the following information should the nurse include? (Select all that apply.)

   A. Older adults are more prone to dehydration than younger adults are.

   B. Older adults need the same amount of most vitamins and minerals as younger adults do.

   C. Many older men and women need calcium supplementation.

   D. Older adults need more calories than they did when they were younger.

   E. Older adults should consume a diet low in carbohydrates.

PRACTICE Active Learning Scenario

A nurse is preparing a presentation in a community center on eating disorders that affect adolescents and young adults. Use the ATI Active Learning Template: Basic Concept to complete this item.

RELATED CONTENT: List two common eating disorders and their characteristics.

Application Exercises Key

1. A. Thin liquids increase the client's risk for aspiration.

   B. **CORRECT:** Tucking the chin when swallowing allows food to pass down the esophagus more easily.

   C. Using a straw increases the client's risk for aspiration.

   D. Sitting for an hour after meals helps prevent gastroesophageal reflux and possible aspiration of stomach contents after a meal.

   Ⓝ *NCLEX® Connection: Reduction of Risk Potential, Potential for Complications of Diagnostic Tests/Treatments/Procedures*

2. A. Although the body gets about half of its energy supply from fat, it is an inefficient means of obtaining energy. It produces end products the body has to excrete, and it requires energy from another source to burn the fat.

   B. Protein can supply energy, but it has other very essential and specific functions that only it can perform. So it is not the body's priority energy source.

   C. Glycogen, which the body stores in the liver, is a backup source of energy, not a primary or priority source.

   D. **CORRECT:** Carbohydrates are the body's greatest energy source; providing energy for cells is their primary function. They provide glucose, which burns completely and efficiently without end products to excrete. They are also a ready source of energy, and they spare proteins from depletion.

   Ⓝ *NCLEX® Connection: Health Promotion and Maintenance, Health Promotion/Disease Prevention*

3. A. Whole grains, such as barley and oats, are high in fiber and thus inappropriate components of a low-residue diet.

   B. Raw and gas-producing vegetables, such as broccoli and the cabbage in coleslaw, are high in fiber and thus inappropriate components of a low-residue diet.

   C. **CORRECT:** A low-residue diet consists of foods that are low in fiber and easy to digest. Dairy products and eggs, such as custard and yogurt, are appropriate for a low-residue diet.

   D. Legumes, such as lentils and black beans, are high in fiber and thus inappropriate components of a low-residue diet.

   Ⓝ *NCLEX® Connection: Basic Care and Comfort, Nutrition and Oral Hydration*

4. BMI = weight (kg) ÷ height (m²).

   Step 1: Client's weight (kg) and height (m) = 80 kg and 1.6 m

   Step 2: $1.6 \times 1.6 = 2.56 \text{ m}^2$

   Step 3: $80 \div 2.56 = 31.25$

   A BMI greater than 30 is considered obese.

   Ⓝ *NCLEX® Connection: Basic Care and Comfort, Nutrition and Oral Hydration*

5. A. **CORRECT:** Sensations of thirst diminish with age, leaving older adults more prone to dehydration.

   B. **CORRECT:** These requirements do not change from middle adulthood to older adulthood.

   C. **CORRECT:** If older adults ingest insufficient calcium in the diet, they need supplements to help prevent bone demineralization (osteoporosis).

   D. Older adults have a slower metabolic rate, so they require less energy (unless they are very active), and therefore need fewer calories.

   E. Many older adults need more carbohydrates for the fiber and bulk they contain. They should, however, reduce their intake of fats and of "empty" calories, such as pastries and soda pop.

   Ⓝ *NCLEX® Connection: Basic Care and Comfort, Nutrition and Oral Hydration*

PRACTICE Answer

Using the ATI Active Learning Template: Basic Concept

RELATED CONTENT

Anorexia nervosa
- Significantly low body weight for gender, age, developmental level, and physical health.
- Fears being fat
- Self-perception of being fat
- Consistent restriction of food intake or repeated behavior that prevents weight gain

Bulimia nervosa
- Cycle of binge eating followed by purging (vomiting, using diuretics or laxatives, exercise, fasting)
- Lack of control during binges
- Average of at least one cycle of binge eating and purging per week for at least 3 months

Binge-eating disorder
- Repeated episodes of binge eating
- Feels a loss of control when binge eating, followed by an emotional response such as guilt, shame, or depression
- Does not use compensatory behaviors, such as purging
- Binge-eating episodes can range from 1 to more than 14 times per week
- Clients are often overweight or obese.

Ⓝ *NCLEX® Connection: Health Promotion and Maintenance, Health Promotion/Disease Prevention*

CHAPTER 40 Mobility and Immobility

Mobility is freedom and independence in purposeful movement. Mobility refers to adapting to and having self-awareness of the environment. Functional musculoskeletal and nervous systems are essential for mobility.

Immobility is the inability to move freely and independently at will. The risk of complications increases with the degree of immobility and the length of time of immobilization. Periods of immobility or prolonged bed rest can cause major physiological and psychosocial effects.

Cutaneous stimulation in the form of cold and heat applications helps relieve pain and promotes healing. Promoting venous return is another key component of reducing the complications of immobility.

Mobility and immobility

Immobility can be the following.
- **Temporary**, such as following knee arthroplasty
- **Permanent**, such as paraplegia
- **Sudden onset**, such as a fractured arm and leg following a motor-vehicle crash
- **Slow onset**, such as multiple sclerosis

Body mechanics involves coordination between the musculoskeletal and nervous systems, and the use of alignment, balance, gravity, and friction.

Movement depends on an intact skeletal system, skeletal muscles, and nervous system.

Assessment focuses on mobility, range of motion (ROM), gait, exercise status, activity tolerance, and body alignment while standing, sitting, and lying.

FACTORS AFFECTING MOBILITY Qpcc
- Alterations in muscles
- Injury to the musculoskeletal system
- Poor posture
- Impaired central nervous system
- Health status and age

BODY SYSTEM CHANGES

Integumentary

- Increased pressure on skin, which is aggravated by metabolic changes
- Decreased circulation to tissue causing ischemia, which can lead to pressure ulcers

Respiratory

- Decreased respiratory movement resulting in decreased oxygenation and carbon dioxide exchange
- Stasis of secretions and decreased and weakened respiratory muscles, resulting in atelectasis and hypostatic pneumonia
- Decreased cough response

Cardiovascular

- Orthostatic hypotension
- Less fluid volume in the circulatory system
- Stasis of blood in the legs
- Diminished autonomic response
- Decreased cardiac output leading to poor cardiac effectiveness, which results in increased cardiac workload
- Increased oxygenation requirement
- Increased risk of thrombus development

Metabolic

- Altered endocrine system
- Decreased basal metabolic rate
- Changes in protein, carbohydrate, and fat metabolism
- Decreased appetite with altered nutritional intake
- Negative nitrogen balance
- Decreased protein resulting in loss of muscle
- Loss of weight
- Alterations in calcium, fluid, and electrolytes
- Resorption of calcium from bones
- Decreased urinary elimination of calcium resulting in hypercalcemia

Elimination

GENITOURINARY

- Urinary stasis
- Change in calcium metabolism with hypercalcemia resulting in renal calculi
- Decreased fluid intake, poor perineal care, and indwelling urinary catheters resulting in urinary tract infections

GASTROINTESTINAL

- Decreased peristalsis
- Decreased fluid intake
- Constipation, then fecal impaction, then diarrhea

Musculoskeletal

- Decreased muscle endurance, strength, and mass
- Impaired balance
- Atrophy of muscles
- Decreased stability
- Altered calcium metabolism
- Osteoporosis
- Pathological fractures
- Contractures
- Foot drop
- Altered joint mobility

Neurological/Psychosocial

- Altered sensory perception
- Ineffective coping

CHANGES IN EMOTIONAL STATUS: depression, alteration in self-concept, and anxiety

BEHAVIORAL CHANGES: withdrawal, altered sleep/wake pattern, hostility, inappropriate laughter, and passivity

Developmental

INFANTS, TODDLERS, AND PRESCHOOLERS

- Slower progression in gross motor skills and intellectual and musculoskeletal development
- Body aligned with line of gravity, resulting in unbalanced posture

ADOLESCENTS

- Imbalanced growth spurt possibly altered with immobility
- Delayed development of independence
- Social isolation

ADULTS

- Alterations in every physiological system
- Alterations in family and social systems
- Alterations in job identity and self-esteem

OLDER ADULTS

- Alterations in balance resulting in a major risk for falls and injuries
- Steady loss of bone mass resulting in weakened bones
- Decreased coordination
- Slower walk with smaller steps
- Alterations in functional status
- Increased dependence on staff and family

ASSESSMENT/DATA COLLECTION AND PATIENT-CENTERED CARE

Integumentary

Maintain intact skin.

ASSESSMENT

- Observe the skin for breakdown, warmth, and change in color.
- Look for pallor or redness in fair-skinned clients, and purple or blue discoloration in dark-skinned clients.
- Observe bony prominences.
- Check skin turgor.
- Use a pressure ulcer risk scale such as Norton or Braden.
- Assess at least every 2 hr.
- Observe for urinary or bowel incontinence.

NURSING INTERVENTIONS

- Identify clients at risk for pressure ulcer development.
- Position using corrective devices such as pillows, foot boots, trochanter rolls, splints, and wedge pillows.
- Turn every 1 to 2 hr, and use devices for support or per protocol.
- Teach clients who can move independently to turn at least every 15 min.
- Provide clients who are sitting in a chair with a device to decrease pressure.
- Limit sitting in a chair to 1 hr. Instruct clients to shift their weight every 15 min.
- Use a therapeutic bed or mattress for clients in bed for an extended time.
- Monitor nutritional intake.
- Provide skin and perineal care.

Respiratory

Maintain airway patency, achieve optimal lung expansion and gas exchange, and mobilize airway secretions.

ASSESSMENT
Complete every 2 hr.
- Observe chest wall movement for symmetry.
- Auscultate lungs and identify diminished breath sounds, crackles, or wheezes.
- Observe for productive cough, and note the color, amount, and consistency of secretions.

NURSING INTERVENTIONS
- Reposition every 1 to 2 hr.
- Instruct clients to turn, cough, and breathe deeply every 1 to 2 hr while awake.
- Instruct clients to yawn every hr while awake.
- Instruct clients to use an incentive spirometer while awake.
- Remove abdominal binders every 2 hr and replace correctly.
- Use chest physiotherapy.
- Auscultate the lungs to determine the effectiveness of chest physiotherapy or other respiratory therapy.
- Instruct clients to consume at least 2,000 mL fluid per day, unless intake is restricted.
- Monitor the ability to expectorate secretions.
- Use suction if unable to expectorate secretions.

Cardiovascular

Maintain cardiovascular function, increase activity tolerance, and prevent thrombus formation.

ASSESSMENT
- Measure orthostatic blood pressure and pulse (lying to sitting to standing), and assess for dizziness.
- Palpate the apical and peripheral pulses.
- Auscultate the heart at the apex for S3 (an early sign of heart failure). Older adult clients might not adapt well to immobility.
- Palpate for edema in the sacrum, legs, and feet.
- Palpate the skin for warmth in peripheral areas to include the nose, ear lobes, hands, and feet.
- Assess for deep-vein thrombosis by observing the calves for redness and palpating for warmth and tenderness.
- Measure the circumference of both calves and thighs and compare in size.

NURSING INTERVENTIONS
- Increase activity as soon as possible by dangling feet on side of bed or transferring to a chair.
- Instruct clients to perform isometric exercises to increase activity tolerance.
- Change position as often as possible.
- Move the client gradually during position changes.
- Instruct clients to avoid the Valsalva maneuver.
- Give a stool softener to prevent straining.
- Teach range of motion (ROM) and antiembolic exercises such as ankle pumps, foot circles, and knee flexion.

- Instruct clients to avoid placing pillows under the knees or lower extremities, crossing the legs, wearing tight clothes around the waist or on the legs, sitting for long periods of time, and massaging the legs.
- Use elastic stockings.
- Use sequential compression devices (SCD) or intermittent pneumatic compression (IPC).
- Increase fluid intake if no restrictions.
- Administer low-dose heparin or enoxaparin subcutaneously prophylactically.
- Contact the provider immediately if there is absence of a peripheral pulse in the lower extremities or assessment data that indicates venous thrombosis.

Metabolic

Reduce skin injury and maintain metabolism.

ASSESSMENT
- Record anthropometric measurements of height, weight, and skinfolds.
- Assess I&O.
- Assess food intake.
- Review urinary and bowel elimination status.
- Assess wound healing.
- Auscultate bowel sounds.
- Check skin turgor.
- Review laboratory values for electrolytes, serum total protein, and BUN.

NURSING INTERVENTIONS
- Provide a high-calorie, high-protein diet with vitamin B and C supplements.
- Monitor and evaluate oral intake. For clients who cannot eat or drink, provide enteral or parenteral nutritional therapy.

Elimination

Maintain urinary and bowel elimination.

ASSESSMENT
- Assess I&O.
- Assess the bladder for distention.
- Observe urine for color, amount, clarity, and frequency.
- Auscultate bowel sounds.
- Observe feces for color, amount, frequency, and consistency.

NURSING INTERVENTIONS
- Maintain hydration (at least 2,000 mL/day unless fluid is restricted).
- Instruct clients to consume a diet that includes fruits and vegetables and is high in fiber.
- Give a stool softener, laxative, or enema as needed.
- Provide perineal care.
- Teach bladder and bowel training.
- Insert a straight or indwelling catheter to relieve or manage bladder distention.
- Promote urination by pouring warm water over the perineal area.

Musculoskeletal

Maintain or regain body alignment and stability, decrease skin and musculoskeletal system changes, achieve full or optimal ROM, and prevent contractures.

ASSESSMENT
- Assess ROM capability.
- Assess muscle tone and mass.
- Observe for contractures.
- Monitor gait.
- Monitor nutritional intake of calcium.
- Monitor use of assistive devices to assist with ADLs.

NURSING INTERVENTIONS
- Make sure clients change position in bed at least every 2 hr and perform weight shifts in the wheelchair every 15 min.
- Encourage active or provide passive ROM two or three times/day.
- Instruct clients to perform ROM while bathing, eating, grooming, and dressing.
- A continuous passive motion (CPM) device might be prescribed. Develop an individualized program for each client. Older adult clients can require a program that addresses the aging process.
- Cluster care to promote a proper sleep-wake cycle.
- Request physical therapy for clients who have decreased mobility.
- Assist client with ambulation. Use assistive devices such as gait belts, walkers, canes, or crutches, as needed.

CANE INSTRUCTIONS
- Maintain two points of support on the ground at all times.
- Keep the cane on the stronger side of the body.
- Support body weight on both legs.
- Move the cane forward 15 to 25 cm (6 to 10 inches).
- Then move the weaker leg forward toward the cane.
- Next, advance the stronger leg past the cane.

CRUTCH INSTRUCTIONS
- Do not alter crutches after fitting.
- Follow the prescribed crutch gait.
- Support body weight at the hand grips with elbows flexed at 20° to 30°.
- Hold the crutches in one hand and grasp the arm of the chair with the other hand for balance while sitting and rising from a chair.

Psychosocial

Maintain an acceptable sleep/wake pattern, achieve socialization, and complete self-care independently.

ASSESSMENT
- Assess emotional status.
- Assess mental status.
- Assess behavior and decision-making skills.
- Monitor mobility status.
- Observe for unusual alterations in sleep/wake pattern.
- Assess coping skills, especially for loss.
- Monitor activities of daily living (ADLs).
- Assess for family support and relationships.
- Monitor social activities.

NURSING INTERVENTIONS
- Assist in using usual coping skills or in developing new coping skills.
- Maintain orientation to time (clock and calendar with date), person (call by name and introduce self), and place (talk about treatments, therapy, and length of stay).
- Develop a schedule of therapies, and place it on a calendar for clients.
- Arrange for clients who have limited mobility to be in a semiprivate room with an alert roommate.
- Involve clients in daily care.
- Provide stimuli such as books, crafts, television, newspapers, and radio.
- Help clients maintain body image by performing or assisting with hygiene and grooming tasks such as shaving or applying makeup.
- Have nurses and other staff interact on a routine and informal social basis.
- Recommend a referral for consultation (psychological, spiritual, or social worker) for clients who are not coping well.

Developmental

Continue expected development and achieve physical and mental stimulation.

Infancy through school age
- ASSESSMENT
  - Gross motor skills, and intellectual and musculoskeletal development
  - Body alignment and posture
  - Developmental tasks specific to age
- NURSING INTERVENTIONS
  - Initiate events that stimulate physical and psychosocial systems. Increase mobility, and involve play therapists in age-appropriate activities.
  - Use measures to prevent falls.
  - Develop strategies for maintaining or enhancing the developmental process.
  - Teach families that their perception of immobility can affect progress and ability to cope.
  - Encourage parents to stay with children.
  - Incorporate children's involvement, if it is age-appropriate, in their treatments.
  - Place children in a room with others who are age-appropriate.

Adolescents

- ASSESSMENT
  - Growth and development specific to age
  - Level of independence
  - Social activities
- NURSING INTERVENTIONS
  - Initiate care that facilitates independence.
  - Involve adolescents in decision-making for ADLs.
  - Provide stimuli to promote socialization (interaction with peers, use of adolescents' activity room).

Adults

- ASSESSMENT
  - All physical systems
  - Family relationships
  - Social status
  - Meaning of career/job
- NURSING INTERVENTIONS
  - Provide care that promotes activity in all physical systems.
  - Discuss with families the importance of interaction with clients.
  - Discuss social involvement.
  - Discuss the meaning of career/job.

Older adults

- ASSESSMENT
  - Balance
  - Coordination
  - Gait
  - Functional status
  - Level of independence
  - Social isolation
- NURSING INTERVENTIONS
  - Plan care with clients and families to increase independence with ADLs and decision-making skills.
  - Teach the staff to facilitate clients' independence in all activities.
  - Provide stimuli such as a clock, newspaper, calendar, and weather status.
  - Encourage families to visit to maintain socialization.
  - Plan for staff to spend some time talking and listening to clients.

Application of heat and cold

THERAPEUTIC EFFECTS

HEAT
- Increases blood flow
- Increases tissue metabolism
- Relaxes muscles
- Eases joint stiffness and pain

COLD
- Decreases inflammation
- Prevents swelling
- Reduces bleeding
- Reduces fever
- Diminishes muscle spasms
- Decreases pain by decreasing the velocity of nerve conduction

PATIENT-CENTERED CARE

NURSING CONSIDERATIONS

FOR CLIENTS AT RISK FOR INJURY FROM HEAT/COLD
- Use extreme caution with clients who are very young or fair-skinned, and older adults because they have fragile skin. ⑥
- Clients who are immobile might not be able to move away from the application if it becomes uncomfortable. They are at risk for skin injuries.
- Clients who have impaired sensory perception might not feel numbness, pain, or burning.
- Use minor temperature changes and short-term applications of heat or cold for best results.
- Avoid long applications of either heat or cold because this can result in tissue damage, burns, and reflex vasodilation (with cold therapy).
- Do not use cold applications for clients who have cold intolerance, vascular insufficiency, open wounds, and disorders aggravated by cold, such as Raynaud's phenomenon.
- Make sure the provider has written a prescription that includes the following.
  - Location
  - Duration and frequency
  - Specific type (moist or dry)
  - Temperature to use

HEAT
- Monitor bony prominences carefully because they are more sensitive to heat applications. Qs
- Avoid the use of heat applications over metal devices (pacemakers, prosthetic joints) to prevent deep tissue burns.
- Do not apply heat to the abdomen of a client who is pregnant to prevent harm to the fetus.
- Do not place a heat application under a client who is immobile because this can increase the risk of burns.
- Do not use heat applications during the first 24 hr after a traumatic injury, for active bleeding, for noninflammatory edema, or for some skin disorders.

SUPPLIES

Heat application

MOIST
- Warm compresses: towel, bath thermometer, hot water, plastic covering, hot pack or aquathermia pad (with distilled water), tape
- Warm soaks: water, bath thermometer, basin, waterproof pads
- Sitz baths: specific chair, tub, or basin (disposable or built-in), bath thermometer, bath blanket, towels

DRY
- Hot pack (disposable or reusable) or an aquathermia pad with distilled water, and a pillowcase
- Warming blanket

Cold application

MOIST
- Cold water compresses
- Cold soaks

DRY
- Ice bag, ice collar, ice glove, or a cold pack
- Cooling blanket

NURSING ACTIONS

- Apply to the area.
- Make sure the call light is within reach, and instruct clients to report any discomfort.
- Assess the site every 5 to 10 min to check for the following.
  - Redness or pallor
  - Pain or burning Qs
  - Numbness
  - Shivering (with cold applications)
  - Blisters
  - Decreased sensation
  - Mottling of the skin
  - Cyanosis (with cold applications)
- Discontinue the application if any of the above occur, or remove the application at the predetermined time (usually 15 to 30 min).
- Document the following.
  - Location, type, and length of the application
  - Condition of the skin before and after the application
  - Client's tolerance of the application

Promoting venous return

- Elastic (antiembolic) stockings cause external pressure on the muscles of the lower extremities to promote blood return to the heart.
- SCDs and IPC have plastic or fabric sleeves that wrap around the leg and secure with hook-and-loop closures. The sleeves are then attached to an electric pump that alternately inflates and deflates the sleeve around the leg. These machines are set to cycle, typically a 10- to 15-second inflation and a 45- to 60-second deflation. QEBP
- Positioning techniques reduce compression of leg veins.
- ROM exercises cause skeletal muscle contractions, which promote blood return. Specific exercises that help prevent thrombophlebitis include ankle pumps, foot circles, and knee flexion.
- Antiembolic stockings, SCDs, and IPC require a prescription.
- Clients who are immobile should perform leg exercises, increase their fluid intake, and change positions frequently.
- When suspecting poor venous return or possible thrombus, notify the provider, elevate the leg, and do not apply pressure or massage the thrombus to avoid dislodging it.

PATIENT-CENTERED CARE

Antiembolic stockings

EQUIPMENT: Tape measure

PROCEDURE
- Perform hand hygiene.
- Assess skin, circulation, and presence of edema in the legs.
- Measure the calf and/or thigh circumference and the length of the leg to select the correct size stocking.
- Turn the stockings inside to the heel.
- Put the stocking on the foot.
- Pull the remainder of the stocking over the heel and up the leg.
- Smooth any creases or wrinkles.
- Remove the stockings every 8 hr to assess for redness, warmth, or tenderness.
- Make sure the stockings are not too tight over the toes.
- Keep the stockings clean and dry. Clients who are postoperative or have specific needs can need a second pair of hose.
- Document the application and removal of the stockings.

SCD and IPC

EQUIPMENT
- Tape measure
- Sequential stockings

PROCEDURE
- Perform hand hygiene.
- Assess circulation and skin prior to application.
- Measure around the largest part of the thigh to determine the stocking size.
- Apply the sleeves to each leg. Position the opening at the client's knees.
- Attach the sleeves to the inflator.
- Turn on the device.
- Monitor circulation and skin after application.
- Remove every 8 hr for assessment of calves.
- Document the application and removal of the stockings.

Positioning techniques

To reduce compression of leg veins

PROCEDURE
Instruct clients to avoid the following.
- Crossing legs
- Sitting for long periods
- Wearing restrictive clothing on the lower extremities
- Putting pillows behind the knees
- Massaging legs

ROM exercises

Hourly while awake.

PROCEDURE
Instruct clients to perform the following.
- **Ankle pumps:** Point the toes toward the head and then away from the head.
- **Foot circles:** Rotate the feet in circles at the ankles.
- **Knee flexion:** Flex and extend the legs at the knees.

COMPLICATIONS

Thrombophlebitis, deep-vein thrombosis

Thrombophlebitis and deep-vein thrombosis are inflammation of a vein (usually in the lower extremities) that result in clot formation.

MANIFESTATIONS: Pain, edema, warmth, and erythema at the site Qpcc

ASSESSMENT: Another assessment method for clients prone to thrombosis is to measure bilateral calf and thigh circumference daily. Unilateral increase is early indication of thrombosis.

NURSING ACTIONS
- Notify the provider immediately.
- Position the client in bed with the leg elevated.
- Avoid any pressure at the site of the inflammation.
- Anticipate giving anticoagulants.

Pulmonary embolism

A pulmonary embolism is a potentially life-threatening occlusion of blood flow to one or more of the pulmonary arteries by a clot. The clot or embolus often originates in the venous system of the lower extremities.

MANIFESTATIONS: Shortness of breath, chest pain, hemoptysis (coughing up blood), decreased blood pressure, and rapid pulse

NURSING ACTIONS
- Prepare to give thrombolytics or anticoagulants.
- Position client in a high-Fowler's position.
- Obtain pulse oximetry.
- Administer oxygen.
- Prepare to obtain blood gas analysis.
- Monitor frequent vital signs.

PRACTICE Active Learning Scenario

A nurse is reviewing the effects of immobility on various body systems with a group of newly licensed nurses. Use the ATI Active Learning Template: Basic Concept to complete this item.

RELATED CONTENT: List at least two effects of immobility on the cardiovascular system and at least two on the respiratory system.

PRACTICE Answer

Using the ATI Active Learning Template: Basic Concept

RELATED CONTENT
Cardiovascular system
- Orthostatic hypotension
- Less fluid volume in the circulatory system
- Stasis of blood in the legs
- Diminished autonomic response
- Decreased cardiac output leading to poor cardiac effectiveness, which results in increased cardiac workload
- Increased oxygenation requirement
- Increased risk of thrombus development

Respiratory system
- Decreased respiratory movement resulting in decreased oxygenation and carbon dioxide exchange
- Stasis of secretions and decreased and weakened respiratory muscles, resulting in atelectasis and hypostatic pneumonia
- Decreased cough response

Ⓝ *NCLEX® Connection: Basic Care and Comfort, Mobility/Immobility*

Application Exercises

1. A nurse is caring for a client who has been sitting in a chair for 1 hr. Which of the following complications is the greatest risk to the client?

   A. Decreased subcutaneous fat

   B. Muscle atrophy

   C. Pressure ulcer

   D. Fecal impaction

2. A nurse is caring for a client who is postoperative. Which of the following interventions should the nurse take to reduce the risk of thrombus development? (Select all that apply.)

   A. Instruct the client not to perform the Valsalva maneuver.

   B. Apply elastic stockings.

   C. Review laboratory values for total protein level.

   D. Place pillows under the client's knees and lower extremities.

   E. Assist the client to change position often.

3. A nurse is planning care for a client who is on bed rest. Which of the following interventions should the nurse plan to implement?

   A. Encourage the client to perform antiembolic exercises every 2 hr.

   B. Instruct the client to cough and deep breathe every 4 hr.

   C. Restrict the client's fluid intake.

   D. Reposition the client every 4 hr.

4. A nurse is evaluating teaching on a client who has a new prescription for a sequential compression device. Which of the following client statements should indicate to the nurse the client understands the teaching?

   A. "This device will keep me from getting sores on my skin."

   B. "This thing will keep the blood pumping through my leg."

   C. "With this thing on, my leg muscles won't get weak."

   D. "This device is going to keep my joints in good shape."

5. A nurse is instructing a client, who has an injury of the left lower extremity, about the use of a cane. Which of the following instructions should the nurse include? (Select all that apply.)

   A. Hold the cane on the right side.

   B. Keep two points of support on the floor.

   C. Place the cane 38 cm (15 in) in front of the feet before advancing.

   D. After advancing the cane, move the weaker leg forward.

   E. Advance the stronger leg so that it aligns evenly with the cane.

Application Exercises Key

1. A. The client is at risk for decreased subcutaneous fat due to altered mobility. However, there is another risk that is the priority.

   B. The client is at risk for muscle atrophy due to altered mobility. However, there is another risk that is the priority.

   C. **CORRECT:** The greatest risk to this client is injury from skin breakdown due to unrelieved pressure over a bony prominence from prolonged sitting in a chair. The nurse should instruct the client to shift his weight every 15 min and reposition the client after 1 hr.

   D. The client is at risk for fecal impaction due to altered mobility. However, there is another risk that is the priority.

   Ⓝ *NCLEX® Connection: Basic Care and Comfort, Mobility/Immobility*

2. A. The Valsalva maneuver increases the workload of the heart, but it does not affect peripheral circulation.

   B. **CORRECT:** Elastic stockings promote venous return and prevent thrombus formation.

   C. A review of the client's total protein level is important for evaluating his ability to heal and prevent skin breakdown.

   D. Placing pillows under the knees and lower extremities can impair circulation of the lower extremities.

   E. **CORRECT:** Frequent position changes prevents venous stasis.

   Ⓝ *NCLEX® Connection: Basic Care and Comfort, Mobility/Immobility*

3. A. **CORRECT:** The nurse should encourage the client to perform antiembolic exercises every 1 to 2 hr to promote venous return and reduce the risk of thrombus formation.

   B. The nurse should instruct the client to cough and deep breathe every 1 to 2 hr to reduce the risk of atelectasis.

   C. The nurse should increase the client's intake of fluids, unless contraindicated, to reduce the risk of thrombus formation, constipation, and urinary dysfunction.

   D. The nurse should reposition the client every 1 to 2 hr to reduce the risk for pressure ulcers.

   Ⓝ *NCLEX® Connection: Basic Care and Comfort, Mobility/Immobility*

4. A. The nurse should assess the skin under the sequential pressure device every 8 hr to check for manifestations of a thrombus and skin breakdown.

   B. **CORRECT:** Sequential pressure devices promote venous return in the deep veins of the legs and thus help prevent thrombus formation.

   C. Continuous passive motion machines, not sequential pressure devices, provide some muscle movement that can assist in preserving some muscle strength.

   D. Continuous passive motion machines, not sequential pressure devices, exercise the knee joint after arthroplasty.

   Ⓝ *NCLEX® Connection: Basic Care and Comfort, Mobility/Immobility*

5. A. **CORRECT:** The client should hold the cane on the uninjured side to provide support for the injured left leg.

   B. **CORRECT:** The client should keep two points of support on the ground at all times for stability.

   C. The client should place the cane 15 to 25 cm (6 to 10 in) in front of her feet before advancing.

   D. **CORRECT:** The client should advance the weaker leg first, followed by the stronger leg.

   E. The client should advance the stronger leg past the cane.

   Ⓝ *NCLEX® Connection: Basic Care and Comfort, Mobility/Immobility*

CHAPTER 41 *Pain Management*

Effective pain management includes the use of pharmacological and nonpharmacological pain management therapies. Invasive therapies such as nerve ablation can be appropriate for intractable cancer-related pain.

Clients have a right to adequate assessment and management of pain. Nurses are accountable for the assessment of pain. The nurse's role is that of an advocate and educator for effective pain management.

Nurses have a priority responsibility to measure the client's pain level on a continual basis and to provide individualized interventions. Nurses should assess the effectiveness of the interventions 30 to 60 min after implementation.

Assessment challenges can occur with clients who have cognitively impairment, who speak a different language than the nurse, or who receive prescribed mechanical ventilation.

Undertreatment of pain is a serious health care problem. Consequences of undertreatment of pain include physiological and psychological components. Acute/chronic pain can cause anxiety, fear, and depression. Poorly managed acute pain can lead to chronic pain syndrome. Q EBP

PHYSIOLOGY OF PAIN

Transduction is the conversion of painful stimuli to an electrical impulse through peripheral nerve fibers (nociceptors).

Transmission occurs as the electrical impulse travels along the nerve fibers, where neurotransmitters regulate it.

Pain threshold is the point at which a person feels pain.

Pain tolerance is the amount of pain a person is willing to bear.

Perception or awareness of pain occurs in various areas of the brain, with influences from thought and emotional processes.

Modulation occurs in the spinal cord, causing muscles to contract reflexively, moving the body away from painful stimuli.

SUBSTANCES THAT INCREASE PAIN TRANSMISSION AND CAUSE AN INFLAMMATORY RESPONSE
- Substance P
- Prostaglandins
- Bradykinin
- Histamine

SUBSTANCES THAT DECREASE PAIN TRANSMISSION AND PRODUCE ANALGESIA
- Serotonin
- Endorphins

PAIN CATEGORIES

Pain is categorized by duration (acute or chronic) or by origin (nociceptive or neuropathic).

Acute pain

- Acute pain is protective, temporary, usually self-limiting, has a direct cause, and resolves with tissue healing.
- Physiological responses (sympathetic nervous system) are fight-or-flight responses (tachycardia, hypertension, anxiety, diaphoresis, muscle tension).
- Behavioral responses include grimacing, moaning, flinching, and guarding.
- Interventions include treatment of the underlying problem.
- Can lead to chronic pain if unrelieved.

Chronic pain

- Chronic pain is not protective. It is ongoing or recurs frequently, lasting longer than 6 months and persisting beyond tissue healing.
- Physiological responses do not usually alter vital signs, but clients can have depression, fatigue, and a decreased level of functioning. It is not usually life-threatening.
- Psychosocial implications can lead to disability.
- Management aims at symptomatic relief. Pain does not always respond to interventions.
- Chronic pain can be malignant or nonmalignant.
- **Idiopathic pain** is a form of chronic pain without a known cause, or pain that exceeds typical pain levels associated with the client's condition.

Nociceptive pain

- Nociceptive pain arises from damage to or inflammation of tissue, which is a noxious stimulus that triggers the pain receptors called nociceptors and causes pain.
- It is usually throbbing, aching, and localized.
- This pain typically responds to opioids and nonopioid medications.

TYPES OF NOCICEPTIVE PAIN
- **Somatic:** In bones, joints, muscles, skin, or connective tissues.
- **Visceral:** In internal organs such as the stomach or intestines. It can cause referred pain in other body locations separate from the stimulus.
- **Cutaneous:** In the skin or subcutaneous tissue.

Neuropathic pain

- Neuropathic pain arises from abnormal or damaged pain nerves.
- It includes phantom limb pain, pain below the level of a spinal cord injury, and diabetic neuropathy.
- Neuropathic pain is usually intense, shooting, burning, or described as "pins and needles."
- This pain typically responds to adjuvant medications (antidepressants, antispasmodic agents, skeletal muscle relaxants).

ASSESSMENT/DATA COLLECTION

- Noted pain experts agree that pain is whatever the person experiencing it says it is, and it exists whenever the person says it does. The client's report of pain is the most reliable diagnostic measure of pain. **Q**pcc
- Self-report using standardized pain scales is useful for clients over the age of 7 years. Specialized pain scales are available for use with younger children or individuals who have difficulty communicating verbally.
- Assess and document pain (the fifth vital sign) frequently.
- Use a symptom analysis to obtain subjective data. **(41.1)**

RISK FACTORS

UNDERTREATMENT OF PAIN **Q**pcc
- Cultural and societal attitudes
- Lack of knowledge
- Fear of addiction
- Exaggerated fear of respiratory depression

POPULATIONS AT RISK FOR UNDERTREATMENT OF PAIN
- Infants
- Children
- Older adults **G**
- Clients who have substance use disorder

CAUSES OF ACUTE AND CHRONIC PAIN
- Trauma
- Surgery
- Cancer (tumor invasion, nerve compression, bone metastases, associated infections, immobility)
- Arthritis
- Fibromyalgia
- Neuropathy
- Diagnostic or treatment procedures (injection, intubation, radiation)

FACTORS THAT AFFECT THE PAIN EXPERIENCE
- **Age**
  - Infants cannot verbalize or understand their pain.
  - Older adult clients can have multiple pathologies that cause pain and limit function. **G**
- **Fatigue:** Can increase sensitivity to pain.
- **Genetic sensitivity:** Can increase or decrease pain tolerance.
- **Cognitive function:** Clients who have cognitively impairment might not be able to report pain or report it accurately.
- **Prior experiences:** Can increase or decrease sensitivity depending on whether clients obtained adequate relief.
- **Anxiety and fear:** Can increase sensitivity to pain.
- **Support systems and coping styles:** Presence of these can decrease sensitivity to pain.
- **Culture:** Cam influence how clients express pain or the meaning they give to pain.

41.1 Symptom analysis

Use anatomical terminology and landmarks to describe location (superficial deep, referred, or radiating).

QUESTIONS

"Where is your pain? Does it radiate anywhere else?"

Ask clients to point to the location.

Quality refers to how the pain feels: sharp, dull, aching, burning, stabbing, pounding, throbbing, shooting, gnawing, tender, heavy, tight, tiring, exhausting, sickening, terrifying, torturing, nagging, annoying, intense, or unbearable.

QUESTIONS

"What does the pain feel like?"

Give more than two choices: "Is the pain throbbing, burning, or stabbing?"

Intensity, strength, and severity are "measures" of the pain. Use a pain intensity scale (visual analog, description, or number rating scales) to measure pain, monitor pain, and evaluate the effectiveness of interventions.

QUESTIONS

"How much pain do you have now?"

"What is the worst/best the pain has been?"

"Rate your pain on a scale of 0 to 10."

Timing: onset, duration, frequency

QUESTIONS

"When did it start?"

"How long does it last?"

"How often does it occur?"

"Is it constant or intermittent?"

Setting: how the pain affects daily life or how activities of daily living (ADLs) affect the pain

QUESTIONS

"Where are you when the symptoms occur?"

"What are you doing when the symptoms occur?"

"How does the pain affect your sleep?"

"How does the pain affect your ability to work or interact with others?"

Document associated findings: fatigue, depression, nausea, anxiety.

QUESTIONS

"What other symptoms do you have when you are feeling pain?"

Aggravating/relieving factors

QUESTIONS

"What makes the pain better?"

"What makes the pain worse?"

"Are you currently taking any prescription, herbal, or over-the-counter medications?"

EXPECTED FINDINGS

- Behaviors complement self-report and assist in pain assessment of nonverbal clients.
  - Facial expressions (grimacing, wrinkled forehead), body movements (restlessness, pacing, guarding)
  - Moaning, crying
  - Decreased attention span
- Blood pressure, pulse, and respiratory rate increase temporarily with acute pain. Eventually, increases in vital signs will stabilize despite the persistence of pain. Therefore, physiologic indicators might not be an accurate measure of pain over time.

PATIENT-CENTERED CARE

NONPHARMACOLOGICAL PAIN MANAGEMENT STRATEGIES

Nonpharmacological strategies should not replace pharmacological pain measures, but can be used along with them.

Cognitive-behavioral measures: changing the way a client perceives pain, and physical approaches to improve comfort

Cutaneous (skin) stimulation: transcutaneous electrical nerve stimulation (TENS), heat, cold, therapeutic touch, and massage **Qᴇʙᴘ**
- Interruption of pain pathways
- Cold for inflammation
- Heat to increase blood flow and to reduce stiffness

Distraction
- Includes ambulation, deep breathing, visitors, television, games, prayer, and music
- Decreased attention to the presence of pain can decrease perceived pain level.

Relaxation: Includes meditation, yoga, and progressive muscle relaxation

Imagery
- Focusing on a pleasant thought to divert focus
- Requires an ability to concentrate

Acupuncture and acupressure: Stimulating subcutaneous tissues at specific points using needles (acupuncture) or the digits (acupressure)

Reduction of pain stimuli in the environment

Elevation of edematous extremities to promote venous return and decrease swelling

PHARMACOLOGICAL INTERVENTIONS

Analgesics are the mainstay for relieving pain. The three classes of analgesics are nonopioids, opioids, and adjuvants.

Nonopioid analgesics

Nonopioid analgesics (acetaminophen, nonsteroidal anti-inflammatory drugs [NSAIDs], including salicylates) are appropriate for treating mild to moderate pain.
- Be aware of the hepatotoxic effects of acetaminophen. Clients who have a healthy liver should take no more than 4 g/day. Make sure clients are aware of opioids that contain acetaminophen, such as hydrocodone bitartrate 5 mg/acetaminophen 500 mg. **Qs**
- Monitor for salicylism (tinnitus, vertigo, decreased hearing acuity).
- Prevent gastric upset by administering the medication with food or antacids.
- Monitor for bleeding with long-term NSAID use.

Opioid analgesics

Opioid analgesics, such as morphine sulfate, fentanyl, and codeine, are appropriate for treating moderate to severe pain (postoperative pain, myocardial infarction pain, cancer pain).
- Managing acute severe pain with short-term (24 to 48 hr) around-the-clock administration of opioids is preferable to following a PRN schedule.
- The parenteral route is best for immediate, short-term relief of acute pain. The oral route is better for chronic, no fluctuating pain.
- Consistent timing and dosing of opioid administration provide consistent pain control.
- It is essential to monitor and intervene for adverse effects of opioid use.
  - **Sedation:** Monitor level of consciousness and take safety precautions. Sedation usually precedes respiratory depression.
  - **Respiratory depression:** Monitor respiratory rate prior to and following administration of opioids (especially for clients who have little previous exposure to opioid medications). Initial treatment of respiratory depression and sedation is generally a reduction in opioid dose. If necessary, slowly administer diluted naloxone to reverse opioid effects until the client can deep breathe with a respiratory rate of at least 8/min.
  - **Orthostatic hypotension:** Advise clients to sit or lie down if lightheadedness or dizziness occur. Instruct clients to avoid sudden changes in position by slowly moving from a lying to a sitting or standing position. Provide assistance with ambulation.
  - **Urinary retention:** Monitor I&O, assess for distention, administer bethanechol, and catheterize.
  - **Nausea/vomiting:** Administer antiemetics, advise clients to lie still and move slowly, and eliminate odors.
  - **Constipation:** Use a preventative approach (monitoring of bowel movements, fluids, fiber intake, exercise, stool softeners, stimulant laxatives, enemas).

Adjuvant analgesics

Adjuvant analgesics enhance the effects of nonopioids, help alleviate other manifestations that aggravate pain (depression, seizures, inflammation), and are useful for treating neuropathic pain. Qs

Anticonvulsants: carbamazepine, gabapentin

Antianxiety agents: diazepam, lorazepam

Tricyclic antidepressants: amitriptyline, nortriptyline

Anesthetics: infusional lidocaine

Antihistamine: hydroxyzine

Glucocorticoids: dexamethasone

Antiemetics: ondansetron

Bisphosphonates and calcitonin: for bone pain

Patient-controlled analgesia

Patient-controlled analgesia (PCA) is a medication delivery system that allows clients to self-administer safe doses of opioids.
- Small, frequent dosing ensures consistent plasma levels.
- Clients have less lag time between identified need and delivery of medication, which increases their sense of control and can decrease the amount of medication they need.
- Morphine, hydromorphone, and fentanyl are typical opioids for PCA delivery.
- Clients should let the nurse know if using the pump does not control the pain.

To prevent inadvertent overdosing, the client is the only person who should push the PCA button. Qpcc

Other interventions

ADDITIONAL PHARMACOLOGICAL PAIN INTERVENTIONS: Local and regional anesthesia and topical analgesia

OTHER STRATEGIES FOR EFFECTIVE PAIN MANAGEMENT
- Take a proactive approach by giving analgesics before pain becomes too severe. It takes less medication to prevent pain than to treat pain.
- Instruct clients to report developing or recurrent pain and not wait until pain is severe (for PRN pain medication).
- Explain misconceptions about pain (medication dependence, pain measurement and perception). Qpcc
- Help clients reduce fear and anxiety.
- Create a treatment plan that includes both nonpharmacological and pharmacological pain-relief measures.

Chronic pain relief strategies

Strategies specific for relieving chronic pain include the above interventions, plus the following.
- Administering long-acting or controlled-release opioid analgesics (including the transdermal route).
- Administering analgesics around the clock rather than PRN.

COMPLICATIONS AND NURSING IMPLICATIONS

Undertreatment of pain is a serious complication and can lead to increased anxiety with acute pain and depression with chronic pain. Assess clients for pain frequently, and intervene as appropriate.

Sedation, respiratory depression, and coma can occur as a result of overdosing. Sedation always precedes respiratory depression. Qs
- Identify high-risk clients (older adult clients, clients who are opioid-naïve). Ⓖ
- Carefully titrate client dose while closely monitoring respiratory status.
- Stop the opioid and give the antagonist naloxone if respiratory rate is below 8/min and shallow, or the client is difficult to arouse.
- Identify the cause of sedation.
- Use a sedation scale in addition to a pain rating scale to assess pain, especially when administering opioids.

Application Exercises

1. A nurse at a clinic is collecting data about pain from of a client who reports severe abdominal pain. The nurse asks the client whether he has nausea and has been vomiting. Which of the following pain characteristics is the nurse attempting to determine?

   A. Presence of associated manifestations

   B. Location of the pain

   C. Pain quality

   D. Aggravating and relieving factors

2. A nurse is collecting data from a client who is reporting pain despite taking analgesia. Which of the following actions should the nurse take to determine the intensity of the client's pain?

   A. Ask the client what precipitates the pain.

   B. Question the client about the location of the pain.

   C. Offer the client a pain scale to measure his pain.

   D. Use open-ended questions to identify the client's pain sensations.

3. A nurse is discussing the care of a group of clients with a newly licensed nurse. Which of the following clients should the newly licensed nurse identify as experiencing chronic pain?

   A. A client who has a broken femur and reports hip pain.

   B. A client who has incisional pain 72 hr following pacemaker insertion.

   C. A client who has food poisoning and reports abdominal cramping.

   D. A client who has episodic back pain following a fall 2 years ago.

4. A nurse is monitoring a client who is receiving opioid analgesia for adverse effects of the medication. Which of the following effects should the nurse anticipate? (Select all that apply.)

   A. Urinary incontinence

   B. Diarrhea

   C. Bradypnea

   D. Orthostatic hypotension

   E. Nausea

5. A nurse is caring for a client who is receiving morphine via a patient-controlled analgesia (PCA) infusion device after abdominal surgery. Which of the following statements indicates that the client knows how to use the device?

   A. "I'll wait to use the device until it's absolutely necessary."

   B. "I'll be careful about pushing the button too much so I don't get an overdose."

   C. "I should tell the nurse if the pain doesn't stop while I am using this device."

   D. "I will ask my adult child to push the dose button when I am sleeping."

PRACTICE Active Learning Scenario

A nurse on a medical-surgical unit is reviewing with a group of newly licensed nurses the various types of pain the clients on the unit have. Use the ATI Active Learning Template: Basic Concept to complete this item.

UNDERLYING PRINCIPLES: List the four different types of pain, their definitions, and characteristics.

1. A. **CORRECT:** The nurse should attempt to identify manifestations that occur along with the client's pain, such as nausea, fatigue, or anxiety.

   B. The nurse should ask the client to point out where he feels pain to determine the location.

   C. The nurse should ask the client if his pain is throbbing, dull, or aching to determine the pain quality.

   D. The nurse should ask the client what makes the pain better or worse to determine aggravating and relieving factors.

   (N) *NCLEX® Connection: Pharmacological and Parenteral Therapies, Pharmacological Pain Management*

2. A. The nurse should ask what precipitates the client's pain when collecting data to determine the cause of the pain.

   B. The nurse should ask the location of the client's pain to help determine the cause or classify the pain as deep, subcutaneous, or radiating.

   C. **CORRECT:** The nurse should use a pain rating scale to help the client report the intensity of his pain. The nurse should use a numeric, verbal, or visual analog scale appropriate to the client's individual needs.

   D. The nurse should ask open-ended questions about the client's pain sensation to help determine the quality of the pain, such as exhausting, tight, or burning.

   (N) *NCLEX® Connection: Pharmacological and Parenteral Therapies, Pharmacological Pain Management*

3. A. The newly licensed nurse should identify pain from a recent, nonhealed bone fracture as acute pain.

   B. The newly licensed nurse should identify postoperative pain as acute pain.

   C. The newly licensed nurse should identify pain associated with a current illness, such as food poisoning, as acute pain.

   D. **CORRECT:** A client who reports pain that lasts more than 6 months and continues beyond the time of tissue healing is experiencing chronic pain. The nurse should identify this client's pain as chronic, and assist with planning interventions to relieve manifestations associated with the pain.

   (N) *NCLEX® Connection: Pharmacological and Parenteral Therapies, Pharmacological Pain Management*

4. A. The nurse should identify urinary retention as a possible adverse effect of opioid analgesia.

   B. The nurse should identify constipation as a possible adverse effect of opioid analgesia.

   C. **CORRECT:** Opioid analgesia can cause respiratory depression, which causes respiratory rates to drop to dangerously low levels. The nurse should monitor the client's respiratory rate, and administer naloxone if indicated.

   D. **CORRECT:** Opioid analgesia can cause orthostatic hypotension. The nurse should monitor the client for dizziness or lightheadedness when changing positions.

   E. **CORRECT:** Opioid analgesia can cause nausea and vomiting. The nurse should monitor for and treat these complications as needed.

   (N) *NCLEX® Connection: Pharmacological and Parenteral Therapies, Pharmacological Pain Management*

5. A. The nurse should remind the client to use the PCA when he begins to feel pain to achieve better pain control.

   B. The nurse should remind the client the PCA has a timing control or lockout mechanism, which enforces a preset minimum interval between medication doses. The client cannot self-administer another dose of medication until that time interval has passed, even if the button is pressed.

   C. **CORRECT:** PCA allows the client to self-administer pain medication on an as-needed basis. If the client is not achieving adequate pain control, he should let the nurse know so that she can initiate a reevaluation of the client's pain management plan and possible dosage change.

   D. The nurse should warn the client he is the only one who should operate the PCA pump. In situations where a client is not able to do so, a provider may authorize a nurse or a family member to operate the pump.

   (N) *NCLEX® Connection: Pharmacological and Parenteral Therapies, Pharmacological Pain Management*

PRACTICE Answer

Using the ATI Active Learning Template: Basic Concept

UNDERLYING PRINCIPLES

Acute pain
- Definition: Protective, temporary, usually self-limiting, resolves with tissue healing
- Physiological responses: Tachycardia, hypertension, anxiety, diaphoresis, muscle tension
- Behavioral responses: Grimacing, moaning, flinching, guarding

Chronic pain
- Definition: Not protective; ongoing or recurs frequently, lasts longer than 6 months, persists beyond tissue healing, can be malignant or nonmalignant
- Physiological responses: No change in vital signs; depression; fatigue; decreased level of functioning; disability

Nociceptive pain
- Definition: Arises from damage to or inflammation of tissue, which is a noxious stimulus that triggers the pain receptors called nociceptors and causes pain, is usually throbbing, aching, localized; pain typically responds to opioids and nonopioid medications
- Types of nociceptive pain:
  ○ Somatic: In bones, joints, muscles, skin, or connective tissues
  ○ Visceral: In internal organs such as the stomach or intestines, can cause referred pain
  ○ Cutaneous: In skin or subcutaneous tissue

Neuropathic pain
- Definition: Arises from abnormal or damaged pain nerves (phantom limb pain, pain below the level of a spinal cord injury, diabetic neuropathy), usually intense, shooting, burning, or "pins and needles"
- Physiological responses to adjuvant medications (antidepressants, antispasmodic agents, skeletal muscle relaxants).

(N) *NCLEX® Connection: Pharmacological and Parenteral Therapies, Pharmacological Pain Management*

CHAPTER 42 Complementary and Alternative Therapies

In combination with allopathic therapies (conventional Western medicine), complementary and alternative therapies comprise integrative health care, which focuses on optimal health of the whole person. Another term for these therapies is complementary and alternative medicine (CAM).

Alternative therapies are unconventional treatment approaches that become the primary treatment and replace allopathic medical care. Complementary therapies are unconventional treatment approaches used in addition to or to enhance conventional medical care.

Many health care entities are developing programs of integrative medicine or integrative therapies to provide clients with conventional and unconventional health care choices, particularly for chronic health problems. Qpcc

The number of clients using CAM is considerably rising. This interest is related to a desire for more natural treatments to add to or replace ineffective allopathic treatment, increased awareness of alternative medicine, and from clients who desire to take a more active role in the treatment process.

An important prerequisite for implementing complementary or alternative therapies is the client's acceptance of and involvement in the therapeutic intervention.

CATEGORIES OF CAM

Alternative medical philosophies: Complete medical systems outside of allopathic medicinal beliefs (traditional Chinese medicine, Ayurveda, homeopathy)

Biological and botanical therapies: Involve the use of natural products to affect health (diets, vitamins, minerals, herbal preparations, probiotics)

Body-based and manipulative methods: Involve external touch to affect body systems (massage, touch, chiropractic therapy, acupressure)

Mind-body therapies: Connect the physiological function to the mind and emotions (acupuncture, breathwork, biofeedback, art therapy, meditation, guided imagery, yoga, psychotherapy, tai chi)

Energy therapies: Involve use of the body's energy fields (Reiki, therapeutic touch, magnet therapy)

Movement therapies: Use exercise or activity to promote physical and emotional well-being (Pilates, dance therapy)

TYPES OF CAM

Specialized licensed or certified practitioners may provide complementary or alternative therapies.

Acupuncture/acupressure: Needles or pressure along meridians to alter body function or produce analgesia

Homeopathic medicine: Administering doses of substances (remedies) that would produce manifestations of the disease state in a well person to ill clients to bring about healing

Naturopathic medicine: Diet, exercise, environment, and herbal remedies to promote natural healing

Chiropractic medicine: Spinal manipulation for healing

Massage therapy: Stretching and loosening muscles and connective tissue for relaxation and circulation

Biofeedback: Using technology to increase awareness of various neurological body responses to minimize extremes

Therapeutic touch: Using hands to help bring energy fields into balance

NATURAL PRODUCTS AND HERBAL REMEDIES

- Natural products include herbal medicines, minerals and vitamins, essential oils, and dietary supplements.
- Clients use nonvitamin, nonmineral natural products to prevent disease and illness, and to promote health.
- Herbal remedies are derived from plant sources and are the oldest form of medicine.
- The FDA does not regulate many of these products.
- Some herbal agents have been deemed safe or effective by nongovernment agencies. However, even safe or commonly used substances can have adverse effects and interfere with prescription medication efficacy. Qs

Aloe: Wound healing

Chamomile: Anti-inflammatory, calming

Echinacea: Enhances immunity

Garlic: Inhibits platelet aggregation

Ginger: Antiemetic

Ginkgo biloba: Improves memory

Ginseng: Increases physical endurance

Valerian: Promotes sleep, reduces anxiety

NURSING AND CAM

Nurses should do the following.

- Understand the varieties of therapies available and any safety precautions associated with their use.
- Be receptive to learning about clients' alternative health beliefs and practices (home remedies, cultural practices, vitamin use, modification of prescriptions).
- Identify clients' needs for complementary or alternative therapies, along with the client's values and treatment preferences. Qpcc
- Incorporate complementary or alternative therapies into clients' care plans.
- Evaluate client's responses to CAM interventions.
- Assist with evaluating the safety of herbal and natural products the client may be using. Provide the client with reliable information, and determine possible interactions with prescription medicines and therapies.

THERAPIES

Nursing interventions can provide some aspects of complementary alternative therapies, including the following.

Guided imagery/visualization therapy: Encourages healing and relaxation of the body by having the mind focus on images

Healing intention: Uses caring, compassion, and empathy in the context of prayer to facilitate healing

Breathwork: Reduces stress and increases relaxation through various breathing patterns

Humor: Reduces tension and improves mood to foster coping

Meditation: Uses rhythmic breathing to calm the mind and body

Simple touch: Communicates presence, appreciation, and acceptance

Music or art therapy: Provides distraction from pain and allows the client to express emotions; earphones improve concentration

Therapeutic communication: Allows clients to verbalize and become aware of emotions and fears in a safe, nonjudgmental environment

Relaxation techniques: Promotes relaxation using breathing techniques while thinking peaceful thoughts (passive relaxation) or while tensing and relaxing specific muscle groups (progressive relaxation)

Application Exercises

1. A nurse is caring for a client scheduled for abdominal surgery. The client reports being worried. Which of the following actions should the nurse take?

   A. Offer information on a relaxation technique and ask the client if he is interested in trying it.

   B. Request a social worker see the client to discuss meditation.

   C. Attempt to use biofeedback techniques with the client.

   D. Tell the client many people feel the same way before surgery and to think of something else.

2. A nurse is assessing a client as part of an admission history. The client reports drinking an herbal tea every afternoon at work to relieve stress. The nurse should suspect the tea includes which of the following ingredients?

   A. Chamomile

   B. Ginseng

   C. Ginger

   D. Echinacea

3. A nurse is reviewing complementary and alternative therapies with a group of nursing students. The nurse should classify which of the following interventions as a mind-body therapy? (Select all that apply.)

   A. Art therapy

   B. Acupressure

   C. Yoga

   D. Therapeutic touch

   E. Biofeedback

4. A nurse is teaching a group of nursing students on complementary and alternative therapies they can incorporate into their practice without the need for specialized licensing or certification. Which of the following should the nurse encourage the students to use? (Select all that apply.)

   A. Guided imagery

   B. Massage therapy

   C. Meditation

   D. Music therapy

   E. Therapeutic touch

5. A nurse is planning to use healing intention with a client who is recovering from a lengthy illness. Which of the following is the priority action the nurse should take before attempting this particular mind-body intervention?

   A. Tell the client the goal of the therapy is to promote healing.

   B. Ask whether the client is comfortable with using prayer.

   C. Encourage the client participate actively for best results.

   D. Instruct the client to relax during the therapy.

PRACTICE Active Learning Scenario

A nurse is reviewing the various categories of complementary and alternative therapies with a group of newly licensed nurses. Use the ATI Active Learning Template: Basic Concept to complete this item.

RELATED CONTENT: List at least four different types of therapies with examples of each.

Application Exercises Key

1. A. **CORRECT:** It is appropriate for the nurse to recommend a noninvasive technique to facilitate coping, and to allow the client to make an informed decision about participating.

   B. Meditation does not require specialized training. The nurse can use this therapy and does not need to request a social worker consult.

   C. The nurse should recognize that biofeedback requires specialized training and licensing or certification. It is not appropriate for the nurse to attempt to use these techniques.

   D. This response by the nurse is nontherapeutic because it uses stereotyping and dismisses the client's feelings. The nurse should use therapeutic communication techniques to allow the client to further verbalize fears.

   Ⓝ *NCLEX® Connection: Basic Care and Comfort,*
   Non-Pharmacological Comfort Interventions

2. A. **CORRECT:** The nurse should suspect the tea might contain chamomile, which produces a calming effect, or valerian, which reduces anxiety. The nurse should attempt to gain further information to confirm the ingredients of any herbal or natural products the client may use.

   B. The nurse should expect a client to use ginseng tea to improve physical endurance.

   C. The nurse should expect a client to use ginger tea to prevent or relieve nausea.

   D. The nurse should expect a client to use Echinacea tea to boost the immune system.

   Ⓝ *NCLEX® Connection: Management of Care,*
   Concepts of Management

3. A. **CORRECT:** The nurse should classify art therapy as a mind-body therapy because it allows the client to express unconscious emotions or concerns about their health.

   B. The nurse should classify acupressure is a body-based therapy because it focuses specifically on body structures and systems.

   C. **CORRECT:** The nurse should classify yoga as a mind-body therapy because it focuses on achieving well-being through exercise, posture, breathing, and meditation.

   D. The nurse should classify therapeutic touch as an energy therapy because it involves using the hands to balance energy fields.

   E. **CORRECT:** The nurse should classify biofeedback because it increases mental awareness of the body responses to stress.

   Ⓝ *NCLEX® Connection: Basic Care and Comfort,*
   Non-Pharmacological Comfort Interventions

4. A. **CORRECT:** Nurses may use guided imagery with clients once they understand the general principles of this therapy.

   B. The nurse should inform the students that massage therapists undergo training as well as certification and/or licensure.

   C. **CORRECT:** Nurses may use meditation with clients once they understand the general principles of this therapy.

   D. **CORRECT:** Nurses may use music therapy with clients once they understand the general principles.

   E. The nurse should inform the students that therapeutic touch practitioners undergo specific training.

   Ⓝ *NCLEX® Connection: Basic Care and Comfort,*
   Non-Pharmacological Comfort Interventions

5. A. The nurse should tell the client the goals of therapy to provide information to the client. However, there is another action the nurse should take first.

   B. **CORRECT:** The first action the nurse should take using the nursing process is to assess or collect data from the client. Because people can have personal, cultural, or religious sensitivities or aversions to religious practices such as prayer, the nurse must first determine that the client is comfortable with a therapy that involves prayer.

   C. The nurse should encourage the client to participate to improve the effectiveness of the therapy. However, there is another action the nurse should take first.

   D. The nurse should instruct the client relax to promote the client's ability to focus during the therapy. However, there is another action the nurse should take first.

   Ⓝ *NCLEX® Connection: Basic Care and Comfort,*
   Non-Pharmacological Comfort Interventions

PRACTICE Answer

Using the ATI Active Learning Template: Basic Concept

RELATED CONTENT

- Alternative medical philosophy: traditional Chinese medicine, Ayurvedic medicine, homeopathy
- Biological and botanical therapies: diets, vitamins, minerals, herbal preparations
- Body manipulation: massage, touch, chiropractic therapy
- Mind-body therapies: biofeedback, art therapy, meditation, yoga, psychotherapy, tai chi
- Energy therapies: Reiki, therapeutic touch

Ⓝ *NCLEX® Connection: Basic Care and Comfort, Non-Pharmacological Comfort Interventions*

CHAPTER 43 *Bowel Elimination*

Many factors can alter bowel function. Interventions such as surgery, immobility, medications, and therapeutic diets can affect bowel elimination. Various disease processes necessitate the creation of bowel diversions to allow fecal elimination to continue.

Stool specimens are collected both for screening and for diagnostic tests, such as for the detection of occult blood, bacteria, or parasites.

Alterations in bowel pattern include infrequent, difficult stools (constipation) or an increased number of loose, liquid stools (diarrhea).

BOWEL ELIMINATION PATTERNS

There are objective ways to assess a client's bowel pattern, but individual bowel patterns vary greatly. Q𝐩𝐜𝐜

FACTORS AFFECTING BOWEL ELIMINATION

Age

INFANTS
- Breast milk stools: watery and yellow brown
- Formula stools: pasty and brown

TODDLERS: Bowel control at 2 to 3 years old

OLDER ADULTS: Decreased peristalsis, relaxation of sphincters

Diet

Fiber requirement: 25 to 30 g/day

Lactose intolerance: Difficulty digesting milk products

Fluid intake

Fluid requirement: 2,000 to 3,000 mL/day from fluid and food sources

Physical activity

Stimulates intestinal activity

Psychosocial factors

Emotional distress increasing peristalsis and exacerbating chronic conditions (colitis, Crohn's disease, ulcers, irritable bowel syndrome)

Depression decreases peristalsis and can lead to constipation.

Personal habits

Willingness to use public toilets, false perception of the need for "one-a-day" bowel movements, lack of privacy when hospitalized

Positioning

NORMAL: Squatting

IMMOBILIZED CLIENT: Difficulty defecating

Pain

- Normal defecation is painless. Discomfort leads to suppression of the urge to defecate.
- Opioid use contributes to constipation.

Pregnancy

- Growing fetus compromising intestinal space
- Slower peristalsis
- Straining increasing the risk of hemorrhoids

Surgery and anesthesia

Temporary slowing of intestinal activity (rationale for auscultating bowel sounds before advancing diet)

Medications

Laxatives: To soften stool

Cathartics: To promote peristalsis

Laxative overuse: Chronic use of laxatives causes a weakening of the bowel's expected response to distention from feces resulting in the development of chronic constipation.

INCONTINENCE

Fecal incontinence is the inability to control defecation, often caused by diarrhea.

- Determine causes, such as medications, infections, or impaction.
- Provide perineal care after each stool, and apply a moisture barrier.
- The provider can prescribe an anal bag or other bowel management system to collect stool and prevent it from coming into contact with the skin.

FLATULENCE

Flatulence results from distention of the bowel from gas accumulation (can cause cramping or a feeling of fullness).

- Check for abdominal distention and the ability to pass gas through the anus.
- Encourage ambulation to promote the passage of flatus.

HEMORRHOIDS

Hemorrhoids are engorged, dilated blood vessels in the rectal wall from difficult defecation, pregnancy, liver disease, and heart failure.

- Hemorrhoids can be itchy, painful, and bloody after defecation.
- Use moist wipes for cleansing the perianal area, and apply ointments or creams as prescribed.
- Use a sitz bath or ice pack to promote relief from hemorrhoid discomfort.

OSTOMIES

- Some bowel disorders prevent the normal elimination of stool from the body. Bowel diversions through ostomies are temporary or permanent openings (stomas) surgically created in the abdominal wall to allow fecal matter to pass.
- Ostomies are created in either the large intestine or the small intestine. **Colostomies** end in the colon, and **ileostomies** end in the ileum.
  - **End stomas** are a result of colorectal cancer or some types of bowel disease.
  - **Loop colostomies** help resolve a medical emergency and are temporary. In a loop colostomy, a loop of bowel is supported on the abdomen with a proximal stoma draining stool and a distal stoma draining mucus. It is usually constructed in the transverse colon.
  - **Double-barrel colostomies** consist of two abdominal stomas: one proximal and one distal. The proximal stoma drains stool and the distal stoma leads to inactive intestine. After the injured area of the intestine heals, the colostomy is often reversed by reattaching the two ends.

Constipation and diarrhea

For healthy clients, constipation and diarrhea are not serious. For older adult clients and clients who have pre-existing medical problems, constipation and diarrhea can have a significant impact on the client's health. Qs

Constipation

Constipation is a bowel pattern of difficult and infrequent evacuation of hard, dry feces.

Paralytic ileus is an intestinal obstruction caused by reduced motility following bowel manipulation during surgery, electrolyte imbalance, wound infection, or by the effects of medication.

CAUSES OF CONSTIPATION

- Frequent use of laxatives
- Advanced age
- Inadequate fluid intake
- Inadequate fiber intake
- Immobilization due to injury
- Sedentary lifestyle
- Pregnancy
- Medication effects

Diarrhea

Diarrhea is a bowel pattern of frequent loose or liquid stools.

CAUSES OF DIARRHEA

- Viral gastroenteritis
- Bacterial gastroenteritis
- Antibiotic therapy
- Inflammatory bowel disease
- Irritable bowel syndrome

ASSESSMENT/DATA COLLECTION

- Perform a routine physical examination of the abdomen (bowel sounds, tenderness).
- Check for fluid deficit.
- Inspect skin integrity around the anal area.
- Collect a detailed history of diet, exercise, and bowel habits.
- Monitor for constipation.
  - Abdominal bloating
  - Abdominal cramping
  - Straining at defecation
  - Presence of dry, hard feces at defecation.
  - Irregular bowel movements, or reduced frequency from client's normal pattern.]
- Monitor for diarrhea.
  - Frequent loose stools
  - Abdominal cramping
  - Stool of watery consistency
- Perform specimen collection for diagnostic testing as indicated.
- Perform a digital rectal examination for impaction.
  - Position on the left side with the knees flexed.
  - Monitor vital signs and response.

DIAGNOSTIC PROCEDURES

Stool samples should come from fresh stools. Avoid contaminating with water or urine.

Fecal occult blood (guaiac) test: Obtain a fecal sample using medical asepsis while wearing gloves. Collect stool specimens for serial guaiac testing three times from three different defecations. Some foods (red meat, citrus fruit, raw vegetables) and medications can cause false positive results. Bleeding can be an indication of cancer. QEBP

Specimens for stool cultures: Obtain using medical asepsis while wearing gloves. Label the specimen, and promptly send it to the laboratory.

Specimen collection

EQUIPMENT
- Specimen container
- Soap/cleansing solution or wipe
- Clean gloves
- Specimen label
- Fecal occult blood test cards
- Wooden applicator or tongue depressor
- Developer solution
- Stool collection container (bedside commode, bedpan, receptacle in toilet)

PROCEDURE
- **Fecal occult blood testing (guaiac test)**
  ○ Explain the procedure to the client.
  ○ Ask the client to collect a specimen in the toilet receptacle, bedpan, or bedside commode.
  ○ Don gloves.
  ○ With a wooden applicator, place small amounts of stool on the windows of the test card or as directed.
  ○ Follow the facility's procedures for handling.
    ▪ Apply a label to the cards and send them to the laboratory for processing.
    ▪ Alternatively, if for point-of-care testing, place a couple of drops of developer on the opposite side of the card. A blue color indicates the stool is positive for blood.
  ○ Remove the gloves and perform hand hygiene.
- **Stool for culture, parasites, and ova**
  ○ Explain the procedure to the client.
  ○ Ask the client to collect the specimen in the toilet receptacle, bedside commode, or bedpan.
  ○ Don gloves.
  ○ Use a wooden tongue depressor to transfer the stool to a specimen container.
  ○ Label the container with the client's identifying information.
  ○ Remove the gloves.
  ○ Perform hand hygiene.
  ○ Transport the specimen to the laboratory.

Colonoscopy

Use of a lighted instrument by the provider to visualize and collect tissue samples for biopsy or remove polyps from the colon or lower small bowel

Sigmoidoscopy

Use of a lighted instrument by the provider to visualize and collect tissue for biopsy or remove polyps from the sigmoid colon and rectum

CLIENT PREPARATION
- Protocols vary with the provider and the facility, but generally include clear liquids only and a bowel cleanser.
- Clients receive moderate (conscious) sedation and may not drive home afterwards.

PATIENT-CENTERED CARE

NURSING CARE

- Closely monitor fluid status and elimination pattern.
- Record food and fluid intake and output. For diarrhea, measure the volume of the stools.
- Observe and document the character of bowel movements. Carefully check for blood or pus.
- Promote regular bowel elimination through several measures. QEBP
  ○ Adequate fiber in the diet
  ○ Adequate fluid intake: Minimum of 1,500 mL/day of water and/or juices
  ○ Adequate activity: Walking 15 to 20 min/day if mobile and exercises in bed or chair (pelvic tilt, single leg lifts, lower trunk rotation)

Constipation

- Increase fiber and water consumption (unless contraindicated) before more invasive interventions.
- Give bulk-forming products before stool softeners, stimulants, or suppositories.
- Enemas are a last resort for stimulating defecation.

Diarrhea

- Help determine and treat the cause.
- Administer medications to slow peristalsis.
- Provide perineal care after each stool, and apply a moisture barrier.
- After diarrhea stops, suggest eating yogurt to help re-establish an intestinal balance of beneficial bacteria.

Meeting needs of older adults ©

- Older adult clients are more susceptible to developing constipation as bowel tone decreases with age. Therefore, they are more at risk for developing fecal impaction. Adequate fluid, fiber intake, and exercise decrease the likelihood of developing constipation or fecal impaction.
- Older adult clients are less able to compensate for fluid lost due to diarrhea. Monitor older adults who have diarrhea for diarrhea-associated complications such as electrolyte imbalances and skin breakdown.

Promoting healthy bowel elimination

EQUIPMENT
- Bedpans
  - Fracture pan: for supine clients and clients in body casts or leg casts
  - Regular pan: for seated clients
- Beside commode
- Toilet

PROCEDURE
- Encourage the client to set aside time to defecate. Sometimes, after a meal works best.
- If not contraindicated or restricted, encourage the client to drink plenty of fluids and to consume a diet high in fiber to prevent constipation.
- Wear gloves when addressing toileting needs.
- Provide privacy.
- Assist the client to a sitting position whether using a regular bedpan, commode, or toilet.
- For clients using a fracture pan, raise the head of the bed to 30°.
- If the client cannot lift his hips to get the bedpan under him, roll him onto one side, position the bedpan over his buttocks, and roll the client back onto the bedpan.
- Encourage the client to decrease stress when sitting or rising by using an elevated toilet seat or a footstool.
- Never leave a client lying flat on a regular bedpan.
- After the client defecates, provide skin care to the perianal area.

Cleansing enema

The height of the bag above the rectum determines the depth of cleansing.

EQUIPMENT
- Gloves
- Lubricant
- Absorbent, waterproof pads
- Bedpan, beside commode, or toilet
- IV pole
- Enema bag with tubing or prepackaged enema
- Solutions and additives: vary with the type of enema
  - Tap water or hypotonic solution
    - Stimulates evacuation
    - Never repeated due to potential water toxicity
  - Soapsuds
    - Pure castile soap in tap water or normal saline
    - Acts as an irritant to promote bowel peristalsis
  - Normal saline
    - Safest due to equal osmotic pressure
    - Volume stimulates peristalsis
  - Low-volume hypertonic
    - Used by clients who cannot tolerate high-volume enemas
    - Commercially prepared
  - Oil retention: Lubricates the rectum and colon for easier passage of stool
  - Medicated enema: Contains medications, such as antibiotics or antihelmintics, to retain for a period of time (1 to 3 hr).

PROCEDURE
- Perform hand hygiene.
- Prepare and warm the enema solution.
- Pour the solution into the enema bag, allowing it to fill the tubing, and then close the clamp.
- Explain the procedure to the client.
- Provide privacy.
- Provide quick access to a commode or bedpan.
- Place absorbent pads under the client to protect the bed linens.
- Position the client on the left side with the right leg flexed forward.
- Put on gloves.
- Lubricate the rectal tube or nozzle.
- Slowly insert the rectal tube 7.5 to 10 cm (3 to 4 in). For a child, insert the tube 5 to 7.5 cm (2 to 3 in).
- With the bag level with the client's hip, open the clamp.
- Raise the bag 30 to 45 cm (12 to 18 in) above the anus, depending on the level of cleansing desired.
- Slow the flow of solution by lowering the container if the client reports cramping, or if fluid leaks around the tube at the anus.
- If using a prepackaged solution, insert the lubricated tip into the rectum, and squeeze the container to instill all of the solution.
- Ask the client to retain the solution for the prescribed amount of time, or until the client is no longer able to retain it.
- Discard the enema bag and tubing.
- Assist the client to the appropriate position to defecate.
- Remove the gloves.
- Perform hand hygiene.
- For clients who have little or no sphincter control, administer the enema on a bedpan.
- Document the results and the client's tolerance of the procedure.

Ostomy care

EQUIPMENT
- Pouch system (skin barrier and pouch)
- Pouch closure clamp
- Barrier pastes (optional)
- Gloves
- Washcloths
- Towel
- Warm water
- Scissors
- Pen

PROCEDURE
- If a wound ostomy continence nurse is not available, educate the client about stoma care.
- Perform hand hygiene.
- Put on gloves.
- Remove the pouch from the stoma.
- Inspect the stoma. It should appear moist, shiny, and pink. The peristomal area should be intact, and the skin should appear healthy.
- Use mild soap and water to cleanse the skin, then dry it gently and completely. Moisturizing soaps can interfere with adherence of the pouch.
- Apply paste if necessary.

- Measure and mark the desired size for the skin barrier.
- Cut the opening 0.15 to 0.3 cm (1/18 to 1/8 in) larger, allowing only the stoma to appear through the opening.
- If necessary, apply barrier pastes to creases.
- Apply the skin barrier and pouch.
- Fold the bottom of the pouch and place the closure clamp on the pouch.
- Dispose of the used pouch. Remove the gloves and perform hand hygiene.

COMPLICATIONS

Complications of constipation

Fecal impaction: Stool becomes wedged in the rectum, and can involve diarrhea fluid leaking around the impacted stool.
- Administer enemas and suppositories or stool softeners as prescribed to promote relief of fecal impaction. If necessary, manually remove fecal impactions that do not respond to other interventions.
- Use a gloved, lubricated finger for digital removal of stool.
- Loosen the stool around the edges and then remove it in small pieces, allowing the client to rest as necessary.
- When evacuating the rectum, be careful to avoid stimulating the vagus nerve.
- Stop the procedure if the heart rate drops significantly or the heart rhythm changes. Qs

Hemorrhoids and rectal fissures

Bradycardia, hypotension, syncope
- Associated with the Valsalva maneuver (occurs with straining/bearing down).
- Instruct clients not to strain to have bowel movements. Qs
- Encourage measures to treat and prevent constipation.

Complications of diarrhea

Dehydration

Fluid and electrolyte disturbances: Metabolic acidosis from excessive loss of bicarbonate
- Monitor for manifestations of dehydration (weak, rapid pulse, hypotension, poor skin turgor, elevated body temperature).
- Monitor for manifestations of electrolyte imbalance.
- Replace fluid and electrolytes as prescribed.

Skin breakdown around the anal area: Provide treatment for skin breakdown as prescribed.

PRACTICE Active Learning Scenario

A nurse is explaining to a group of nursing students the various factors that alter bowel elimination patterns. Use the ATI Active Learning Template: Basic Concept to complete this item.

UNDERLYING PRINCIPLES: List at least eight factors that affect bowel elimination, along with a brief example or description of each.

Application Exercises

1. A nurse is caring for a client who will perform fecal occult blood testing at home. Which of the following information should the nurse include when explaining the procedure to the client?

   A. Eating more protein is optimal prior to testing.

   B. One stool specimen is sufficient for testing.

   C. A red color change indicates a positive test.

   D. The specimen cannot be contaminated with urine.

2. A nurse is talking with a client who reports constipation. When the nurse discusses dietary changes that can help prevent constipation, which of the following foods should the nurse recommend?

   A. Macaroni and cheese

   B. Fresh fruit and whole wheat toast

   C. Bread pudding and yogurt

   D. Roast chicken and white rice

3. A nurse is caring for a client who has had diarrhea for 4 days. When assessing the client, the nurse should expect which of the following findings? (Select all that apply.)

   A. Bradycardia

   B. Hypotension

   C. Elevated temperature

   D. Poor skin turgor

   E. Peripheral edema

4. While a nurse is administering a cleansing enema, the client reports abdominal cramping. Which of the following actions should the nurse take?

   A. Have the client hold his breath briefly and bear down.

   B. Discontinue the fluid instillation.

   C. Remind the client that cramping is common at this time.

   D. Lower the enema fluid container.

5. A nurse is preparing to administer a cleansing enema to an adult client in preparation for a diagnostic procedure. Which of the following steps should the nurse take? (Select all that apply.)

   A. Warm the enema solution prior to instillation.

   B. Position the client on the left side with the right leg flexed forward.

   C. Lubricate the rectal tube or nozzle.

   D. Slowly insert the rectal tube about 5 cm (2 in).

   E. Hang the enema container 61 cm (24 in) above the client's anus.

1. A. Some proteins can alter the test results. The nurse should instruct the client not to consume red meat, fish, and poultry prior to testing.

    B. The nurse should instruct the client to obtain three specimens from three different bowel movements.

    C. The nurse should inform the client to look for a blue color on the card to indicate positive blood in the stool.

    D. **CORRECT:** For fecal occult blood testing, the nurse should warn the client not to contaminate the stool specimens with water or urine.

    (N) *NCLEX® Connection: Reduction of Risk Potential, Therapeutic Procedures*

2. A. The nurse should identify macaroni and cheese as a low-residue option that could actually worsen constipation.

    B. **CORRECT:** A high-fiber diet promotes normal bowel elimination. The nurse should recommend the client consume fresh fruits and vegetables with whole-grain carbohydrates to provide the highest fiber option.

    C. The nurse should identify bread pudding and yogurt as low-residue options that could actually worsen constipation.

    D. The nurse should identify roast chicken and white rice as low-residue options that could actually worsen constipation.

    (N) *NCLEX® Connection: Basic Care and Comfort, Elimination*

3. A. The nurse should expect the client who has prolonged diarrhea to have tachycardia.

    B. **CORRECT:** Prolonged diarrhea leads to dehydration. The nurse should expect the client to have a decrease in blood pressure.

    C. **CORRECT:** Prolonged diarrhea leads to dehydration. The nurse should expect the client to have an increased temperature.

    D. **CORRECT:** Prolonged diarrhea leads to dehydration. The nurse should expect the client to have poor skin turgor.

    E. The nurse should expect the client who has prolonged diarrhea to possibly have weakened peripheral pulses. Peripheral edema results from a fluid overload.

    (N) *NCLEX® Connection: Physiological Adaptation, Illness Management*

4. A. The nurse should have the client take slow, deep breaths to relax and ease discomfort.

    B. The nurse should stop the instillation if the client's abdomen becomes rigid and distended or if the nurse notes bleeding from the rectum.

    C. This action by the nurse is nontherapeutic because it implies that the client must tolerate the discomfort and that the nurse cannot or will not do anything to ease it.

    D. **CORRECT:** To relieve the client's discomfort, the nurse should slow the rate of instillation by reducing the height of the enema solution container.

    (N) *NCLEX® Connection: Reduction of Risk Potential, Potential for Complications of Diagnostic Tests/Treatments/Procedures*

5. A. **CORRECT:** The nurse should warm the enema solution because cold fluid can cause abdominal cramping, and hot fluid can injure the intestinal mucosa.

    B. **CORRECT:** The nurse should place the client in this position to promote a downward flow of solution by gravity along the natural anatomical curve of the sigmoid colon.

    C. **CORRECT:** The nurse should lubricate the tubing to prevent trauma or irritation to the rectal mucosa.

    D. The correct length of insertion for a child is 5 cm (2 in). For an adult client, the nurse should insert the tube 7.6 to 10.2 cm (3 to 4 in).

    E. The maximum recommended height is 46 cm (18 in). The height of the fluid container affects the speed of instillation. The nurse should hang the container within the recommended height range to prevent rapid instillation and possibly painful distention of the colon.

    (N) *NCLEX® Connection: Reduction of Risk Potential, Diagnostic Tests*

PRACTICE Answer

Using the ATI Active Learning Template: Basic Concept

UNDERLYING PRINCIPLES

- Age
  - Infants
    - Breast milk stools: Watery and yellow brown
    - Formula stools: Pasty and brown
  - Toddlers: Bowel control at 2 to 3 years old
  - Older adults: Decreased peristalsis, relaxation of sphincters
- Diet
  - Fiber requirement: 25 to 30 g/day
  - Lactose intolerance: Difficulty digesting milk products
  - Fluid requirement: 2,000 to 3,000 mL/day from fluid and food sources

- Physical activity: Stimulates intestinal activity
- Psychosocial factors
  - Emotional distress increasing peristalsis and exacerbating chronic conditions (colitis, Crohn's disease, ulcers, irritable bowel syndrome)
  - Depression decreasing peristalsis
- Personal habits: Use of public toilets, false perception of the need for "one-a-day" bowel movements, lack of privacy when hospitalized
- Positioning
  - Normal: Squatting
  - Immobilized client: Difficulty defecating

- Pain
  - Discomfort leading to suppression of the urge to defecate
  - Opioid use contributing to constipation
- Pregnancy
  - Growing fetus compromising intestinal space
  - Slower peristalsis
  - Straining increasing the risk of hemorrhoids
- Surgery and anesthesia
  - Temporary slowing of intestinal activity
  - Paralytic ileus
- Medications
  - Laxatives: To soften stool; overuse leads to chronic constipation
  - Cathartics: To promote peristalsis

(N) *NCLEX® Connection: Physiological Adaptation, Pathophysiology*

CHAPTER 44 *Urinary Elimination*

Urinary elimination is a precise system of filtration, reabsorption, and excretion. These processes help maintain fluid and electrolyte balance while filtering and excreting water-soluble wastes.

The primary organs of urinary elimination are the kidneys, with the nephrons performing most of the functions of filtration and elimination. Most adults produce 1,500 to 2,000 mL/day of urine.

After filtration, the urine passes through the ureters into the bladder, the storage reservoir for urine. Once an adequate amount of urine (150 to 200 mL) collects in the bladder, stretch receptors in the bladder wall send a signal to the brain to indicate the need to urinate. The person then relaxes the internal and external sphincters at the bottom of the bladder and the urethra. Urine passes from the bladder through the urethra, from which it exits the body.

Interventions such as surgery, immobility, medications, and therapeutic diets can affect urinary elimination.

URINARY DIVERSIONS

- Urinary diversions are the surgical creation of a stoma, either temporary or permanent, for the drainage of urine. Surgeons create urinary diversions for clients who have bladder cancer or injury. Qᴘᴄᴄ
- Urinary diversions have many similarities to bowel diversions. Clients who have urinary diversions often share similar body image concerns as those who have bowel diversions.
- Diversions are either continent (with controlled elimination of urine from the body) or incontinent (with urine draining continuously without control).
- Continent diversions have a reservoir in the abdomen that allows clients to control the elimination of urine.

Ureterostomy: An incontinent urinary diversion for which the surgeon attaches one or both ureters via a stoma to the surface of the abdominal wall

Nephrostomy: An incontinent urinary diversion for which the surgeon attaches a tube from the renal pelvis via a stoma to the surface of the abdominal wall

FACTORS AFFECTING URINARY ELIMINATION

- Poor abdominal and pelvic muscle tone
- Acute and chronic disorders
- Spinal cord injury

Age

- Children achieve full bladder control by 4 to 5 years of age.
- The prostate enlarges after 40 years of age, leading to urinary frequency, hesitancy, retention, incontinence, and urinary tract infections (UTIs).
- Childbirth and gravity weaken the pelvic floor, putting clients at risk for prolapse of the bladder, leading to stress incontinence, which clients can help manage with pelvic floor (Kegel) exercises.

OLDER ADULT CLIENTS Ⓖ
- Fewer nephrons
- Loss of muscle tone of the bladder leading to frequency
- Inefficient emptying of the bladder: residual urine increasing the risk for UTIs
- Increase in nocturia

Pregnancy

- A growing fetus compromises bladder space and compresses the bladder.
- There is a 30% to 50% increase in circulatory volume, which increases renal workload and output.
- The hormone relaxin causes relaxation of the sphincter.

Diet

- An increase in sodium leads to decreased urination.
- Caffeine and alcohol intake lead to increased urination.

Immobility

Incontinence is not a result of aging, but of neurological or mobility impairments.

Psychosocial factors

- Emotional stress and anxiety
- Having to use public toilets
- Lack of privacy during hospital stays
- Not having enough time to urinate (predetermined bathroom breaks in elementary schools)

Pain

- Suppression of the urge to urinate when there is pain in the urinary tract
- Obstruction in the ureter leading to renal colic
- Arthritis or painful joints causing immobility and leading to delayed urination

Surgical procedures

- Alterations in glomerular filtration rate from anesthesia and opioid analgesics, resulting in decreased urine output
- Lower abdominal surgery creating obstructive edema and inflammation

Medications

- Diuretics preventing reabsorption of water
- Antihistamines and anticholinergics causing urinary retention
- Chemotherapy creating a toxic environment for the kidneys

MEDICATIONS THAT CHANGE URINE COLOR
- Phenazopyridine: orange, red
- Amitriptyline: green–blue
- Levodopa: dark

DIAGNOSTIC TESTS

Bedside sonography with a bladder scanner: Noninvasive portable ultrasound scanner for measuring bladder volume and residual volume after urination

Kidneys, ureters, bladder: X-ray to determine size, shape, and position of these structures

Intravenous pyelogram: Injection of contrast media (iodine) for viewing of ducts, renal pelvis, ureters, bladder, and urethra

> ! Allergy to shellfish contraindicates the use of this contrast medium.

Renal scan: View of renal blood flow and anatomy of the kidneys without contrast

Renal ultrasound: View of gross renal structures and structural abnormalities using high-frequency sound waves

Cystoscopy: Use of a lighted instrument to visualize, treat, and obtain specimens from the bladder and urethra

Urodynamic testing: Test for bladder muscle function by filling the bladder with CO_2 or 0.9% sodium chloride and comparing pressure readings with reported sensations

CONSIDERATIONS

Promoting healthy urinary elimination

EQUIPMENT
- Urinal for men
- Toilet, bedpan, or commode
  - Fracture pan: For clients who must remain supine and clients in body or leg casts
  - Regular pan: For clients who can sit up

PROCEDURE NURSING CONSIDERATIONS
- Have clients sit when possible.
- Provide for privacy needs with adequate time for urinating.

I&O

EQUIPMENT
- Hard plastic urometer on an indwelling catheter drainage bag
- Graduated cylinders, urinal, or toilet receptacle

PROCEDURE NURSING CONSIDERATIONS
- Measure output from a bedpan, commode, or collection bag into a graduated container.
- Use a receptacle to measure urine clients void into the toilet.
- Use markings on the side of the urinal to measure urine.

> ! Less than 30 mL/hr for more than 2 hr is a cause for concern.

Bladder retraining for treating urge incontinence

EQUIPMENT: Clock

PROCEDURE NURSING CONSIDERATIONS
- Use timed voiding to increase intervals between urination.
- Have clients perform pelvic floor (Kegel) exercises.
- Assist clients to perform relaxation techniques.
- Offer undergarments while clients are retraining.
- Teach clients not to ignore the urge to urinate.
- Provide positive reinforcement as clients remain continent.
- Tell clients to eliminate or decrease caffeine drinks.
- Instruct clients to take diuretics in the morning.

Specimen collection

EQUIPMENT
- Specimen container
  - Nonsterile for urinalysis
  - Sterile for clean-catch midstream and specimens from a catheter
- Soap or cleansing solution and towel
- Gloves (for contact with any body fluids)
- Specimen label
- Urine collection container (catheter, urinal, receptacle in toilet, commode)

Urinalysis: random nonsterile specimen
NURSING CONSIDERATIONS
- Explain the procedure.
- Label the container with clients' identifying information, and follow the facility's policy for transporting the specimen to the laboratory.

Clean-catch midstream for culture and sensitivity (C&S)
NURSING CONSIDERATIONS
- Teach the technique for obtaining the specimen.
- After thorough cleansing of the urethral meatus, clients catch the urine sample midstream.

Catheter urine specimen for C&S
NURSING CONSIDERATIONS: Obtain a sterile specimen from a straight or indwelling catheter using surgical asepsis (sterile technique).

Timed urine specimens
NURSING CONSIDERATIONS
- Collect for 24 hr or other duration.
- Discard the first voiding.
- Collect all other urine. Refrigerate, label, and transport the specimen.

Straight or indwelling catheter insertion

EQUIPMENT
- Usual size and type of catheter
  - 8 to 10 Fr for children
  - 14 to 16 Fr for women
  - 16 to 18 Fr for men
  - Use silicon or Teflon products for clients who have latex allergies.
- Catheterization kit with a sterile drainage bag for indwelling catheter insertion
- Soap and water
- Collection container for straight catheterization

PROCEDURE NURSING CONSIDERATIONS
- Explain the procedure, and provide for privacy.
- Use the correct technique for inserting an indwelling catheter or for straight catheterization.

Closed intermittent irrigation

Use the correct technique to perform closed intermittent irrigation.

Routine catheter care

EQUIPMENT
- Soap and water
- Washcloth
- Gloves

PROCEDURE NURSING CONSIDERATIONS
- Use soap and water at the insertion site.
- Cleanse the catheter at least three times a day and after defecation.
- Monitor the patency of the catheter.
  - For reports of fullness in the bladder area, check for kinks in the tubing, and check for sediment in the tubing.
  - Make sure the collection bag is at a level below the bladder to avoid reflux.

Condom catheter application

EQUIPMENT
- Gloves
- Condom catheter
- Elastic tape
- Leg or standard collection bag

PROCEDURE NURSING CONSIDERATIONS
- Explain the procedure.
- Use the correct technique for application of a condom catheter.

COMPLICATIONS

Urinary tract infections

Most due to *Escherichia coli*

RISK FACTORS
- In women, close proximity of the urethral meatus to the anus
- Frequent sexual intercourse
- Menopause: decreasing estrogen levels
- Uncircumcised males
- Use of indwelling catheters Q EBP

NURSING CONSIDERATIONS
- Cleanse female clients from front to back.
- Cleanse beneath the foreskin in males.
- Provide catheter care regularly.

Urinary incontinence

Urinary incontinence is a significant contributing factor to skin breakdown and falls, especially in older adults. ⊙

MAJOR TYPES

Stress: Loss of small amounts of urine from increased abdominal pressure without bladder muscle contraction with laughing, sneezing, or lifting

Urge: Inability to stop urine flow long enough to reach the bathroom due to an overactive detrusor muscle with increased bladder pressure

Overflow: Urinary retention from bladder overdistention and frequent loss of small amounts of urine due to obstruction of the urinary outlet or an impaired detrusor muscle

Reflex: Involuntary loss of a moderate amount of urine usually without warning due to hyperreflexia of the detrusor muscle, usually from spinal cord dysfunction

Functional: Loss of urine due to factors that interfere with responding to the need to urinate, such as cognitive, mobility, and environmental barriers

Total: Unpredictable, involuntary loss of urine that generally does not respond to treatment

ASSESSMENT/DATA COLLECTION

RISK FACTORS

- Female gender
- History of multiple pregnancies and vaginal births, aging, chronic urinary retention, urinary bladder spasm, renal disease, chronic bladder infection (cystitis)
- Neurological disorders: Parkinson's disease, cerebrovascular accident, spinal cord injury, multiple sclerosis
- Medication therapy: Diuretics, opioids, anticholinergics, calcium channel blockers, sedative/hypnotics, adrenergic antagonists
- Obesity
- Confusion, dementia, immobility, depression
- Physiological changes of aging ⊙
- Decreased estrogen levels and decreased pelvic-muscle tone
- Immobility, chronic degenerative diseases, dementia, diabetes mellitus, cerebrovascular accident
- Urinary incontinence increasing the risk for falls, fractures, pressure ulcers, and depression Qs

EXPECTED FINDINGS

- Loss of urine when laughing, coughing, sneezing
- Enuresis (bed-wetting)
- Bladder spasms
- Urinary retention
- Frequency, urgency, nocturia

LABORATORY TESTS

Urinalysis and urine culture and sensitivity: To identify UTI (presence of RBCs, WBCs, micro-organisms)

Serum creatinine and BUN: To assess renal function (elevated with renal dysfunction)

DIAGNOSTIC PROCEDURES

Ultrasound: Detects bladder abnormalities and/or residual urine

Voiding cystourethrography: Identifies the size, shape, support, and function of the urinary bladder, obstruction (prostate), residual urine

Urodynamic testing
- **Cystourethroscopy:** Visualizes the inside of the bladder
- **Uroflowmetry:** Measures the rate and degree of bladder emptying

Electromyography: Measures the strength of pelvic muscle contractions

PATIENT-CENTERED CARE

NURSING CARE

- Establish a toileting schedule.
- Monitor and increase fluid intake during the daytime, and decrease fluid intake prior to bedtime.
- Remove or control barriers to toileting.
- Provide incontinence garments.
- Apply an external or condom catheter for men.
- Avoid the use of indwelling urinary catheters.
- Provide incontinence care.
- Teach clients the following.
  - How to keep an incontinence diary.
  - How to perform Kegel exercises: Tighten pelvic muscles for a count of 10, relax slowly for a count of 10, and repeat in sequences of 15 in the lying-down, sitting, and standing positions.
  - Bladder compression techniques (Credé, Valsalva, double voiding, splinting) to help manage reflex incontinence.
  - To avoid caffeine and alcohol consumption because these produce diuresis and the urge to urinate.
  - Adverse effects of medications that affect urination.
  - Vaginal cone therapy to strengthen pelvic muscles (for stress incontinence).

MEDICATIONS

Antibiotics

Gentamicin and cephalexin for infection

NURSING CONSIDERATIONS: Administer medication with food to decrease gastrointestinal distress.

CLIENT EDUCATION
- Inform clients that antibiotics might change the urine's odor.
- Instruct clients to report loose stools.
- Tell clients to complete the full course of therapy even if symptoms resolve.

Tricyclic antidepressants

Nortriptyline has anticholinergic effects that help relieve urinary incontinence.

NURSING CONSIDERATIONS
- Monitor for dizziness.
- Evaluate blood pressure for orthostatic hypotension.
- Do not administer to clients taking an MAOI.

CLIENT EDUCATION: Encourage clients to get up slowly. Qs

Urinary antispasmodics or anticholinergic agents

Oxybutynin and dicyclomine decrease urgency and help alleviate pain from a neurogenic or overactive bladder.

NURSING CONSIDERATIONS
- Ask clients about a history of glaucoma. These medications increase intraocular pressure.
- Monitor for dizziness, tachycardia, and urinary retention.

CLIENT EDUCATION
- Instruct clients to report dysuria, palpitations, and constipation.
- Inform clients that dizziness and dry mouth are common with these medications.

Phenazopyridine

This bladder analgesic treats the symptoms of UTIs.

NURSING CONSIDERATIONS
- This medication will not treat infection but will help relieve bladder discomfort.
- Monitor for decreases in Hgb and Hct.
- Hepatic disorders and renal insufficiency are contraindications.

CLIENT EDUCATION
- Encourage clients to take the medication with food.
- Inform clients that the medication turns urine orange.
- Instruct clients to notify the provider immediately if their skin becomes yellowish.

Hormone replacement therapy

This is controversial, but it increases the blood supply to the pelvis.

THERAPEUTIC PROCEDURES

Bladder-retraining program

Urinary bladder retraining increases the bladder's ability to hold urine and clients' ability to suppress urination.

NURSING CONSIDERATIONS
- Clients should urinate at scheduled intervals.
- Clients should gradually increase urination intervals after no incontinence episodes for 3 days, working toward the optimal 4-hr intervals.

CLIENT EDUCATION
- Remind clients to hold urine until the scheduled toileting time.
- Encourage clients to keep track of urination times.

Urinary habit training

Urinary habit training helps clients who have limited cognitive ability to establish a predictable pattern of bladder emptying.

NURSING CONSIDERATIONS: Clients should urinate at scheduled intervals.

CLIENT EDUCATION
- Inform clients that urination patterns determine the toileting schedule.
- Encourage clients to follow a toileting schedule according to the pattern with which they have no incontinence.

Intermittent urinary catheterization

Intermittent urinary catheterization is periodic catheterization to empty the bladder. It reduces the risk of infection from indwelling catheterization, which is a temporary intervention for clients at risk for skin breakdown, or when other options have failed.

NURSING CONSIDERATIONS
- Adjust the frequency of catheterization to keep output at 300 mL or less.
- Explain the procedure.

CLIENT EDUCATION: Encourage clients to follow a toileting schedule according to the pattern with which they have no incontinence.

Anterior vaginal repair, retropubic suspension, pubovaginal sling, insertion of an artificial sphincter

- Catheters (suprapubic or urinary) remain until clients have a post-void residual of less than 50 mL. Traction (with tape) helps prevent movement of the bladder.
- Surgeons insert suprapubic catheters into the abdomen above the pubic bone and in the bladder and suture the catheter in place. The care for the catheter tubing and drainage bag is the same as for an indwelling catheter.

NURSING ACTIONS
- Monitor output and for any signs of infection (color of urine, sediment, level of output).
- Keep the catheter patent at all times.
- Determine clients' ability to detect the urge to urinate.

CLIENT EDUCATION
- Teach skin care around the insertion site.
- Teach care and emptying of the catheter bag.

Periurethral collagen injections to the bladder neck

CARE AFTER DISCHARGE
- To alleviate stress incontinence, consult nutritional services for dietary modifications for clients who are obese.
- Consult home care services to provide intermittent catheters, portable commodes, or stool risers. Suggest installing handrails to assist clients who have bathroom needs. Q𝗧𝗖

CLIENT EDUCATION Q𝗘𝗕𝗣

- Instruct clients to drink 2 to 3 L of fluid daily.
- Instruct clients to try to hold urine, and stay on schedule with bladder retraining.
- Advise clients to drink cranberry juice to decrease the risk of infection.
- Encourage clients who are obese to participate in a weight-reduction program to help resolve stress incontinence.
- Instruct clients to take medications to help resolve incontinence.
- Teach intermittent catheterization if necessary.
- Encourage clients to express their feelings about incontinence.

COMPLICATIONS

Skin breakdown (from chronic exposure to urine)

NURSING ACTIONS
- Keep the skin clean and dry.
- Assess for signs of breakdown.
- Apply protective barrier creams.
- Implement a bladder-retraining program.

Social isolation

NURSING ACTIONS
- Assist with measures to conceal urinary leaking (perineal pads, external catheters, adult incontinence garments).
- Offer emotional support.

Application Exercises

1. A nurse in a provider's office is evaluating a client who reports losing control of urine whenever she coughs, laughs, or sneezes. The client relates a history of three vaginal births, but no serious accidents or illnesses. Which of the following interventions should the nurse suggest for helping to control or eliminate the client's incontinence? (Select all that apply.)

   A. Limit total daily fluid intake.
   B. Decrease or avoid caffeine.
   C. Take calcium supplements.
   D. Avoid drinking alcohol.
   E. Use the Credé maneuver.

2. A client who has an indwelling catheter reports a need to urinate. Which of the following actions should the nurse take?

   A. Check to see whether the catheter is patent.
   B. Reassure the client that it is not possible for her to urinate.
   C. Recatheterize the bladder with a larger-gauge catheter.
   D. Collect a urine specimen for analysis.

3. A nurse is caring for a client who has a prescription for a 24-hr urine collection. Which of the following actions should the nurse take?

   A. Discard the first voiding.
   B. Keep the urine in a single container at room temperature.
   C. Ask the client to urinate and pour the urine into a specimen container.
   D. Ask the client to urinate into the toilet, stop midstream, and finish urinating into the specimen container.

4. A nurse is reviewing factors that increase the risk of urinary tract infections (UTIs) with a client who has recurrent UTIs. Which of the following factors should the nurse include? (Select all that apply.)

   A. Frequent sexual intercourse
   B. Lowering of testosterone levels
   C. Wiping from front to back
   D. Location of the urethra in relation to the anus
   E. Frequent catheterization

5. A nurse is preparing to initiate a bladder-retraining program for a client who has incontinence. Which of the following actions should the nurse take? (Select all that apply.)

   A. Establish a schedule of urinating prior to meal times.
   B. Have the client record urination times.
   C. Gradually increase the urination intervals.
   D. Remind the client to hold urine until the next scheduled urination time.
   E. Provide a sterile container for urine.

PRACTICE Active Learning Scenario

A nurse is teaching a group of nursing students about the various types of urinary incontinence. Use the ATI Active Learning Template: System Disorder to complete this item.

ALTERATION IN HEALTH (DIAGNOSIS): List at least four of the six types of urinary incontinence, along with a brief example or description of each.

RISK FACTORS: List at least 10 common risk factors for urinary incontinence.

Application Exercises Key

1. A. Because stress incontinence results from weak pelvic muscles and other structures, limiting fluids will not resolve the problem.

   B. **CORRECT:** Caffeine is a bladder irritant and can worsen stress incontinence.

   C. Calcium has no effect on stress incontinence.

   D. **CORRECT:** Alcohol is a bladder irritant and can worsen stress incontinence.

   E. The Credé maneuver helps manage reflex incontinence, not stress incontinence.

   Ⓝ *NCLEX® Connection: Basic Care and Comfort, Elimination*

2. A. **CORRECT:** A clogged or kinked catheter causes the bladder to fill and stimulates the need to urinate.

   B. Reassuring the client that it is not possible to urinate is a nontherapeutic response because it dismisses the client's concern.

   C. There are less invasive approaches the nurse can try before replacing the catheter.

   D. Although it might become necessary to collect a urine specimen, there is a simpler approach the nurse can take to assess and possibly resolve the client's problem.

   Ⓝ *NCLEX® Connection: Reduction of Risk Potential, Potential for Complications of Diagnostic Tests/Treatments/Procedures*

3. A. **CORRECT:** The nurse should discard the first voiding of the 24-hr urine specimen, and note the time.

   B. The nurse should keep the urine in a refrigerated container.

   C. For a urinalysis, the nurse should ask the client to urinate and pour the urine into a specimen container.

   D. For a culture specimen, the nurse should ask the client to urinate first into the toilet, then stop midstream, and finish urinating in the specimen container.

   Ⓝ *NCLEX® Connection: Reduction of Risk Potential, Diagnostic Tests*

4. A. **CORRECT:** Having frequent sexual intercourse increases the risk of UTIs in both men and women.

   B. The decrease in estrogen levels during menopause increases a woman's susceptibility to UTIs.

   C. Wiping from front to back decreases a woman's risk of UTIs.

   D. **CORRECT:** The close proximity of the female urethra to the anus is a factor that increases the risk of UTIs.

   E. **CORRECT:** Frequent catheterization and the use of indwelling catheters are risk factors for UTIs.

   Ⓝ *NCLEX® Connection: Reduction of Risk Potential, Potential for Complications of Diagnostic Tests/Treatments/Procedures*

5. A. Bladder training involves voiding at scheduled frequent intervals and gradually increasing these intervals to 4 hr. Meal times are not regular, and the intervals can be longer than every 4 hr.

   B. **CORRECT:** The nurse should ask the client to keep track of urination times as a record of progress toward the goal of 4-hr intervals between urination.

   C. **CORRECT:** Gradually increasing the urination intervals helps the client progress toward the goal of 4-hr intervals between urination.

   D. **CORRECT:** The nurse should remind the client to hold urine until the next scheduled urination time as part of progressing toward the goal of 4-hr intervals between urination.

   E. A bladder-retraining program does not involve collecting sterile urine specimens.

   Ⓝ *NCLEX® Connection: Reduction of Risk Potential, Potential for Complications of Diagnostic Tests/Treatments/Procedures*

PRACTICE Answer

Using the ATI Active Learning Template: System Disorder

ALTERATION IN HEALTH (DIAGNOSIS)

- Stress: The loss of small amounts of urine from increased abdominal pressure without bladder muscle contraction with laughing, sneezing, or lifting
- Urge: The inability to stop urine flow long enough to reach the bathroom due to an overactive detrusor muscle with increased bladder pressure
- Overflow: Urinary retention from bladder overdistention and frequent loss of small amounts of urine due to obstruction of the urinary outlet or an impaired detrusor muscle
- Reflex: The involuntary loss of a moderate amount of urine usually without warning due to hyperreflexia of the detrusor muscle, usually from spinal cord dysfunction
- Functional: The loss of urine due to factors that interfere with responding to the need to urinate, such as cognitive, mobility, and environmental barriers
- Total: The unpredictable, involuntary loss of urine that does not generally respond to treatment

Ⓝ *NCLEX® Connection: Physiological Adaptation, Pathophysiology*

RISK FACTORS

- Female gender
- History of multiple pregnancies and vaginal births, aging, chronic urinary retention, urinary bladder spasm, renal disease, chronic bladder infection
- Neurological disorders: Parkinson's disease, cerebrovascular accident, spinal cord injury, multiple sclerosis
- Medications: diuretics, opioids, anticholinergics, calcium channel blockers, sedative/hypnotics, adrenergic antagonists
- Obesity
- Confusion, dementia, immobility, depression
- Physiological changes of aging
- Decreased estrogen levels, decreased pelvic-muscle tone
- Immobility, chronic degenerative diseases, dementia, diabetes mellitus, cerebrovascular accident
- Urinary incontinence increasing the risk for falls, fractures, pressure ulcers, and depression

CHAPTER 45 *Sensory Perception*

Sensory perception is the ability to receive and interpret sensory impressions through sight (visual), hearing (auditory), touch (tactile), smell (olfactory), taste (gustatory), and movement or position (kinesthetic). Sensory input affects consciousness, arousal, awareness, memory, affect, judgment, awareness of reality, and language.

A sensory deficit is a change in reception and/or perception. Deficits can affect any of the senses. When a sensory deficit develops gradually, the body often compensates for the deficit.

Sensory deprivation is reduced sensory input from the internal or external environment. It can result from illness, trauma, or isolation. Manifestations of sensory deprivation can be cognitive (decreased ability to learn, disorientation), affective (restlessness, anxiousness), or perceptual (decreased coordination, decreased color perception).

Sensory overload is excessive, sustained, and unmanageable multisensory stimulation. Manifestations are similar to those of sensory deprivation and include racing thoughts, anxiousness, and restlessness.

CONTRIBUTING FACTORS

Vision loss: Presbyopia, cataracts, glaucoma, diabetic retinopathy, macular degeneration, infection, inflammation, injury, brain tumor

Conductive hearing loss: Obstruction, wax accumulation, tympanic membrane perforation, ear infections, otosclerosis Qᴇʙᴘ

Sensorineural hearing loss: Exposure to loud noises, ototoxic medications, aging, acoustic neuroma

PATIENT-CENTERED CARE

NURSING CARE

- Check for communication deficits, and adjust care accordingly.
- Collect equipment necessary to care for any assistive devices clients have (corrective lenses, hearing aids). Make sure these devices are available for use.
- Make every effort to communicate with clients who have sensoriperceptual losses because they tend to withdraw from interactions with others.

NURSING CONSIDERATIONS
EQUIPMENT
- Assistive devices
- Orientation tools (clocks, calendars)
- Radio, television, CD/DVD player, digital audio player
- Large-print materials

NURSING CONSIDERATIONS
- Keep clients safe and free from injury. Qs
  - Make sure the call light is easily accessible.
  - Orient clients to the room.
  - Keep furniture clear from the path to the bathroom.
  - Keep personal items within reach.
  - Place the bed in its lowest position.
  - Make sure IV poles, drainage tubes, and bags are easy to maneuver.
- Learn clients' preferred method of communication, and make accommodations.
- FOR CLIENTS WHO HAVE HEARING LOSS
  - Sit and face the clients.
  - Avoid covering your mouth while speaking.
  - Encourage the use of hearing devices.
  - Speak slowly and clearly.
  - Do not shout.
  - Try lowering vocal pitch before increasing volume.
  - Use brief sentences with simple words.
  - Write down what clients do not understand.
  - Minimize background noise.
  - Ask for a sign-language interpreter if necessary.
  - Do not shout. Qᴘᴄᴄ
- FOR CLIENTS WHO HAVE VISION LOSS
  - Call clients by name before approaching to avoid startling them.
  - Identify yourself.
  - Stay within clients' visual field if they have a partial loss.
  - Give specific information about the location of items or areas of the building.
  - Explain interventions before touching clients.
  - Before leaving, inform clients of your departure.
  - Carefully appraise clients' clothing, and suggest changes if soiled or torn.
  - Make a radio, television, CD player, or digital audio player available.
  - Describe the arrangement of the food on the tray before leaving the room.

- FOR CLIENTS WHO HAVE APHASIA
  - Greet clients, and call them by name.
  - Make sure only one person speaks at a time.
  - Speak clearly and slowly using short sentences and simple words.
  - Do not shout. Qpcc
  - Pause between statements to allow time for clients to understand.
  - Check for comprehension.
  - Tell clients when you do not understand them.
  - Ask questions that require simple answers.
  - Reinforce verbal with nonverbal communication (gestures, body language).
  - Allow plenty of time for clients to respond.
  - Use methods speech therapists implement, such as a picture chart, to improve communication.
  - Acknowledge any frustration in communicating.
- FOR CLIENTS WHO ARE DISORIENTED
  - Call clients by name, and identify yourself.
  - Maintain eye contact at eye level.
  - Use brief, simple sentences.
  - Ask only one question at a time.
  - Allow plenty of time for clients to respond.
  - Give directions one step at a time.
  - Avoid lengthy conversations.
  - Provide for adequate sleep and pain management.
- Encourage clients to verbalize feelings about sensoriperceptual loss.
- Orient clients to time, person, place, and situation.
  - Keep a clock in the room.
  - Post a calendar, or write the date where it is visible.
- Provide and use assistive devices.
- Provide care clients cannot perform (reading menus, opening containers).

INTERPROFESSIONAL CARE

- Determine which assistive devices clients need, and plan for their procurement.
- Consult with rehabilitation therapists for restorative potential.
- Refer clients to community-based support groups and organizations for additional resources.

COMPLICATIONS

Risk for injury in the home environment Qs

Teach ways to reduce hazards at home.

VISUAL
- Remove throw rugs to prevent tripping hazards.
- Keep walking pathways clear.
- Ensure that stairways are well lit with secure handrails.

AUDITORY: Use flashing lights vs. a warning sound for alarms and doorbells.

OLFACTORY: Make sure smoke and carbon monoxide detectors are functioning to sense odors and odorless gases (burning food, natural gas, carbon monoxide).

GUSTATORY: Read expiration dates on food packages to avoid consuming contaminated or spoiled food products.

TACTILE: Protect and inspect body parts that lack sensation (burns, pressure ulcers, frostbite). Avoid the use of hot water bottles; label faucets "hot" and "cold" with words or colors; and set hot water heaters to avoid excessively hot water. Sources vary, but an upper limit of 48.8° C (120° F) is generally acceptable.

Sensory deprivation and overload

Minimize overall stimuli and provide meaningful stimulation.
- Provide a private room.
- Minimize glare.
- Manage pain effectively.
- Allow for adequate sleep and rest periods.
- Provide large-print materials or electronic players for audio books.
- Amplify phones.
- Season foods.
- Reduce unpleasant odors.
- Provide pleasant aromas.
- Increase touch (if acceptable) with back rubs, hand holding, range-of-motion exercises, and hair care.
- Organize care to minimize the activity surrounding the bed when possible.

Vision loss

- Visual acuity is the degree of detail clients can perceive in an image.
- Reduced visual acuity can be unilateral (one eye) or bilateral (both eyes).

HEALTH PROMOTION AND DISEASE PREVENTION

- Advise clients to wear sunglasses while outside and protective eyewear while working in areas and at tasks with a risk for eye injury. Q PCC
- Instruct clients to avoid rubbing eyes.
- Tell clients to get an eye examination regularly, especially after age 40.

ASSESSMENT/DATA COLLECTION

RISK FACTORS

- Age is the most significant risk factor for visual sensory alterations. C
- Eye infection, inflammation, or injury
- Brain tumor

Presbyopia: Age-related loss of the eye's ability to focus on close objects due to decreased elasticity of the lens

Cataracts: Opacity of the lens, which blocks the entry of light rays into the eye

Glaucoma: Structural damage within the eye resulting from elevated pressure within the eye leading to blindness

Diabetic retinopathy: Noninflammatory changes in the eye's blood vessels leading to blindness

Macular degeneration: Loss of central vision from deterioration of the center of the retina

EXPECTED FINDINGS

- Frequent headaches
- Frequent eye strain
- Blurred vision
- Poor judgment of depth
- Diplopia: double vision
- Tendency to close or favor one eye
- Poor hand–eye coordination

DIAGNOSTIC PROCEDURES

Ophthalmoscopy: Allows visualization of the back part of the eyeball (fundus), including the retina, optic disc, macula, and blood vessels

Visual acuity tests: Snellen and Rosenbaum eye charts

Tonometry: Measures intraocular pressure (expected range 10 to 21 mm Hg), which is elevated with glaucoma, especially angle-closure glaucoma

Gonioscopy: Allows visualization of the iridocorneal angle or anterior chamber of the eyes

Slit lamp examination: Allows visualization of the anterior portion of the eye, such as the cornea, anterior chamber, and lens

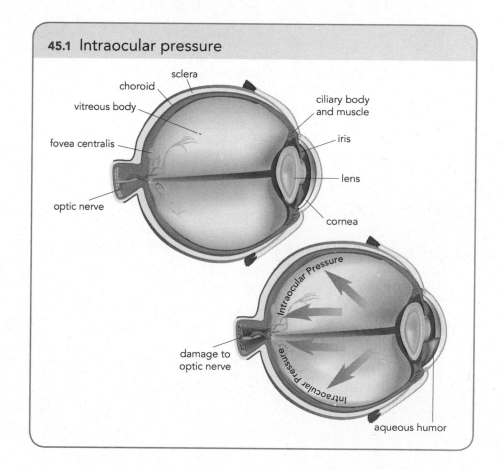

45.1 Intraocular pressure

PATIENT-CENTERED CARE

NURSING CARE

- Monitor the following.
  - Visual acuity using Snellen and Rosenbaum eye charts.
    - Both measure distance vision.
    - The Snellen method has clients stand 20 ft away.
    - The Rosenbaum method has clients hold the chart 14 inches away from their eyes.
  - External and internal eye structures (ophthalmoscope)
  - Functional ability
- Assess how clients adapt to the environment to maintain safety.
  - Increase the amount of light in a room.
  - Arrange the home to remove hazards, such as eliminating throw rugs. Qs
  - Use phones with large numbers and auto dial.
- Suggest adaptive devices that accommodate for reduced vision.
  - Magnifying lens and large-print books and newspapers
  - Talking devices, such as clocks and watches

MEDICATIONS

Anticholinergics

Anticholinergics, such as atropine ophthalmic solution, provide mydriasis (dilation of the pupil) and cycloplegia (ciliary paralysis) for examinations and surgery.

CLIENT EDUCATION: Adverse effects include reduced accommodation, blurred vision, and photophobia. With systemic absorption, there could be anticholinergic effects (tachycardia, decreased secretions).

CLIENT EDUCATION

- Wash hands before and after instilling eye medication.
- Quit smoking.
- Limit alcohol intake.
- Keep blood pressure, blood glucose, and cholesterol under control.
- Eat foods rich in antioxidants, such as green leafy vegetables.

CARE AFTER DISCHARGE: Initiate referrals to social services, support groups, and reduced-vision resources.

COMPLICATIONS

Risk for injury

Reduced vision increases injury risk, especially for older adults. ©

NURSING ACTIONS: Monitor for safety risks, such as the ability to drive safely, and intervene to reduce risks.

Hearing loss

Hearing loss is difficulty in hearing or interpreting speech and other sounds due to a problem in the middle or inner ear.

Conductive hearing loss is an alteration in the middle ear that blocks sound waves before they reach the cochlea of the inner ear.

Sensorineural hearing loss is an alteration in the inner ear, auditory nerve, or hearing center of the brain.

Mixed hearing loss is a combination of conductive and sensorineural hearing loss.

HEALTH PROMOTION AND DISEASE PREVENTION

- Advise clients not to place any objects in the ear, including cotton-tipped swabs.
- Tell clients to have an otologist remove any object lodged in the ear. Use a commercial ceruminolytic (ear drops that soften cerumen) for impactions, and follow with warm-water irrigation.
- Instruct clients to wear ear protection during exposure to high-intensity noise and risk for ear trauma. Qs
- Tell clients to blow the nose gently and with both nostrils unobstructed.
- Advise clients to keep the volume as low as possible when wearing headphones.

ASSESSMENT/DATA COLLECTION

RISK FACTORS

- Advancing age ©
- Use of ototoxic medications (aminoglycosides, monobactams)

Conductive hearing loss

- History of middle ear infections
- Older age (otosclerosis)

Sensorineural hearing loss

- Prolonged exposure to loud noises
- Ototoxic medications
- Infectious processes
- Older age (presbycusis: decreased ability to hear high-pitched sounds)

EXPECTED FINDINGS

Conductive hearing loss

- Hears better in a noisy environment
- Speaks softly
- Obstruction in external canal (packed cerumen)
- Tympanic membrane findings (holes, scarring)
- Rinne test that demonstrates air conduction of sound less than or equal to bone conduction (AC ≤ BC)
- Weber test that lateralizes to the affected ear

Sensorineural hearing loss

- Tinnitus (ringing, roaring, humming in ears)
- Dizziness
- Hears poorly in a noisy environment
- Speaks loudly
- No otoscopic findings
- Rinne test that demonstrates expected response of air conduction being greater than bone conduction (AC > BC), but with length of time decreased for both
- Weber test lateralizing to unaffected ear
- Diagnosis of acoustic neuroma (benign tumor cranial nerve VIII)

DIAGNOSTIC PROCEDURES

Audiometry

An audiogram identifies whether hearing loss is sensorineural and/or conductive.

NURSING CONSIDERATIONS

- Use audiometry when screening for hearing loss in a school or older adult setting (after specific training to perform this procedure). Results are more accurate in a quiet room.
- Assess clients' ability to hear various frequencies (high vs. low pitch) at various decibels (soft vs. loud tones).
- Have clients wear audiometer headphones and face away from the examiner.
- Have clients indicate when they hear a tone and in which ear by raising their hand on the corresponding side. Comparing the responses on a graph with expected age and other norms yields information about the type and degree of hearing loss.

Tympanogram Q_PCC

A tympanogram measures the mobility of the tympanic membrane and middle ear structures relative to sound to diagnose disorders of the middle ear.

Otoscopy

An otoscope allows visualization of the external auditory canal, the tympanic membrane (TM), and malleus bone visible through the TM.

NURSING CONSIDERATIONS

- Perform an otoscopic examination when audiometry results indicate a possible impairment or for ear pain.
- Select a speculum according to the size of the ear, then attach it and insert the otoscope into the external ear.
- If the ear canal curves, pull up and back on the auricle of adults and down and back on the auricle of children younger than 3 years to straighten out the canal and enhance visualization.
- The tympanic membrane should be pearly gray and intact. It should provide complete structural separation of the outer and middle ear structures.
- The light reflex should be visible from the center of the TM anteriorly (5 o'clock right ear; 7 o'clock left ear).
- With fluid or infection in the middle ear, the tympanic membrane will become inflamed and can bulge from the pressure of the exudate. This also will displace the light reflex, a significant finding.
- Avoid touching the lining of the ear canal, which causes pain due to sensitivity.

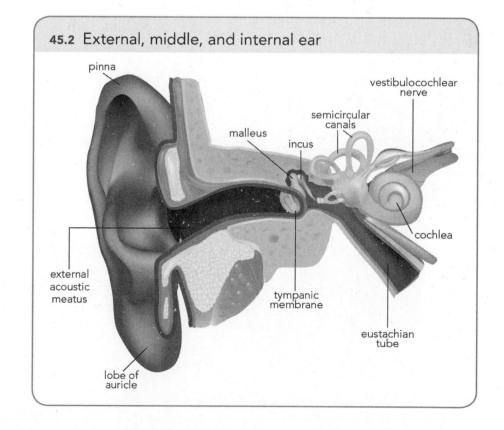

45.2 External, middle, and internal ear

pinna

vestibulocochlear nerve

semicircular canals

malleus

incus

cochlea

external acoustic meatus

tympanic membrane

eustachian tube

lobe of auricle

PATIENT-CENTERED CARE

NURSING CARE

- Monitor functional ability.
- Check the hearing of clients receiving ototoxic medications for more than 5 days. Reduced renal function that occurs with aging increases the risk for ototoxicity.

Ototoxic medications

- Antibiotics: gentamicin, metronidazole
- Diuretics: furosemide
- NSAIDs: aspirin, ibuprofen
- Chemotherapeutic agents: cisplatin

Communication

- Get clients' attention before speaking.
- Stand or sit facing clients in a well-lit, quiet room without distractions.
- Speak clearly and slowly without shouting and without hands or other objects covering the mouth.
- Arrange for communication assistance (sign-language interpreter, closed-captions, phone amplifiers, teletypewriter [TTY] capabilities).

INTERPROFESSIONAL CARE

Refer clients who have audiometry findings to an audiologist for more sensitive testing.

THERAPEUTIC PROCEDURES

Hearing aids

- Hearing aids amplify sounds, but do not help clients interpret what they hear.
- Amplification of sound in a loud environment can be distracting and disturbing.

CLIENT EDUCATION

- Use the lowest setting that allows hearing without feedback.
- To clean the ear mold, use mild soap and water while keeping the hearing aid dry.
- When the hearing aid is not in use for an extended period of time, turn it off and remove the battery to conserve battery power and avoid corrosion of the hearing aid. Keep replacement batteries on hand. Qpcc

Tympanoplasty and myringoplasty

For conductive hearing loss
- Tympanoplasty is a surgical reconstruction of the middle ear structures
- Myringoplasty is an eardrum repair.

NURSING ACTIONS

- Place sterile ear packing postoperatively.
- Position clients flat with the operative ear facing up for 12 hr.

CLIENT EDUCATION

- Tell clients to avoid air travel and forceful straining, coughing, or sneezing with the mouth closed.
- Teach clients to cover the ear with a dressing before washing hair and not to allow water to enter the ear.
- Remind clients that they will hear less while packing is in the ear.

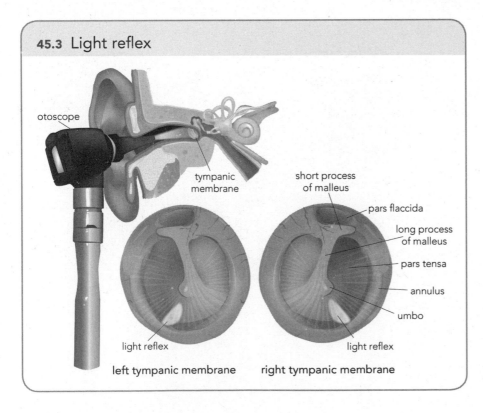

45.3 Light reflex

otoscope

tympanic membrane

short process of malleus

pars flaccida

long process of malleus

pars tensa

annulus

umbo

light reflex

light reflex

left tympanic membrane

right tympanic membrane

Application Exercises

1. A nurse is caring for a client who recently had a cerebrovascular accident and has aphasia. Which of the following interventions should the nurse use to promote communication with this client? (Select all that apply.)

   A. Increase the volume of your voice.

   B. Make sure only one person speaks at a time.

   C. Avoid discouraging the client by saying that you do not understand him.

   D. Allow plenty of time for the client to respond.

   E. Use brief sentences with simple words.

2. A nurse is caring for a client who had an amphetamine overdose and has sensory overload. Which of the following interventions should the nurse implement?

   A. Immediately complete a thorough assessment.

   B. Put the client in a room with a client who has a hearing loss.

   C. Provide a private room, and limit stimulation.

   D. Speak at a higher volume to the client, and encourage ambulation.

3. A nurse is caring for a client who reports difficulty hearing. Which of the following assessment findings indicate a sensorineural hearing loss in the left ear? (Select all that apply.)

   A. Weber test showing lateralization to the right ear

   B. Light reflex at 10 o'clock in the left ear

   C. Indications of obstruction in the left ear canal

   D. Rinne test showing less time for air and bone conduction

   E. Rinne test showing air conduction less than bone conduction in the left ear

4. A nurse is caring for a client who has several risk factors for hearing loss. Which of the following medications, that the client currently takes, should alert the nurse to a further risk for ototoxicity? (Select all that apply.)

   A. Furosemide

   B. Ibuprofen

   C. Cimetidine

   D. Simvastatin

   E. Amiodarone

5. A nurse is reviewing instructions with a client who has a hearing loss and has just started wearing hearing aids. Which of the following statements should the nurse identify as an indication that the client understands the instructions?

   A. "I use a damp cloth to clean the outside part of my hearing aids."

   B. "I clean the ear molds of my hearing aids with rubbing alcohol."

   C. "I keep the volume of my hearing aids turned up so I can hear better."

   D. "I take the batteries out of my hearing aids when I take them off at night."

PRACTICE Active Learning Scenario

A nurse is teaching a group of nursing students how to intervene for clients who have sensory impairment. Use the ATI Active Learning Template: System Disorder to complete this item.

NURSING CARE
- List at least six interventions for clients who have hearing loss.
- List at least six interventions for clients who have vision loss.

Application Exercises Key

1. A. The nurse should speak in a normal tone of voice to a client who had a stroke and has aphasia to promote communication.

   B. **CORRECT:** Trying to understand more than one voice at a time is challenging.

   C. Feigning understanding shows a lack of respect for the client's needs and blocks further communication.

   D. **CORRECT:** Allowing ample time for the client to respond helps enhance communication. Rushing ahead to the next question would be demeaning and could cause frustration.

   E. **CORRECT:** Brief sentences with simple words are generally easiest to understand.

   Ⓝ *NCLEX® Connection: Psychosocial Integrity, Therapeutic Communication*

2. A. Immediately completing a thorough assessment might overwhelm the client at this time. Brief assessments throughout the shift are better.

   B. Rooming with a client who has a hearing loss would increase environmental stimuli.

   C. **CORRECT:** Minimizing stimuli helps clients who have sensory overload.

   D. Talking at a higher volume would increase environmental stimuli.

   Ⓝ *NCLEX® Connection: Basic Care and Comfort, Assistive Devices*

3. A. **CORRECT:** With sensorineural hearing loss, the Weber test demonstrates lateralization to the unaffected ear.

   B. A light reflex at 10 o'clock in the left ear indicates that air or fluid has displaced the tympanic membrane, but it does not indicate sensorineural hearing loss.

   C. Indications of obstruction in the ear canal would indicate conductive hearing loss.

   D. **CORRECT:** With sensorineural hearing loss in the left ear, length of time is decreased for both air and bone conduction.

   E. With sensorineural hearing loss in the left ear, air conduction is greater than bone conduction in the left ear.

   Ⓝ *NCLEX® Connection: Safety and Infection Control, Accident/Error/Injury Prevention*

4. A. **CORRECT:** Furosemide, a loop diuretic, can cause hearing loss as well as blurred vision.

   B. **CORRECT:** Ibuprofen, a nonsteroidal anti-inflammatory agent, can cause hearing loss as well as vision loss.

   C. Cimetidine, a medication that decreases gastric acid secretion, is unlikely to cause hearing loss.

   D. Simvastatin, a medication that helps lower cholesterol, is unlikely to cause hearing loss.

   E. Amiodarone, an antidysrhythmic medication, is more likely to cause blurred vision than hearing loss.

   Ⓝ *NCLEX® Connection: Reduction of Risk Potential, System Specific Assessments*

5. A. The client should keep the hearing aids completely dry at all times.

   B. The client should clean the ear molds with mild soap and water.

   C. To avoid feedback, the client should keep the volume on the lowest setting that allows her to hear.

   D. **CORRECT:** To conserve battery power, the client should turn off the hearing aids and remove the batteries when not in use.

   Ⓝ *NCLEX® Connection: Psychosocial Integrity, Sensory/Perceptual Alterations*

PRACTICE Answer

Using the ATI Active Learning Template: System Disorder

NURSING CARE

Hearing loss
- Sit and face the client.
- Avoid covering your mouth while speaking.
- Encourage the use of hearing devices.
- Speak slowly and clearly.
- Do not shout.
- Try lowering vocal pitch before increasing volume.
- Use brief sentences with simple words.
- Write down what clients do not understand.
- Minimize background noises.
- Ask for a sign-language interpreter if necessary.

Vision loss
- Call clients by name before approaching to avoid startling them.
- Identify yourself.
- Stay within the clients' visual field if they have a partial loss.
- Give specific information about the location of items or areas of the building.
- Explain interventions before touching clients.
- Before leaving, inform clients of your departure.
- Carefully appraise clothing and suggest changes if soiled or torn.
- Make a radio, television, CD player, or digital audio player available.
- Describe the arrangement of the food on the tray before leaving the room.

Ⓝ *NCLEX® Connection: Psychosocial Integrity, Sensory/Perceptual Alterations*

ⓝ NCLEX® Connections

When reviewing the following chapters, keep in mind the relevant topics and tasks of the NCLEX outline, in particular:

Client Needs: Management of Care

CLIENT RIGHTS: Recognize the client's right to refuse treatment/procedures.

CONTINUITY OF CARE: Use approved abbreviations and standard terminology when documenting care.

Client Needs: Safety and Infection Control

ACCIDENT/ERROR/INJURY PREVENTION: Ensure proper identification of client when providing care.

Client Needs: Pharmacological and Parenteral Therapies

DOSAGE CALCULATION: Perform calculations needed for medication administration.

EXPECTED ACTIONS/OUTCOMES: Obtain information on a client's prescribed medications.

MEDICATION ADMINISTRATION: Prepare and administer medications, using rights of medication administration.

CHAPTER 46 *Pharmacokinetics and Routes of Administration*

Pharmacokinetics refers to how medications travel through the body. Medications undergo a variety of biochemical processes that result in absorption, distribution, metabolism, and excretion.

PHASES OF PHARMACOKINETICS

Absorption

The transmission of medications from the location of administration (gastrointestinal [GI] tract, muscle, skin, or subcutaneous tissue) to the bloodstream. The most common routes of administration are enteral (through the GI tract) and parenteral (by injection). Each of these routes has a unique pattern of absorption.
- The rate of medication absorption determines how soon the medication takes effect.
- The amount of medication the body absorbs determines its intensity.
- The route of administration affects the rate and amount of absorption.

Route: Oral
- BARRIERS TO ABSORPTION: Medications must pass through the layer of epithelial cells that line the GI tract.
- ABSORPTION PATTERN varies greatly due to
  - Stability and solubility of the medication
  - Gastrointestinal pH and emptying time
  - Presence of food in the stomach or intestines
  - Concurrent medications
  - Forms of medications (enteric-coated pills, liquids)

Route: Subcutaneous and intramuscular
- BARRIERS TO ABSORPTION: The capillary walls have large spaces between cells. Therefore, there is no significant barrier.
- ABSORPTION PATTERN factors determining the rate of absorption
  - Solubility of the medication in water
    - Highly soluble medications have rapid absorption (10 to 30 min).
    - Poorly soluble medications have slow absorption.
  - Blood perfusion at the site of injection
    - Sites with high blood perfusion have rapid absorption.
    - Sites with low blood perfusion have slow absorption.

Route: Intravenous
- BARRIERS TO ABSORPTION: No barriers
- ABSORPTION PATTERN
  - Immediate: enters directly into the blood
  - Complete: reaches the blood in its entirety

Distribution

The transportation of medications to sites of action by bodily fluids.

FACTORS INFLUENCING DISTRIBUTION
- **Circulation:** Conditions that inhibit blood flow or perfusion, such as peripheral vascular or cardiac disease, can delay medication distribution.
- **Permeability of the cell membrane:** The medication must be able to pass through tissues and membranes to reach its target area. Medications that are lipid-soluble or have a transport system can cross the blood–brain barrier and the placenta.
- **Plasma protein binding:** Medications compete for protein binding sites within the bloodstream, primarily albumin. The ability of a medication to bind to a protein can affect how much of the medication will leave and travel to target tissues. Two medications can compete for the same binding sites, resulting in toxicity.

Metabolism (biotransformation)

Changes medications into less active forms or inactive forms by the action of enzymes. This occurs primarily in the liver, but also takes place in the kidneys, lungs, intestines, and blood.

FACTORS INFLUENCING MEDICATION METABOLISM RATE
- **Age:** Infants have a limited medication-metabolizing capacity. The aging process also can influence medication metabolism, but varies with the individual. In general, hepatic medication metabolism tends to decline with age. Older adults require smaller doses of medications due to the possibility of accumulation in the body. ©
- **An increase in some medication-metabolizing enzymes:** This can metabolize a particular medication sooner, requiring an increase in dosage of that medication to maintain a therapeutic level. It can also cause an increase in the metabolism of other concurrent-use medications.
- **First-pass effect:** The liver inactivates some medications on their first pass through the liver. Thus, they require a nonenteral route (sublingual, IV) because of their high first-pass effect.
- **Similar metabolic pathways:** When the same pathway metabolizes two medications, it can alter the metabolism of one or both of them. In this way, the rate of metabolism can decrease for one or both of the medications, leading to medication accumulation.
- **Nutritional status:** Clients who are malnourished can be deficient in the factors that are necessary to produce specific medication-metabolizing enzymes, thus impairing medication metabolism.

Excretion

The elimination of medications from the body, primarily through the kidneys. Elimination also takes place through the liver, lungs, intestines, and exocrine glands (such as in breast milk). Kidney dysfunction can lead to an increase in the duration and intensity of a medication's response.

MEDICATION RESPONSES

- Medication dosing attempts to regulate medication responses to maintain plasma levels between the minimum effective concentration (MEC) and the toxic concentration.
- A plasma medication level is in the therapeutic range when it is effective and not toxic. Nurses use therapeutic levels of many medications to monitor clients' responses.

THERAPEUTIC INDEX (TI)

Medications with a high TI have a wide safety margin; therefore, there is no need for routine serum medication-level monitoring. Medications with a low TI require close monitoring of serum medication levels. Nurses should consider the route of administration when monitoring for peak levels (highest plasma level when elimination = absorption).

- For example, an oral medication can peak from 1 to 3 hr after administration.
- If the route is IV, the peak time might occur within 10 min.
- Refer to a medication reference or a pharmacist for specific medication peak times.
- For trough levels, obtain a blood sample immediately before the next medication dose, regardless of the route of administration.
- A plateau is a medication concentration in plasma during a series of doses.

HALF-LIFE (t$_{1/2}$)

The time for the medication in the body to drop by 50%. Liver and kidney function affect half-life. It usually takes four half-lives to achieve a steady state of serum concentration (medication intake = medication metabolism and excretion).

Short half-life	Long half-life
Medications leave the body quickly: 4 to 8 hr.	Medications leave the body more slowly: over more than 24 hr, with a greater risk for medication accumulation and toxicity.
Short-dosing interval or MEC drops between doses.	Can give medications at longer intervals without a loss of therapeutic effects.
	Medications take a longer time to reach a steady state.

PHARMACODYNAMICS (MECHANISM OF ACTION)

The interactions between medications and target cells, body systems, and organs to produce effects. These interactions result in functional changes that are the mechanism of action of the medication. Qs

Agonist: Medication that can mimic the receptor activity that endogenous compounds regulate. For example, morphine is an agonist because it activates the receptors that produce analgesia, sedation, constipation, and other effects. (Receptors are the medication's target sites on or within the cells.)

Antagonist: Medication that can block the usual receptor activity that endogenous compounds regulate or the receptor activity of other medications. For example, losartan, an angiotensin II receptor blocker, is an antagonist. It works by blocking angiotensin II receptors on blood vessels, which prevents vasoconstriction.

Partial agonists: Medication that acts as an agonist and an antagonist, with limited affinity to receptor sites. For example, nalbuphine acts as an antagonist at mu receptors and an agonist at kappa receptors, causing analgesia at low doses with minimal respiratory depression.

ROUTES OF ADMINISTRATION

Oral or enteral

Tablets, capsules, liquids, suspensions, elixirs, lozenges
- Most common route
- Least expensive
- Convenient

NURSING CONSIDERATIONS
- Contraindications for oral medication administration include vomiting, decreased GI motility, absence of a gag reflex, difficulty swallowing, and a decreased level of consciousness.
- Have clients sit upright at a 90° angle to facilitate swallowing. Qs
- Administer irritating medications, such as analgesics, with small amounts of food.
- Do not mix with large amounts of food or beverages in case clients cannot consume the entire quantity.
- Avoid administration with interacting foods or beverages such as grapefruit juice.
- In general, administer oral medications on an empty stomach (30 min to 1 hr before meals, 2 hr after meals).
- Follow the manufacturer's directions for crushing, cutting, and diluting medications. Break or cut scored tablets only.
- Make sure clients swallow enteric-coated or time-release medications whole.
- Use a liquid form of the medication to facilitate swallowing whenever possible.

Sublingual and buccal

Directly enters the bloodstream and bypasses the liver
• Sublingual: under the tongue
• Buccal: between the cheek and the gum

NURSING CONSIDERATIONS
• Instruct clients to keep the medication in place until complete absorption occurs.
• Clients should not eat or drink while the tablet is in place or until it has completely dissolved.

Liquids, suspensions, and elixirs

NURSING CONSIDERATIONS
• Follow directions for dilution and shaking.
• When administering the medication, pour it into a cup on flat surface. Make sure the base of the meniscus (lowest fluid line) is at the level of the dose. Q EBP

Transdermal

Medication in a skin patch for absorption through the skin, producing systemic effects

CLIENT EDUCATION
• Apply patches as prescribed to ensure proper dosing.
• Wash the skin with soap and water, and dry it thoroughly before applying a new patch.
• Place the patch on a hairless area and rotate sites to prevent skin irritation.

Topical

• Painless
• Limited adverse effects

NURSING CONSIDERATIONS
• Apply with a glove, tongue blade, or cotton-tipped applicator.
• Do not apply with a bare hand.

Instillation (drops, ointments, sprays)

Generally used for eyes, ears, and nose

Eyes
NURSING CONSIDERATIONS
• Use medical aseptic technique when instilling medications in eyes.
• Have clients sit upright or lie supine, tilt their head slightly, and look up at the ceiling.
• Rest your dominant hand on the clients' forehead, hold the dropper above the conjunctival sac about 1 to 2 cm, drop the medication into the center of the sac, avoid placing it directly on the cornea, and have them close the eye gently. If they blink during installation, repeat the procedure.
• Apply gentle pressure with your finger and a clean facial tissue on the nasolacrimal duct for 30 to 60 seconds to prevent systemic absorption of the medication. Qs
• If instilling more than one medication in the same eye, wait at least 5 minutes between them.
• For eye ointment, apply a thin ribbon to the edge of the lower eyelid from the inner to the outer canthus.

Ears
NURSING CONSIDERATIONS
• Use medical aseptic technique when administering medications into the ears.
• Have clients sit upright or lie on their side.
• Straighten the ear canal by pulling the auricle upward and outward for adults or down and back for children. Hold the dropper 1 cm above the ear canal, instill the medication, and then gently apply pressure with your finger to the tragus of the ear unless it is too painful.
• Do not press a cotton ball deep into the ear canal. If necessary, gently place it into the outermost part of the ear canal.
• Have clients remain in the side-lying position if possible for 2 to 3 min after installation of ear drops.

Nose
NURSING CONSIDERATIONS
• Use medical aseptic technique when administering medications into the nose.
• Have clients lie supine with their head positioned to allow the medication to enter the appropriate nasal passage.
• Use your dominant hand to instill the drops, supporting the head with your nondominant hand.
• Instruct clients to breathe through the mouth, stay in a supine position, and not to blow the nose for 5 min after drop instillation.

Inhalation

Administered through metered-dose inhalers (MDI) or dry-powder inhalers (DPI)

MDI
CLIENT INSTRUCTIONS
• Remove the cap from the inhaler's mouthpiece.
• Shake the inhaler vigorously five or six times.
• Hold the inhaler with the mouthpiece at the bottom.
• Hold the inhaler with your thumb near the mouthpiece and your index and middle fingers at the top.
• Hold the inhaler about 2 to 4 cm (1 to 2 in) away from the front of your mouth or close your mouth around the mouthpiece of the inhaler with the opening pointing toward the back of your throat.
• Take a deep breath, and then exhale.
• Tilt your head back slightly, press the inhaler, and, at the same time, begin a slow, deep inhalation breath. Continue to breathe slowly and deeply for 3 to 5 seconds to facilitate delivery to the air passages.
• Hold your breath for 10 seconds to allow the medication to deposit in your airways.
• Take the inhaler out of your mouth and slowly exhale through pursed lips.
• Resume normal breathing.
• A spacer keeps the medication in the device longer, thereby increasing the amount of medication the device delivers to the lungs and decreasing the amount of medication in the oropharynx. Q EBP
• **For clients who use a spacer**
  ○ Remove the covers from the mouthpieces of the inhaler and of the spacer.
  ○ Insert the MDI into the end of the spacer.
  ○ Shake the inhaler five or six times.
  ○ Exhale completely, and then close your mouth around the spacer's mouthpiece. Continue as with an MDI.

DPI
CLIENT INSTRUCTIONS
- Do not shake the device.
- Take the cover off the mouthpiece.
- Follow the manufacturer's directions for preparing the medication, such as turning the wheel of the inhaler or loading a medication pellet.
- Exhale completely.
- Place the mouthpiece between your lips and take a deep inhalation breath through your mouth.
- Hold your breath for 5 to 10 seconds.
- Take the inhaler out of your mouth and slowly exhale through pursed lips.
- Resume normal breathing.
- Clients who need more than one puff should wait the length of time the provider specifies before self-administering the second puff.
- Instruct clients to rinse their mouth out with water or brush their teeth if using a corticosteroid inhaler to reduce the risk of fungal infections of the mouth. Qs
- Instruct clients to remove the canister and rinse the inhaler, cap, and spacer once a day with warm running water and dry them completely before using the inhaler again.

Nasogastric and gastrostomy tubes

NURSING CONSIDERATIONS
- Verify proper tube placement.
- Use a syringe and allow the medication to flow in by gravity or push it in with the plunger of the syringe.

GENERAL GUIDELINES
- Use liquid forms of medications; if not available, consider crushing medications if appropriate guidelines allow.
- Do not administer sublingual medications.
- Do not crush specially prepared oral medications (extended/time-release, fluid-filled, enteric-coated).
- Administer each medication separately.
- Do not mix medications with enteral feedings.
- Completely dissolve crushed tablets and capsule contents in 15 to 30 mL of sterile water prior to administration.
- To prevent clogging, flush the tubing before and after each medication with 15 to 30 mL water.
- Flush with another 15 to 30 mL sterile water after instilling all the medications.

Suppositories

NURSING CONSIDERATIONS
- Follow the manufacturer's directions for storage.
- Wear gloves for the procedure.
- Remove the wrapper, and lubricate the suppository if necessary.

Rectal suppositories (thin, bullet-shaped medication)
NURSING CONSIDERATIONS
- Position clients in the left lateral or Sims' position.
- Insert the suppository just beyond the internal sphincter.
- Instruct clients to remain flat or in the left lateral position for at least 5 min after insertion to retain the suppository. Absorption times vary with the medication.

Vaginal suppositories
NURSING CONSIDERATIONS
- Position clients supine with their knees bent and their feet flat on the bed and close to their hips (modified lithotomy or dorsal recumbent position).
- Use the applicator, if available.
- Insert the suppository along the posterior wall of the vagina 7.5 to 10 cm (3 to 4 in).
- Instruct clients to remain supine for at least 5 min after insertion to retain the suppository.
- If using an applicator, wash it with soap and water. (If it is disposable, discard it.)

Parenteral

NURSING CONSIDERATIONS
- The vastus lateralis is best for infants 1 year and younger.
- The ventrogluteal site is preferable for IM injections and for injecting volumes exceeding 2 mL. QEBP
- The deltoid site has a smaller muscle mass and can only accommodate up to 1 mL of fluid.
- Use a needle size and length appropriate for the type of injection and the client's size. Syringe size should approximate the volume of medication.
- Use a tuberculin syringe for solution volumes less than 0.5 mL.
- Rotate injection sites to enhance medication absorption, and document each site.
- Do not use injection sites that are edematous, inflamed, or have moles, birthmarks, or scars.
- For IV administration, immediately monitor clients for therapeutic and adverse effects.
- Discard all sharps (broken ampule bottles, needles) in leak- and puncture-proof containers.

Intradermal

NURSING CONSIDERATIONS
- Use for tuberculin testing or checking for medication or allergy sensitivities.
- Use small amounts of solution (0.01 to 0.1 mL) in a tuberculin syringe with a fine-gauge needle (26- to 27-gauge) in lightly pigmented, thin-skinned, hairless sites (the inner surface of the mid-forearm or scapular area of the back) at a 10° to 15° angle.
- Insert the needle with the bevel up. A small bleb should appear.
- Do not massage the site after injection.

Subcutaneous

NURSING CONSIDERATIONS
- Use for small doses of nonirritating, water-soluble medications, such as insulin and heparin.
- Use a 3/8- to 5/8-inch, 25- to 27-gauge needle or a 28- to 31-gauge insulin syringe. Inject no more than 1.5 mL of solution.
- Select sites that have an adequate fat-pad size (abdomen, upper hips, lateral upper arms, thighs).
- For average-size clients, pinch up the skin and inject at a 45° to 90° angle. For clients who are obese, use a 90° angle. QPCC

Intramuscular

NURSING CONSIDERATIONS

- Use for irritating medications, solutions in oils, and aqueous suspensions.
- The most common sites are ventrogluteal, deltoid, and vastus lateralis (pediatric). The dorsogluteal is no longer recommended as a common injection site due to its close proximity to the sciatic nerve.
- Use a needle size 18- to 27-gauge (usually 22- to 25-gauge), 1- to 1.5-inch long, and inject at a 90° angle. Solution volume is usually 1 to 3 mL. Divide larger volumes into two syringes and use two different sites.

Z-track

NURSING CONSIDERATIONS

Use this technique for all IM injections because it is less painful, prevents medication from leaking back into subcutaneous tissue, and prevents skins stains (e.g., iron preparations).

Intravenous

NURSING CONSIDERATIONS

- Use for administering medications, fluid, and blood products.
- Vascular access devices can be for short-term use (catheters) or long-term use (infusion ports).
  - Use 16-gauge devices for clients who have trauma.
  - Use 18-gauge during surgery and blood administration.
  - Use 22- to 24-gauge for children, older adults, and clients who have medical issues or are stable postoperatively.
- Peripheral veins in the arm or hand are preferable. Ask clients which site they prefer. For newborns, use veins in the head, lower legs, and feet. After administration, immediately monitor for therapeutic and adverse effects.

Epidural

NURSING CONSIDERATIONS

- Use for IV opioid analgesia (morphine or fentanyl).
- The clinician advances the catheter through the needle into the epidural space at the level of the fourth or fifth vertebra.
- Use an infusion pump to administer medication.

46.1 Advantages and disadvantages of different routes

	ADVANTAGES	DISADVANTAGES
Oral	Safe Inexpensive Easy and convenient	Oral medications have highly variable absorption. Inactivation can occur by the GI tract or first-pass effect. Clients must be cooperative and conscious. Contraindications include nausea and vomiting.
Subcutaneous and intramuscular (IM)	Use for poorly soluble medications. Use for administering medications that have slow absorption for an extended period of time (depot preparations).	IM injections are more costly. IM injections are inconvenient. There can be pain with the risk for local tissue damage and nerve damage. There is a risk for infection at the injection site.
Intravenous (IV)	Onset is rapid, and absorption into the blood is immediate, which provides an immediate response. This route allows control over the precise amount of medication to administer. It allows for administration of large volumes of fluid. It dilutes irritating medications in free-flowing IV fluid.	IV injections are even more costly. IV injections are inconvenient. Absorption of the medication into the blood is immediate. This is potentially dangerous if giving the wrong dosage or the wrong medication. There is an increased risk for infection or embolism with IV injections. Poor circulation can inhibit the medication's distribution.

Application Exercises

1. A nurse is caring for a client who is 1 day postoperative following a total knee arthroplasty. The client states his pain level is 10 on a scale of 0 to 10. After reviewing the client's medication administration record, which of the following medications should the nurse administer?

   A. Meperidine 75 mg IM

   B. Fentanyl 50 mcg/hr transdermal patch

   C. Morphine 2 mg IV

   D. Oxycodone 10 mg PO

2. A nurse is teaching a client about taking multiple oral medications at home to include time-release capsules, liquid medications, enteric-coated pills, and opioids. Which of the following statements should the nurse identify as an indication that the client understands the instructions?

   A. "I can open the capsule with the beads in it and sprinkle them on my oatmeal."

   B. "If I am having difficulty swallowing, I will add the liquid medication to a batch of pudding."

   C. "I can crush the pills with the coating on them."

   D. "I will eat two crackers with the pain pills."

3. A nurse is teaching a client how to administer medication through a jejunostomy tube. Which of the following instructions should the nurse include?

   A. "Flush the tube before and after each medication."

   B. "Mix your medications with your enteral feeding."

   C. "Push tablets through the tube slowly."

   D. "Mix all the crushed medications prior to dissolving them in water."

4. A nurse is preparing to inject heparin subcutaneously for a client who is postoperative. Which of the following actions should the nurse take?

   A. Use a 22-gauge needle.

   B. Select a site on the client's abdomen.

   C. Spread the skin with the thumb and index finger.

   D. Observe for bleb formation to confirm proper placement.

5. A nurse is teaching an adult client how to administer ear drops. Which of the following statements should the nurse identify as an indication that the client understands the proper technique?

   A. "I will straighten my ear canal by pulling my ear down and back."

   B. "I will gently apply pressure with my finger to the front part of my ear after putting in the drops."

   C. "I will insert the nozzle of the ear drop bottle snug into my ear before squeezing the drops in."

   D. "After the drops are in, I will place a cotton ball all the way into my ear canal."

PRACTICE Active Learning Scenario

A nurse educator is teaching a module on biotransformation as a phase of pharmacokinetics during nursing orientation to a group of newly licensed nurses. Use the ATI Active Learning Template: Basic Concept to complete this item.

RELATED CONTENT: List four areas of the body where biotransformation takes place.

UNDERLYING PRINCIPLES: List at least three factors that influence the rate of biotransformation.

Application Exercises Key

1. A. Although meperidine is a strong analgesic, the IM route of administration can allow for slow absorption, delaying the onset of pain relief. The IM route also can cause additional pain from the injection.

   B. Although fentanyl is a strong analgesic, the transdermal route of administration can allow for slow absorption, delaying the onset of pain relief.

   C. **CORRECT:** The nurse should administer IV morphine because the onset is rapid, and absorption of the medication into the blood is immediate, which provides the optimal response for a client who is reporting pain at a level of 10.

   D. Although oxycodone is a strong analgesic, the oral route of administration of this medication can allow for onset of pain relief in 10 to 15 min, which can be a long time for a client who is reporting pain at a level of 10.

   Ⓝ *NCLEX® Connection: Pharmacological and Parenteral Therapies, Pharmacological Pain Management*

2. A. Although this might help a client who has swallowing issues, it is essential for the client to swallow enteric-coated or time-release medications whole.

   B. Although adding a liquid medication to food is helpful if the client is having difficulty swallowing, he should not mix the medication with large amounts of food or beverages in case he cannot consume the entire quantity.

   C. The client must not crush enteric-coated or time-release preparations. He must swallow them whole.

   D. **CORRECT:** The client should take irritating medications, such as analgesics, with small amounts of food. It can help prevent nausea and vomiting.

   Ⓝ *NCLEX® Connection: Pharmacological and Parenteral Therapies, Pharmacological Pain Management*

3. A. **CORRECT:** The client should flush the tubing before and after each medication with 15 to 30 mL water to prevent clogging of the tube.

   B. To maximize the therapeutic effect of a medication, the client should not mix medications with enteral formula. In addition, if the client does not receive the entire feeding, he does not receive the entire medication. This can also delay the client receiving the medication.

   C. The client should not administer tablets or undissolved medications through a jejunostomy tube because they can clog the tube.

   D. The client should self-administer each medication separately.

   Ⓝ *NCLEX® Connection: Pharmacological and Parenteral Therapies, Medication Administration*

4. A. For a subcutaneous injection, the nurse should use a 25- to 27-gauge needle.

   B. **CORRECT:** For a subcutaneous injection, the nurse should select a site that has an adequate fat-pad size (abdomen, upper hips, lateral upper arms, thighs).

   C. For a subcutaneous injection, the nurse should pinch the skin with her thumb and index finger.

   D. Bleb formation confirms injection into the dermis, not into subcutaneous tissue.

   Ⓝ *NCLEX® Connection: Physiological Adaptation, Pathophysiology*

5. A. The client should straighten his ear canal by pulling the auricle upward and outward to open up the ear canal and allow the medication to reach the eardrum.

   B. **CORRECT:** The client should gently apply pressure with the finger to the tragus of the ear after administering the drops to help the drops go into the ear canal.

   C. The client should never occlude the ear canal with the dropper when instilling ear drops because this can cause pressure that could injure the eardrum.

   D. The client should not place a cotton ball past the outermost part of the ear canal because it could introduce bacteria to the inner or middle ear.

   Ⓝ *NCLEX® Connection: Pharmacological and Parenteral Therapies, Medication Administration*

PRACTICE Answer

Using the ATI Active Learning Template: Basic Concept

RELATED CONTENT: Biotransformation (metabolism) changes medications into less active forms or inactive forms by the action of enzymes. This occurs primarily in the liver, but also takes place in the kidneys, lungs, intestines, and blood.

UNDERLYING PRINCIPLES

- Age: Infants have a limited medication-metabolizing capacity. The aging process also can influence medication metabolism, but varies with the individual. In general, hepatic medication metabolism tends to decline with age. Older adults require smaller doses of medications due to the possibility of accumulation in the body.
- An increase in some medication-metabolizing enzymes: This can metabolize a particular medication sooner, requiring an increase in dosage of that medication to maintain a therapeutic level. It can also cause an increase in the metabolism of other concurrent-use medications.
- First-pass effect: The liver inactivates some medications on their first pass through the liver. Thus, they require a nonenteral route (sublingual, IV) because of their high first-pass effect.
- Similar metabolic pathways: When the same pathway metabolizes two medications, it can alter the metabolism of one or both of them. In this way, the rate of metabolism can decrease for one or both of the medications, leading to medication accumulation.
- Nutritional status: Clients who are malnourished can be deficient in the factors that are necessary to produce specific medication-metabolizing enzymes, thus impairing medication metabolism.

Ⓝ *NCLEX® Connection: Physiological Adaptation, Pathophysiology*

CHAPTER 47 ## Safe Medication Administration and Error Reduction

The providers who may legally write prescriptions in the United States include physicians, advanced practice nurses, dentists, and physician assistants.

PROVIDER RESPONSIBILITIES

- Obtaining clients' medical history and performing a physical examination
- Diagnosing
- Prescribing medications
- Monitoring the response to therapy
- Modifying medication prescriptions as necessary

NURSE RESPONSIBILITIES Qs

- Having knowledge of federal, state (nurse practice acts), and local laws, and facilities' policies that govern the prescribing, dispensing, and administration of medications
- Preparing, administering, and evaluating clients' responses to medications
- Developing and maintaining an up-to-date knowledge base of medications they administer, including uses, mechanisms of action, routes of administration, safe dosage range, adverse and side effects, precautions, contraindications, and interactions
- Maintaining knowledge of acceptable practice and skills competency
- Determining the accuracy of medication prescriptions
- Reporting all medication errors
- Safeguarding and storing medications

MEDICATION CATEGORY AND CLASSIFICATION

NOMENCLATURE

Chemical name: A medication's chemical composition (*N*–acetyl–para–aminophenol).

Generic name: Official or nonproprietary name the United States Adopted Names Council gives a medication. Each medication has only one generic name (acetaminophen).

Trade name: Brand or proprietary name the company that manufacturers the medication gives it. One medication can have multiple trade names (Tylenol, Tempra).

PRESCRIPTION MEDICATIONS

Nurses administer prescription medications under the supervision of providers. These medications can be habit-forming, have potential harmful effects, and require monitoring.

Uncontrolled substances

These medications require monitoring by a provider, but do not generally pose a risk of abuse or addiction. Antibiotics are an example of uncontrolled prescription medications.

Controlled substances

Medications that have a potential for abuse and dependence and have a "schedule" classification. Heroin is in Schedule I and has no medical use in the United States. Medications in Schedules II through V have legitimate applications. Each subsequent level has a decreasing risk of abuse and dependence. For example, morphine is a Schedule II medication that has a greater risk for abuse and dependence than phenobarbital, which is a Schedule IV medication.

Pregnancy Risk Categories

The U.S. Food and Drug Administration's (FDA's) Pregnancy Risk Categories (A, B, C, D, X) classify medications according to their potential harm during pregnancy, with Category A being the safest and Category X the most dangerous. Teratogenesis from unsafe medications is most likely to occur during the first trimester. Before administering any medication to a woman who is pregnant or could be pregnant, determine whether it is safe for administration during pregnancy.

KNOWLEDGE REQUIRED PRIOR TO MEDICATION ADMINISTRATION

Medication category

Medications have a pharmacological action, therapeutic use, body system target, chemical makeup, and classification for use during pregnancy. For example, lisinopril is an angiotensin-converting enzyme inhibitor (pharmacological action) and an antihypertensive (therapeutic use).

Mechanism of action

This is how the medication produces its therapeutic effect. For example, glipizide is an oral hypoglycemic agent that lowers blood glucose levels primarily by stimulating pancreatic islet cells to release insulin.

Therapeutic effect

This is the expected effect for which the nurse administers the medication to a specific client. One medication can have more than one therapeutic effect. For example, one client receives acetaminophen to lower fever, whereas another receives it to relieve pain.

Side effects

These are expected and predictable effects that result at a therapeutic dose. For example, morphine for pain relief usually results in constipation.

Adverse effects

These are undesirable, inadvertent, and unexpected dangerous effects of the medication. Some are immediate, whereas others take weeks or months to develop.

Toxic effects

Medications can have specific risks and manifestations of toxicity. For example, nurses monitor clients taking digoxin for dysrhythmias, a manifestation of cardiotoxicity. Hypokalemia places these clients at greater risk for digoxin toxicity.

Interactions

Medications can interact with each other, resulting in beneficial or harmful effects. For example, giving the beta-blocker atenolol concurrently with the calcium channel blocker nifedipine helps prevent reflex tachycardia. Medications can also increase or decrease the actions of other medications, and food can interact beneficially or harmfully with medications.

Precautions, contraindications

These are conditions (diseases, age, pregnancy, lactation) that make it risky or completely unsafe for clients to take specific medications. For example, tetracyclines can stain developing teeth; therefore, children younger than 8 years should not take these medications. Another example is that heart failure is a contraindication for labetalol, an antihypertensive medication.

Preparation, dosage, administration

It is important to know any specific considerations for preparation, safe dosages, and how to administer the medication. For example, morphine is available in many different formulations. Oral doses of morphine are generally higher than parenteral doses due to extensive first-pass effect. Clients who have chronic severe pain, such as with cancer, generally take oral doses of morphine.

MEDICATION PRESCRIPTIONS

Each facility has written policies for medication prescriptions, including which providers may write, receive, and transcribe medication prescriptions.

TYPES OF MEDICATION PRESCRIPTIONS

Routine or standard prescriptions

- A routine or standard prescription identifies medications nurses give on a regular schedule with or without a termination date. Without a termination date, the prescription will be in effect until the provider discontinues it or discharges the client.
- Providers must re-prescribe some medications, such as opioids and antibiotics, within a specific amount of time or they will automatically discontinue.

Single or one-time prescriptions

A single or one-time prescription is for administration once at a specific time or as soon as possible. These prescriptions are common for preoperative or preprocedural medications. For example, a one-time prescription instructs the nurse to administer warfarin 5 mg PO at 1700.

Stat prescriptions

A stat prescription is only for administration once and immediately. For example, a stat prescription instructs the nurse to administer digoxin 0.125 mg IV bolus stat.

Now prescriptions

A now prescription is only for administration once, but up to 90 min from when the nurse received the prescription. For example, a now prescription instructs the nurse to administer vancomycin 1 g intermittent IV bolus now.

PRN prescriptions

A PRN (*pro re nata*) prescription specifies at what dosage, what frequency, and under what conditions a nurse may administer the medication. The nurse uses clinical judgment to determine the client's need for the medication. For example, a PRN prescription instructs the nurse to administer morphine 2 mg IV bolus every hour PRN for chest pain.

Standing prescriptions

Providers write standing prescriptions for specific circumstances or for specific units. For example, a critical care unit has standing prescriptions for treating clients who have asystole.

COMPONENTS OF A MEDICATION PRESCRIPTION

- The client's full name
- The date and time of the prescription
- The name of the medication (generic or brand)
- The strength and dosage of the medication
- The route of administration
- The time and frequency of administration: exact times or number of times per day (according to the facility's policy or the specific qualities of the medication)
- The quantity to dispense and the number of refills
- The signature of the prescribing provider

COMMUNICATING MEDICATION PRESCRIPTIONS

Origin of medication prescriptions

Providers or nurses who take verbal or telephone prescriptions from a provider write medication prescriptions on the client's medical record. If the nurse writes a medication prescription on the client's medical record, the facility's policy specifies how much time the provider has to sign the prescription. Nurses transcribe medication prescriptions onto the medication administration record (MAR).

Taking a telephone prescription

Only when absolutely necessary
- Ensure that the prescription is complete and correct by reading it back to the provider: the client's name, the name of the medication, the dosage, the time to give it, the frequency, and the route.
- To ensure correct spelling, use aids such as "b as in boy." State numbers separately, such as "one, seven" for 17.
- Remind the provider to verify the prescription and sign it within the amount of time the facility's policy specifies.
- Write or enter the prescription in the client's medical record.

MEDICATION RECONCILIATION Qs

The Joint Commission requires policies and procedures for medication reconciliation. Nurses compile a list of each client's current medications, including all medications with correct dosages and frequency. They compare the list with new medication prescriptions and reconcile it to resolve any discrepancies. This process takes place at admission, when transferring clients between units or facilities, and at discharge.

PREASSESSMENT FOR MEDICATION THERAPY

Nurses obtain the following information before initiating medication therapy, and update it as necessary.

Health history

- Age
- Health problems and the current reason for seeking care
- All medications clients currently take (prescription and nonprescription): the name, dose, route, and frequency of each
- Any unexpected findings possibly from medication therapy
- Use of herbal or "natural" products for medicinal purposes
- Use of caffeine, tobacco, alcohol, or illicit drugs
- Clients' understanding of the purpose of the medications
- All medication and food allergies

Physical examination

A systematic physical examination provides a baseline for evaluating the therapeutic effects of medication therapy and for detecting possible side and adverse effects.

RIGHTS OF SAFE MEDICATION ADMINISTRATION

Right client

Verify clients' identification before each medication administration. The Joint Commission requires two client identifiers. Acceptable identifiers include the client's name, an assigned identification number, telephone number, birth date, or other person-specific identifier, such as a photo identification card. Nurses also use bar-code scanners to identify clients. Check for allergies by asking clients, checking for an allergy bracelet or medal, and checking the MAR.

Right medication

Correctly interpret medication prescriptions, verifying completeness and clarity. Read medication labels and compare them with the MAR three times: before removing the container, when removing the amount of medication from the container, and in the presence of the client before administering the medication. Leave unit-dose medication in its package until administration.

Right dose

Use a unit-dose system to decrease errors. If not available, calculate the correct medication dose; check a drug reference to make sure the dose is within the usual range. Ask another nurse to verify the dose if uncertain of the calculation. Prepare medication dosages using standard measurement devices, such as graduated cups or syringes. Some medication dosages require a second verifier or witness, such as some cytotoxic medications. Automated medication dispensing systems use a machine to control the dispensing of medications. **Qs**

Right time

Administer medication on time to maintain a consistent therapeutic blood level. It is generally acceptable to administer the medication 30 min before or after the scheduled time. Refer to the drug reference or the facility's policy for exceptions.

Right route

The most common routes of administration are oral, topical, subcutaneous, intramuscular (IM), and intravenous (IV). Additional administration routes include sublingual, buccal, intradermal, transdermal, epidural, inhalation, nasal, ophthalmic, otic, rectal, vaginal, intraosseous, and via enteral tubes. Select the correct preparation for the route the provider prescribed (otic vs. ophthalmic topical ointment or drops).

Right documentation

Immediately record pertinent information, including the client's response to the medication. Document the medication after administration, not before.

Right client education

Inform clients about the medication: its purpose, what to expect, how to take it, and what to report. To individualize the teaching, determine what the clients already know about the medication, need to know about the medication, and want to know about the medication.

Right to refuse

Respect clients' right to refuse any medication. Explain the consequences, inform the provider, and document the refusal.

47.1 Error-prone abbreviation list

Some abbreviations cause a high number of medication errors.

DO NOT USE	USE
MS, MSO$_4$	morphine
MgSO$_4$	magnesium sulfate
abbreviated medication names (AZT, KCl, HCT, PTU, HCTZ)	full name of medication
nitro	nitroglycerin
decimal points without a leading zero (.5 mg)	smaller units (500 mcg) or a leading zero (0.5 mg)
trailing zero (1.0 mg, 100.0 g)	without a trailing zero (1 mg, 100 g)
u, U, IU	units
μ, μg	mcg or microgram
x3d	times 3 days
cc	mL
apothecary units	metric units
od, O.D., OD	daily or intended time of administration
q.d, qd, Q.D, QD, q1d, i/d	daily

DO NOT USE	USE
q.o.d., QOD	every other day
Q6PM, etc.	6 p.m. daily or daily at 6 p.m.
TIW, tiw	3 times weekly
mg., mL.	mg, mL (no period)
HS	half-strength, bedtime (hour of sleep)
BT, hs, HS, qhs, qn	bedtime or hour of sleep
SC, SQ, sub q	subcutaneously
IN	intranasal
IJ	injection
OJ	orange juice
> or <	greater than or less than
@	at
&, +	and
/	per
AD, AS, AU	right ear, left ear, both ears
OD, OS, OU	right eye, left eye, both eyes
D/C, dc, d/c	discharge or discontinue

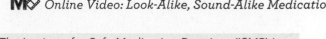

Right assessment

Collect any essential data before and after administering any medication. For example, measure apical heart rate before giving digoxin.

Right evaluation

Follow up with clients to verify therapeutic effects as well as side and adverse effects.

RESOURCES FOR MEDICATION INFORMATION

- Nursing drug handbooks
- Pharmacology textbooks
- Professional journals
- *Physicians' Desk Reference* (PDR)
- Professional websites
- Pharmacists

MEDICATION ERROR PREVENTION

COMMON MEDICATION ERRORS Qs

- Wrong medication or IV fluid
- Incorrect dose or IV infusion rate
- Wrong client, route, or time
- Administration of a medication to which the client is allergic
- Omission of a dose or extra doses
- Incorrect discontinuation of medication or IV fluid
- Inaccurate prescribing

> The Institute for Safe Medication Practices (ISMP) is a nonprofit organization working to educate health care providers and consumers about safe medication practices. The ISMP and the FDA identify the most common medical abbreviations that result in misinterpretation, mistakes, and injury. For a complete list, go to www.ismp.org.

NURSING PROCESS

Use the nursing process to prevent medication errors.

Assessment/data collection

- Ensure knowledge of medication to administer and why.
- Obtain information about the clients' medical diagnoses and conditions that relate to medication administration, such as the ability to swallow, diet, allergies, and heart, liver, and kidney disorders.
  - Identify allergies.
  - Obtain necessary preadministration data (heart rate, blood pressure) to assess the appropriateness of the medication and to obtain baseline data for evaluating the effectiveness of medications.
  - Omit or delay doses according to findings, and notify the provider.
- Determine if the medication prescription is complete: with the client's name, date and time, name of medication, dosage, route of administration, time and frequency, and signature of the prescribing provider.
- Interpret the medication prescription accurately. Refer to the ISMP lists.

47.2 Confused medication name list

Sound-alike and look-alike medication names

ESTABLISHED NAME	RECOMMENDED NAME
acetohexamide	acetoHEXAMIDE
acetazolamide	acetaZOLAMIDE
bupropion	buPROPion
buspirone	busPIRone
chlorpromazine	chlorproMAZINE
chlorpropamide	chlorproPAMIDE
clomiphene	clomiPHENE
clomipramine	clomiPRAMINE
cyclosporine	cycloSPORINE
cycloserine	cycloSERINE
daunorubicin	DAUNOrubicin
doxorubicin	DOXOrubicin
dimenhydrinate	dimenhyDRINATE
diphenhydramine	diphenhydrAMINE
dobutamine	DOBUTamine
dopamine	DOPamine
glipizide	glipiZIDE
glyburide	glyBURIDE

ESTABLISHED NAME	RECOMMENDED NAME
hydralazine	hydrALAZINE
hydromorphone	hYDROmorphone
hydroxyzine	hydrOXYzine
medroxyprogesterone	medroxyPROGESTERone
methylprednisolone	methylPREDNISolone
methyltestosterone	methylTESTOSTERone
mitoxantrone	mitoXANTRONE
nicardipine	niCARdipine
nifedipine	NIFEdipine
prednisone	predniSONE
prednisolone	prednisoLONE
risperidone	risperiDONE
ropinirole	ROPINIRole
sulfadiazine	sulfADIAZINE
sulfisoxazole	sulfiSOXAZOLE
tolazamide	TOLAZamide
tolbutamide	TOLBUTamide
vinblastine	vinBLAStine
vincristine	vinCRIStine

- Question the provider if the prescription is unclear or seems inappropriate for the client's condition. Refuse to administer a medication if it seems unsafe, and notify the charge nurse or supervisor.
- Providers usually make dosage changes gradually. Question the provider about abrupt and excessive changes.
- Determine clients' learning needs.

Planning

- Identify clients' outcomes for medication administration.
- Set priorities.

Implementation

- Avoid distractions during medication preparation (poor lighting, phones). Interruptions increase the risk of error.
- Prepare medications for one client at a time.
- Check the labels for the medication's name and concentration. Read labels carefully. Measure doses accurately, and double-check dosages of high-alert medications, such as insulin and heparin, with a colleague. Check the medication's expiration date.
- Doses are usually one to two tablets or one single-dose vial. Question multiple tablets or vials for a single dose.
- Follow the rights of medication administration consistently. Take the MAR to the bedside.
- Only give medications that you have prepared.
- Encourage clients to become part of the safety net, teaching them about medications and the importance of proper identification before medication administration. Omit or delay a dose when clients question the size of the dose or the appearance of the medication. Qs

- Follow correct procedures for all routes of administration.
- Communicate clearly both in writing and speaking.
- Use verbal prescriptions only for emergencies, and follow the facility's protocol for telephone prescriptions. Nursing students *may not* accept verbal or telephone orders.
- Follow all laws and regulations for preparing and administering controlled substances. Keep them in a secure area. Have another nurse witness the discarding of controlled substances.
- Do not leave medications at the bedside. Some facilities' policies allow exceptions, such as for topical medications.

Evaluation

- Evaluate clients' responses to medications, and document and report them.
- Recognize side and adverse effects, and document and report them.
- Report all errors, and implement corrective measures immediately.
  - Complete an incident report within the specified time frame, usually 24 hr. Include the client's identification, the time and place of the incident, an accurate account of the event, who you notified, what actions you took, and your signature. Do not reference or include this report in the client's medical record.
  - Medication errors relate to systems, procedures, product design, or practice patterns. Report all errors to assist the facility's risk managers to learn how errors occur and what changes to make to avoid similar errors in the future. Qal

---

47.3 High-alert medication list

The following medications and medication categories from the ISMP's list require specific safeguards to reduce the risk of errors. Strategies include limiting access; using auxiliary labels and automated alerts; standardizing the prescription, preparation, and administration; and using automated or independent double checks.

Class or category of medications

- Adrenergic agonists, IV (epinephrine)
- Adrenergic antagonists, IV (propranolol)
- Anesthetic agents, general, inhaled and IV (propofol)
- Cardioplegic solutions
- Chemotherapeutic agents, parenteral and oral
- Dextrose, hypertonic, 20% or greater
- Dialysis solutions, peritoneal and hemodialysis
- Epidural or intrathecal medications
- Glycoprotein IIb/IIIa inhibitors (eptifibatide)
- Hypoglycemics, oral
- Inotropic medications, IV (digoxin, milrinone)
- Liposomal forms of drugs (liposomal amphotericin B)
- Moderate sedation agents, IV (midazolam)
- Moderate sedation agents, oral, for children (chloral hydrate)
- Narcotics/opiates, IV and oral (including liquid concentrates, immediate- and sustained-release)
- Neuromuscular blocking agents (succinylcholine)
- Radiocontrast agents, IV
- Sodium chloride injection, hypertonic, more than 0.9% concentration
- Thrombolytics/fibrinolytics, IV (tenecteplase)
- Total parenteral nutrition solutions

Specific medications

- Epinephrine, subcutaneous
- Epoprostenol, IV
- Heparin, low molecular weight, injection
- Heparin, unfractionated, IV
- Insulin, subcutaneous and IV
- Lidocaine, IV
- Magnesium sulfate injection
- Methotrexate, oral, nononcologic use
- Opium tincture
- Oxytocin, IV
- Nitroprusside for injection
- Potassium chloride for injection concentrate
- Potassium phosphates injection
- Promethazine, IV
- Vasopressin, IV or intraosseous
- Warfarin

Application Exercises

1. A nurse prepares an injection of morphine to administer to a client who reports pain. Prior to administering the medication, the nurse assists another client onto a bedpan. She asks a second nurse to give the injection. Which of the following actions should the second nurse take?

   A. Offer to assist the client who needs the bedpan.

   B. Administer the injection the other nurse prepared.

   C. Prepare another syringe and administer the injection.

   D. Tell the client who needs the bedpan she will have to wait for her nurse.

2. A nurse is preparing to administer a 0900 medication to a client. Which of the following are acceptable administration times for this medication? (Select all that apply.)

   A. 0905

   B. 0825

   C. 1000

   D. 0840

   E. 0935

3. A nurse is working with a newly licensed nurse who is administering medications to clients. Which of the following actions should the nurse identify as an indication that the newly hired nurse understands medication error prevention?

   A. Taking all medications out of the unit-dose wrappers before entering the client's room

   B. Checking with the provider when a single dose requires administration of multiple tablets

   C. Administering a medication, then looking up the usual dosage range

   D. Relying on another nurse to clarify a medication prescription

4. A nurse educator is teaching a module about safe medication administration to newly licensed nurses. Which of the following statements should the nurse identify as an indication that one of the group understands how to implement medication therapy? (Select all that apply.)

   A. "I will observe for side effects."

   B. "I will monitor for therapeutic effects."

   C. "I will prescribe the appropriate dose."

   D. "I will change the dose if adverse effects occur."

   E. "I will refuse to give a medication if I believe it is unsafe."

5. A nurse is preparing to administer digoxin to a client who states, "I don't want to take that medication. I do not want one more pill." Which of the following responses should the nurse make?

   A. "Your physician prescribed it for you, so you really should take it."

   B. "Well, let's just get it over quickly then."

   C. "Okay, I'll just give you your other medications."

   D. "Tell me your concerns about taking this medication."

PRACTICE Active Learning Scenario

A nurse educator is teaching a module about the rights of safe medication administration to a group of newly licensed nurses. Use the ATI Active Learning Template: Basic Concept to complete this item.

RELATED CONTENT: List the rights of safe medication administration.

UNDERLYING PRINCIPLES: List at least three acceptable identifiers to use to verify the client's identity.

Application Exercises Key

1. A. **CORRECT:** The second nurse should offer to assist the client who needs the bedpan. This will allow the nurse who prepared the injection to administer it.

   B. A nurse should only administer medications that she prepared.

   C. Preparing another syringe will delay the administration of the pain medication.

   D. Telling the client to wait is not an acceptable option for a client who needs a bedpan.

   Ⓝ *NCLEX® Connection: Management of Care, Legal Rights and Responsibilities*

2. A. **CORRECT:** The nurse should administer medications within 30 min of the time it is due. 0905 is within 30 min of the time the medication is due.

   B. 0825 is not within 30 min of the time the medication is due.

   C. 1000 is not within 30 min of the time the medication is due.

   D. **CORRECT:** 0840 is within 30 min of the time the medication is due.

   E. 0935 is not within 30 min of the time the medication is due.

   Ⓝ *NCLEX® Connection: Pharmacological and Parenteral Therapies, Medication Administration*

3. A. To prevent errors, the nurse should not take unit-dose medications out of wrappers until at the bedside when performing the third check of medication administration. The nurse can encourage clients' involvement and provide teaching at this time.

   B. **CORRECT:** If a single dose requires multiple tablets, it is possible that an error has occurred in the prescription or transcription of the medication. This action could prevent a medication error.

   C. Reviewing the usual dosage range prior to administration can help the nurse identify an inaccurate dosage.

   D. If the prescription is unclear, the nurse should contact the provider, not another nurse, for clarification.

   Ⓝ *NCLEX® Connection: Pharmacological and Parenteral Therapies, Medication Administration*

4. A. **CORRECT:** The nurse is responsible for observing for side effects. This is within a nurse's scope of practice.

   B. **CORRECT:** The nurse is responsible for monitoring therapeutic effects. This is within a nurse's scope of practice.

   C. The provider is responsible for prescribing the appropriate dose. This is outside of the nurse's scope of practice.

   D. The provider is responsible for changing the dose if adverse effects occur. This is outside of the nurse's scope of practice.

   E. **CORRECT:** The nurse is responsible for identifying when a medication could harm a client. It is within the nurse's scope of practice to refuse to administer the medication and contact the provider.

   Ⓝ *NCLEX® Connection: Pharmacological and Parenteral Therapies, Expected Actions/Outcomes*

5. A. This response dismisses the client's concerns.

   B. The nurse is dismissing the client's concerns about taking the medication by continuing with medication administration.

   C. Although clients have the right to refuse a medication, the nurse should provide information about the risk of refusal instead of proceeding with medication administration.

   D. **CORRECT:** Although clients have the right to refuse a medication, the nurse is correct in determining the reason for refusal by asking the client his concerns. Then the nurse can provide information about the risk of refusal and facilitate an informed decision. At that point, if the client still exercises his right to refuse a medication, the nurse should notify and the provider and document the refusal and the actions the nurse took.

   Ⓝ *NCLEX® Connection: Management of Care, Client Rights*

PRACTICE Answer

Using the ATI Active Learning Template: Basic Concept

RELATED CONTENT: Rights of Safe Medication Administration

- **Right client:** Verify clients' identification before each medication administration. The Joint Commission requires two client identifiers. Acceptable identifiers include the client's name, an assigned identification number, telephone number, birth date, or other person-specific identifier, such as a photo identification card. Nurses also use bar-code scanners to identify clients. Check for allergies by asking clients, checking for an allergy bracelet or medal, and checking the MAR.
- **Right medication:** Correctly interpret medication prescriptions, verifying completeness and clarity. Read medication labels and compare them with the MAR three times: before removing the container, when removing the amount of medication from the container, and in the presence of the client before administering the medication. Leave unit-dose medication in its package until administration.
- **Right dose:** Use a unit-dose system to decrease errors. If not available, calculate the correct medication dose; check a drug reference to make sure the dose is within the usual range. Ask another nurse to verify the dose if uncertain of the calculation. Prepare medication dosages using standard measurement devices, such as graduated cups or syringes. Some medication dosages, such as some cytotoxic medications, require a second verifier or witness. Automated medication dispensing systems use a machine to control the dispensing of medications.
- **Right time:** Administer medication on time to maintain a consistent therapeutic blood level. It is generally acceptable to administer the medication 30 min before or after the scheduled time. Refer to the drug reference or the facility's policy for exceptions.
- **Right route:** The most common routes of administration are oral, topical, subcutaneous, intramuscular, and intravenous. Additional administration routes include sublingual, buccal, intradermal, transdermal, epidural, inhalation, nasal, ophthalmic, otic, rectal, vaginal, intraosseous, and via enteral tubes. Select the correct preparation for the route the provider prescribed (otic vs. ophthalmic topical ointment or drops).
- **Right documentation:** Immediately record pertinent information, including the client's response to the medication. Document the medication after administration, not before.
- **Right client education:** Inform clients about the medication: its purpose, what to expect, how to take it, and what to report. To individualize the teaching, determine what the clients already know, need to know, and want to know about the medication.
- **Right to refuse:** Respect clients' right to refuse any medication. Explain the consequences, inform the provider, and document the refusal.
- **Right assessment:** Collect any essential data before and after administering any medication. For example, measure apical heart rate before giving digoxin.

UNDERLYING PRINCIPLES

- Acceptable identifiers include the client's name, an assigned identification number, telephone number, birth date, or other person-specific identifier.
- The nurse can use bar-code scanners to identify clients.

Ⓝ *NCLEX® Connection: Pharmacological and Parenteral Therapies, Medication Administration*

CHAPTER 48   Dosage Calculation

Basic medication dose conversion and calculation skills are essential for providing safe nursing care.

Nurses are responsible for administering the correct amount of medication by calculating the precise amount of medication to give. Nurses can use three different methods for dosage calculation: ratio and proportion, formula (desired over have), and dimensional analysis.

TYPES OF CALCULATIONS

- Solid oral medication
- Liquid oral medication
- Injectable medication
- Correct doses by weight
- IV infusion rates

STANDARD CONVERSION FACTORS

- 1 mg = 1,000 mcg
- 1 g = 1,000 mg
- 1 kg = 1,000 g
- 1 oz = 30 mL
- 1 L = 1,000 mL
- 1 tsp = 5 mL
- 1 tbsp = 15 mL
- 1 tbsp = 3 tsp
- 1 kg = 2.2 lb
- 1 gr = 60 mg

GENERAL ROUNDING GUIDELINES

ROUNDING UP: If the number to the right is equal to or greater than 5, round up by adding 1 to the number on the left.

ROUNDING DOWN: If the number to the right is less than 5, round down by dropping the number, leaving the number to the left as is.

For dosages less than 1.0: Round to the nearest hundredth.

- For example (rounding up): 0.746 mL = 0.75 mL. The calculated dose is 0.746 mL. Look at the number in the thousandths place (6). Six is greater than 5. To round to hundredths, add 1 to the 4 in the hundredths place and drop the 6. The rounded dose is 0.75 mL.
- Or (rounding down): 0.743 mL = 0.74 mL. The calculated dose is 0.743 mL. Look at the number in the thousandths place (3). Three is less than 5. To round to the hundredth, drop the 3 and leave the 4 as is. The rounded dose is 0.74 mL.

For dosages greater than 1.0: Round to the nearest tenth.

- For example (rounding up): 1.38 = 1.4. The calculated dose is 1.38 mg. Look at the number in the hundredths place (8). Eight is greater than 5. To round to the tenth, add 1 to the 3 in the tenth place and drop the 8. The rounded dose is 1.4 mg.
- Or (rounding down): 1.34 mL = 1.3 mL. The calculated dose is 1.34 mL. Look at the number in the hundredths place (4). Four is less than 5. To round to the tenth, drop the 4 and leave the 3 as is. The rounded dose is 1.3 mL.

Solid dosage

Example: A nurse is preparing to administer phenytoin 0.2 g PO every 8 hr. The amount available is phenytoin 100 mg/capsule. How many capsules should the nurse administer per dose? (Round the answer to the nearest whole number. Use a leading zero if it applies. Do not use a trailing zero.)

USING RATIO AND PROPORTION

STEP 1: What is the unit of measurement the nurse should calculate?

capsules

STEP 2: What is the dose the nurse should administer? Dose to administer = Desired

0.2 g

STEP 3: What is the dose available? Dose available = Have

100 mg

STEP 4: Should the nurse convert the units of measurement? Yes (g ≠ mg)

1 g = 1,000 mg (1 × 1,000)

0.2 g = 200 mg (0.2 × 1,000)

STEP 5: What is the quantity of the dose available? = Quantity

1 capsule

STEP 6: Set up the equation and solve for X.

$$\frac{Have}{Quantity} = \frac{Desired}{X}$$

$$\frac{100 \text{ mg}}{1 \text{ cap}} = \frac{200 \text{ mg}}{X \text{ cap}}$$

$$X = 2$$

STEP 7: Round, if necessary.

STEP 8: Reassess to determine whether the amount to administer makes sense. If there are 100 mg/capsule and the prescription reads 0.2 g (200 mg), it makes sense to administer 2 capsules. The nurse should administer phenytoin 2 capsules PO.

USING DESIRED OVER HAVE

STEP 1: What is the unit of measurement the nurse should calculate?

> capsules

STEP 2: What is the dose the nurse should administer? Dose to administer = Desired

> 0.2 g

STEP 3: What is the dose available? Dose available = Have

> 100 mg

STEP 4: Should the nurse convert the units of measurement? Yes (g ≠ mg)

> 1 g = 1,000 mg (1 × 1,000)

> 0.2 g = 200 mg (0.2 × 1,000)

STEP 5: What is the quantity of the dose available? = Quantity

> 1 capsule

STEP 6: Set up the equation and solve for X.

> $$\frac{Desired \times Quantity}{Have} = X$$

> $$\frac{200\ mg \times 1\ cap}{100\ mg} = X\ cap$$

> $X = 2$

STEP 7: Round, if necessary.

STEP 8: Reassess to determine whether the amount to administer makes sense. If there are 100 mg/capsule and the prescription reads 0.2 g (200 mg), it makes sense to administer 2 capsules. The nurse should administer phenytoin 2 capsules PO.

USING DIMENSIONAL ANALYSIS

STEP 1: What is the unit of measurement the nurse should calculate?

> capsules

STEP 2: What is the quantity of the dose available? = Quantity

> 1 capsule

STEP 3: What is the dose available? Dose available = Have

> 100 mg

STEP 4: What is the dose the nurse should administer? Dose to administer = Desired

> 0.2 g

STEP 5: Should the nurse convert the units of measurement? Yes (g ≠ mg)

> 1,000 mg = 1 g

> 0.2 g = 200 mg (0.2 × 100)

STEP 6: Set up the equation and solve for X.

> $$X = \frac{Quantity}{Have} \times \frac{Conversion\ (Have)}{Conversion\ (Desired)} \times Desired$$

> $$X\ cap = \frac{1\ cap}{100\ mg} \times \frac{1,000\ mg}{1\ g} \times 0.2\ g$$

> $X = 2$

STEP 7: Round, if necessary.

STEP 8: Reassess to determine whether the amount to administer makes sense. If there are 100 mg/capsule and the prescription reads 0.2 g (200 mg), it makes sense to administer 2 capsules. The nurse should administer phenytoin 2 capsules PO.

Liquid dosage

> Example: A nurse is preparing to administer amoxicillin 0.25 g PO every 8 hr. The amount available is amoxicillin oral suspension 250 mg/5 mL. How many mL should the nurse administer per dose? (Round the answer to the nearest tenth. Use a leading zero if it applies. Do not use a trailing zero.)

USING RATIO AND PROPORTION

STEP 1: What is the unit of measurement the nurse should calculate?

> mL

STEP 2: What is the dose the nurse should administer? Dose to administer = Desired

> 0.25 g

STEP 3: What is the dose available? Dose available = Have

> 250 mg

STEP 4: Should the nurse convert the units of measurement? Yes (g ≠ mg)

> 1 g = 1,000 mg (1 × 1,000)

> 0.25 g = 250 mg (0.25 × 1,000)

STEP 5: What is the quantity of the dose available? = Quantity

> 5 mL

STEP 6: Set up the equation and solve for X.

> $$\frac{Have}{Quantity} = \frac{Desired}{X}$$

> $$\frac{250\ mg}{5\ mL} = \frac{250\ mg}{X\ mL}$$

> $X = 5$

STEP 7: Round, if necessary.

STEP 8: Reassess to determine whether the amount to administer makes sense. If there are 250 mg/5 mL and the prescription reads 0.25 g (250 mg), it makes sense to administer 5 mL. The nurse should administer amoxicillin 5 mL PO every 8 hr.

USING DESIRED OVER HAVE

STEP 1: What is the unit of measurement the nurse should calculate?

mL

STEP 2: What is the dose the nurse should administer? Dose to administer = Desired

0.25 g

STEP 3: What is the dose available? Dose available = Have

250 mg

STEP 4: Should the nurse convert the units of measurement? Yes (g ≠ mg)

1 g = 1,000 mg (1 × 1,000)

0.25 g = 250 mg (0.25 × 1,000)

STEP 5: What is the quantity of the dose available? = Quantity

5 mL

STEP 6: Set up the equation and solve for X.

$$\frac{Desired \times Quantity}{Have} = X$$

$$\frac{250 \text{ mg} \times 5 \text{ mL}}{250 \text{ mg}} = X \text{ mL}$$

$$5 = X$$

STEP 7: Round, if necessary.

STEP 8: Reassess to determine whether the amount to administer makes sense. If there are 250 mg/5 mL and the prescription reads 0.25 g (250 mg), it makes sense to administer 5 mL. The nurse should administer amoxicillin 5 mL PO every 8 hr.

USING DIMENSIONAL ANALYSIS

STEP 1: What is the unit of measurement the nurse should calculate?

mL

STEP 2: What is the quantity of the dose available? = Quantity

5 mL

STEP 3: What is the dose available? Dose available = Have

250 mg

STEP 4: What is the dose the nurse should administer? Dose to administer = Desired

0.25 g

STEP 5: Should the nurse convert the units of measurement? Yes (g ≠ mg)

1,000 mg = 1 g

0.25 g = 250 mg (0.25 × 1,000)

STEP 6: Set up the equation and solve for X.

$$X = \frac{Quantity}{Have} \times \frac{Conversion\ (Have)}{Conversion\ (Desired)} \times Desired$$

$$X \text{ mL} = \frac{5 \text{ mL}}{250 \text{ mg}} \times \frac{1,000 \text{ mg}}{1 \text{ g}} \times 0.25 \text{ g}$$

$$X = 5$$

STEP 7: Round, if necessary.

STEP 8: Reassess to determine whether the amount to administer makes sense. If there are 250 mg/5 mL and the prescription reads 0.25 g (250 mg), it makes sense to administer 5 mL. The nurse should administer amoxicillin 5 mL PO every 8 hr.

Injectable dosage

Example: A nurse is preparing to administer heparin 8,000 units subcutaneously every 12 hr. Available is heparin injection 10,000 units/mL. How many mL should the nurse administer per dose? (Round the answer to the nearest tenth. Use a leading zero if it applies. Do not use a trailing zero.)

USING RATIO AND PROPORTION

STEP 1: What is the unit of measurement the nurse should calculate?

mL

STEP 2: What is the dose the nurse should administer? Dose to administer = Desired

8,000 units

STEP 3: What is the dose available? Dose available = Have

10,000 units

STEP 4: Should the nurse convert the units of measurement? No

STEP 5: What is the quantity of the dose available? = Quantity

1 mL

STEP 6: Set up the equation and solve for X.

$$\frac{Have}{Quantity} = \frac{Desired}{X}$$

$$\frac{10,000 \text{ units}}{1 \text{ mL}} = \frac{8,000 \text{ units}}{X \text{ mL}}$$

$$X = 0.8$$

STEP 7: Round, if necessary.

STEP 8: Reassess to determine whether the amount to administer makes sense. If there are 10,000 units/mL and the prescription reads 8,000 units, it makes sense to administer 0.8 mL. The nurse should administer heparin injection 0.8 mL subcutaneously every 12 hr.

USING DESIRED OVER HAVE

STEP 1: What is the unit of measurement the nurse should calculate?

mL

STEP 2: What is the dose the nurse should administer? Dose to administer = Desired

8,000 units

STEP 3: What is the dose available? Dose available = Have

10,000 units

STEP 4: Should the nurse convert the units of measurement? No

STEP 5: What is the quantity of the dose available? = Quantity

1 mL

STEP 6: Set up an equation and solve for X.

$$\frac{Desired \times Quantity}{Have} = X$$

$$\frac{8,000 \text{ units} \times 1 \text{ mL}}{10,000 \text{ units}} = X \text{ mL}$$

$$0.8 = X$$

STEP 7: Round, if necessary.

STEP 8: Reassess to determine whether the amount to administer makes sense. If there are 10,000 units/mL and the prescription reads 8,000 units, it makes sense to administer 0.8 mL. The nurse should administer heparin injection 0.8 mL subcutaneously every 12 hr.

USING DIMENSIONAL ANALYSIS

STEP 1: What is the unit of measurement the nurse should calculate?

mL

STEP 2: What is the quantity of the dose available? = Quantity

1 mL

STEP 3: What is the dose available? Dose available = Have

10,000 units

STEP 4: What is the dose the nurse should administer? Dose to administer = Desired

8,000 units

STEP 5: Should the nurse convert the units of measurement? No

STEP 6: Set up an equation and solve for X.

$$X = \frac{Quantity}{Have} \times \frac{Conversion\ (Have)}{Conversion\ (Desired)} \times Desired$$

$$X \text{ mL} = \frac{1 \text{ mL}}{10,000 \text{ units}} \times 8,000 \text{ units}$$

$$X = 0.8$$

STEP 7: Round, if necessary.

STEP 8: Reassess to determine whether the amount to administer makes sense. If there are 10,000 units/mL and the prescription reads 8,000 units, it makes sense to administer 0.8 mL. The nurse should administer heparin injection 0.8 mL subcutaneously every 12 hr.

Dosages by weight

Example: A nurse is preparing to administer cefixime 8 mg/kg/day PO to divide equally every 12 hr to a toddler who weighs 22 lb. Available is cefixime suspension 100 mg/5 mL. How many mL should the nurse administer per dose? (Round the answer to the nearest tenth. Use a leading zero if it applies. Do not use a trailing zero.)

STEP 1: What is the unit of measurement the nurse should calculate?

kg

STEP 2: Set up an equation and solve for X.

$$\frac{2.2 \text{ lb}}{1 \text{ kg}} = \frac{client's\ desired\ weight\ in\ lb}{X \text{ kg}}$$

$$\frac{2.2 \text{ lb}}{1 \text{ kg}} = \frac{22 \text{ lb}}{X \text{ kg}}$$

$$X = 10$$

STEP 3: Round, if necessary.

STEP 4: Reassess to determine whether the equivalent makes sense. If 1 kg = 2.2 lb, it makes sense that 22 lb = 10 kg.

STEP 5: What is the unit of measurement the nurse should calculate?

mg

STEP 6: Set up an equation and solve for X.

$$mg \times kg/day = X$$

$$\frac{8 \text{ mg} \times 10 \text{ kg}}{1 \text{ day}} = 80 \text{ mg}$$

STEP 7: Round, if necessary.

STEP 8: Reassess to determine whether the amount makes sense. If the prescription reads 8 mg/kg/day to divide equally every 12 hr and the toddler weighs 10 kg, it makes sense to give 80 mg/day, or 40 mg every 12 hr.

USING RATIO AND PROPORTION

STEP 9: What is the unit of measurement the nurse should calculate?

mL

STEP 10: What is the dose the nurse should administer? Dose to administer = Desired

40 mg

STEP 11: What is the dose available? Dose available = Have

100 mg

STEP 12: Should the nurse convert the units of measurement? No

STEP 13: What is the quantity of the dose available? = Quantity

5 mL

STEP 14: Set up the equation and solve for X.

$$\frac{Have}{Quantity} = \frac{Desired}{X}$$

$$\frac{100\ mg}{5\ mL} = \frac{40\ mg}{X\ mL}$$

$$X = 2$$

STEP 15: Round, if necessary.

STEP 16: Reassess to determine whether the amount to give makes sense. If there are 100 mg/5 mL and the prescription reads 40 mg, it makes sense to give 2 mL. The nurse should administer cefixime suspension 2 mL PO every 12 hr.

USING DESIRED OVER HAVE

STEP 9: What is the unit of measurement the nurse should calculate?

mL

STEP 10: What is the dose the nurse should administer? Dose to administer = Desired

40 mg

STEP 11: What is the dose available? Dose available = Have

100 mg

STEP 12: Should the nurse convert the units of measurement? No

STEP 13: What is the quantity of the dose available? = Quantity

5 mL

STEP 14: Set up an equation and solve for X.

$$\frac{Desired \times Quantity}{Have} = X$$

$$\frac{40\ mg \times 5\ mL}{100\ mg} = X\ mL$$

$$2 = X$$

STEP 15: Round, if necessary.

STEP 16: Reassess to determine whether the amount to give makes sense. If there are 100 mg/5 mL and the prescription reads 40 mg, it makes sense to give 2 mL. The nurse should administer cefixime suspension 2 mL PO every 12 hr.

USING DIMENSIONAL ANALYSIS

STEP 9: What is the unit of measurement the nurse should calculate?

mL

STEP 10: What is the quantity of the dose available? = Quantity

5 mL

STEP 11: What is the dose available? Dose available = Have

100 mg

STEP 12: What is the dose the nurse should administer? Dose to administer = Desired

40 mg

STEP 13: Should the nurse convert the units of measurement? No

STEP 14: Set up an equation and solve for X.

$$X = \frac{Quantity}{Have} \times \frac{Conversion\ (Have)}{Conversion\ (Desired)} \times Desired$$

$$X\ mL = \frac{5\ mL}{100\ mg} \times 40\ mg$$

$$X = 2$$

STEP 15: Round, if necessary.

STEP 16: Reassess to determine whether the amount to give makes sense. If there are 100 mg/5 mL and the prescription reads 40 mg, it makes sense to give 2 mL. The nurse should administer cefixime suspension 2 mL PO every 12 hr.

IV flow rates

Nurses calculate IV flow rates for large-volume continuous IV infusions and intermittent IV bolus infusions using electronic infusion pumps (mL/hr) and manual IV tubing (gtt/min).

IV INFUSIONS WITH ELECTRONIC INFUSION PUMPS

Infusion pumps control an accurate rate of fluid infusion. Infusion pumps deliver a specific amount of fluid during a specific amount of time. For example, an infusion pump can deliver 150 mL in 1 hr or 50 mL in 20 min.

> Example: A nurse is preparing to administer dextrose 5% in water (D_5W) 500 mL IV to infuse over 4 hr. The nurse should set the IV infusion pump to deliver how many mL/hr? (Round the answer to the nearest whole number. Use a leading zero if it applies. Do not use a trailing zero.)

STEP 1: What is the unit of measurement the nurse should calculate?

> mL/hr

STEP 2: What is the volume the nurse should infuse?

> 500 mL

STEP 3: What is the total infusion time?

> 4 hr

STEP 4: Should the nurse convert the units of measurement? No

STEP 5: Set up the equation and solve for X.

> $$\frac{Volume \text{ (mL)}}{Time \text{ (hr)}} = X \text{ mL/hr}$$
>
> $$\frac{500 \text{ mL}}{4 \text{ hr}} = X \text{ mL/hr}$$
>
> $125 = X$

STEP 6: Round, if necessary.

STEP 7: Reassess to determine whether the IV flow rate makes sense. If the prescription reads 500 mL to infuse over 4 hr, it makes sense to administer 125 mL/hr. The nurse should set the IV pump to deliver D_5W 500 mL IV at 125 mL/hr.

> Example: A nurse is preparing to administer cefotaxime 1 g intermittent IV bolus over 45 min. Available is cefotaxime 1 g in 100 mL 0.9% sodium chloride (0.9% NaCl). The nurse should set the IV infusion pump to deliver how many mL/hr? (Round the answer to the nearest whole number.)

STEP 1: What is the unit of measurement the nurse should calculate?

> mL/hr

STEP 2: Should the nurse convert the units of measurement? Yes (min ≠ hr) Yes (g ≠ mL)

> $$\frac{60 \text{ min}}{45 \text{ min}} = \frac{1 \text{ hr}}{X \text{ hr}} \qquad\qquad \frac{100 \text{ mL}}{1 \text{ g}} = \frac{X \text{ mL}}{1 \text{ g}}$$
>
> $X = 0.75 \qquad\qquad\qquad\qquad\qquad X = 100$

STEP 3: What is the total infusion time?

> 45 min

STEP 4: What is the volume the nurse should infuse?

> 100 mL

STEP 5: Set up an equation and solve for X.

> $$\frac{Volume \text{ (mL)}}{Time \text{ (hr)}} = X \text{ mL/hr}$$
>
> $$\frac{100 \text{ mL}}{0.75 \text{ hr}} = X \text{ mL/hr}$$
>
> $133.3333 = X$

STEP 6: Round, if necessary.

> $133.3333 = 133$

STEP 7: Reassess to determine whether the IV flow rate makes sense. If the prescription reads 100 mL to infuse over 45 min (0.75 hr), it makes sense to administer 133 mL/hr. The nurse should set the IV pump to deliver cefotaxime 1 g in 100 mL of 0.9% NaCl IV at 133 mL/hr.

MANUAL IV INFUSIONS

If an electronic infusion pump is not available, regulate the IV flow rate using the roller clamp on the IV tubing. When setting the flow rate, count the number of drops that fall into the drip chamber over 1 min. Then calculate the flow rate using the drop factor on the manufacturer's package containing the administration set. The drop factor is the number of drops per milliliter of solution.

> Example: A nurse is preparing to administer lactated Ringer's (LR) 1,500 mL IV to infuse over 10 hr. The drop factor of the manual IV tubing is 15 gtt/mL. The nurse should adjust the manual IV infusion to deliver how many gtt/min? (Round the answer to the nearest whole number. Use a leading zero if it applies. Do not use a trailing zero.)

USING RATIO AND PROPORTION AND DESIRED OVER HAVE

STEP 1: What is the unit of measurement the nurse should calculate?

> gtt/min

STEP 2: What is the quantity of the drop factor that is available?

> 15 gtt/mL

STEP 3: What is the volume the nurse should infuse?

> 1,500 mL

STEP 4: What is the total infusion time?

> 10 hr

STEP 5: Should the nurse convert the units of measurement? No (mL = mL) Yes (hr ≠ min)

> $$\frac{1\ hr}{60\ min} = \frac{10\ hr}{X\ min}$$

> $X = 600$ min

STEP 6: Set up the equation and solve for X.

> $$\frac{Volume\ \text{(mL)}}{Time\ \text{(min)}} \times Drop\ factor\ \text{(gtt/mL)} = X$$

> $$\frac{1,500\ mL}{600\ min} \times 15\ gtt/mL = X\ gtt/min$$

> $37.5 = X$

STEP 7: Round, if necessary.

> 37.5 = 38

STEP 8: Reassess to determine whether the IV flow rate makes sense. If the prescription reads 1,500 mL to infuse over 10 hr (600 min), it makes sense to administer 38 gtt/min. The nurse should adjust the manual IV infusion to deliver LR 1,500 mL IV at 38 gtt/min.

USING DIMENSIONAL ANALYSIS

STEP 1: What is the unit of measurement the nurse should calculate?

> gtt/min

STEP 2: What is the quantity of the drop factor that is available?

> 15 gtt/mL

STEP 3: What is the total infusion time?

> 10 hr

STEP 4: What is the volume the nurse should infuse?

> 1,500 mL

STEP 5: Should the nurse convert the units of measurement? No (mL = mL) Yes (hr ≠ min)

> $$\frac{1\ hr}{60\ min} = \frac{10\ hr}{X\ min}$$

> $X = 600$ min

STEP 6: Set up the equation and solve for X.

> $$X = \frac{Quantity}{1\ mL} \times \frac{Conversion\ (Have)}{Conversion\ (Desired)} \times \frac{Volume}{Time}$$

> $$X\ gtt/min = \frac{15\ gtt}{1\ mL} \times \frac{1\ hr}{60\ min} \times \frac{1,500\ mL}{10\ hr}$$

> $X = 37.5$

STEP 7: Round, if necessary.

> 37.5 = 38

STEP 8: Reassess to determine whether the IV flow rate makes sense. If the prescription reads 1,500 mL to infuse over 10 hr (600 min), it makes sense to administer 38 gtt/min. The nurse should adjust the manual IV infusion to deliver LR 1,500 mL IV at 38 gtt/min.

Example: A nurse is preparing to administer ranitidine 150 mg by intermittent IV bolus. Available is ranitidine 150 mg in 100 mL of 0.9% sodium chloride (0.9% NaCl) to infuse over 30 min. The drop factor of the manual IV tubing is 10 gtt/mL. The nurse should adjust the manual IV infusion to deliver how many gtt/min? (Round the answer to the nearest whole number. Use a leading zero if it applies. Do not use a trailing zero.)

USING RATIO AND PROPORTION AND DESIRED OVER HAVE

STEP 1: What is the unit of measurement the nurse should calculate?

gtt/min

STEP 2: Should the nurse convert the units of measurement? Yes (mg ≠ mL)

$$\frac{150 \text{ mg}}{100 \text{ mL}} = \frac{150 \text{ mg}}{X \text{ mL}}$$

$X = 100$

STEP 3: What is the total infusion time?

30 min

STEP 4: What is the quantity of the drop factor that is available?

10 gtt/mL

STEP 5: What is the volume the nurse should infuse?

100 mL

STEP 6: Set up an equation and solve for X.

$$\frac{Volume \text{ (mL)}}{Time \text{ (min)}} \times Drop\ factor \text{ (gtt/mL)} = X$$

$$\frac{100 \text{ mL}}{30 \text{ min}} \times 10 \text{ gtt/mL} = X \text{ gtt/min}$$

$33.3333 = X$

STEP 7: Round, if necessary.

$33.3333 = 33$

STEP 8: Reassess to determine whether the IV flow rate makes sense. If the amount prescribed is 100 mL to infuse over 30 min, it makes sense to administer 33 gtt/min. The nurse should adjust the manual IV infusion to deliver ranitidine 150 mg in 100 mL of 0.9% NaCl IV at 33 gtt/min.

USING DIMENSIONAL ANALYSIS

STEP 1: What is the unit of measurement to calculate?

gtt/min

STEP 2: What is the quantity of the drop factor that is available?

10 gtt/mL

STEP 3: What is the total infusion time?

30 min

STEP 4: Should the nurse convert the units of measurement? Yes (mg ≠ mL)

$$\frac{150 \text{ mg}}{100 \text{ mL}} = \frac{150 \text{ mg}}{X \text{ mL}}$$

$X = 100$

STEP 5: What is the volume the nurse should infuse?

100 mL

STEP 6: Set up an equation and solve for X.

$$X = \frac{Quantity}{1 \text{ mL}} \times \frac{Conversion\ (Have)}{Conversion\ (Desired)} \times \frac{Volume}{Time}$$

$$X \text{ gtt/min} = \frac{10 \text{ gtt}}{1 \text{ mL}} \times \frac{100 \text{ mL}}{30 \text{ min}}$$

$X = 33.3333$

STEP 7: Round, if necessary.

$33.3333 = 33$

STEP 8: Reassess to determine whether the IV flow rate makes sense. If the amount prescribed is 100 mL to infuse over 30 min, it makes sense to administer 33 gtt/min. The nurse should adjust the manual IV infusion to deliver ranitidine 150 mg in 100 mL of 0.9% NaCl IV at 33 gtt/min.

Application Exercises

1. A nurse is preparing to administer methylprednisolone 10 mg by IV bolus. The amount available is methylprednisolone injection 40 mg/mL. How many mL should the nurse administer? (Round the answer to the nearest tenth. Do not use a trailing zero.)

2. A nurse is preparing to administer lactated Ringer's (LR) IV 100 mL over 15 min. The nurse should set the IV infusion pump to deliver how many mL/hr? (Round the answer to the nearest whole number. Do not use a trailing zero.)

3. A nurse is preparing to administer 0.9% sodium chloride (0.9% NaCl) 250 mL IV to infuse over 30 min. The drop factor of the manual IV tubing is 10 gtt/mL. The nurse should adjust the manual IV infusion to deliver how many gtt/min? (Round the answer to the nearest whole number. Do not use a trailing zero.)

4. A nurse is preparing to administer metoprolol 200 mg PO daily. The amount available is metoprolol 100 mg/tablet. How many tablets should the nurse administer? (Round the answer to the nearest whole number. Do not use a trailing zero.)

5. A nurse is preparing to administer ketorolac 0.5 mg/kg IV bolus every 6 hr to a school-age child who weighs 66 lb. The amount available is ketorolac injection 30 mg/mL. How many mL should the nurse administer per dose? (Round the answer to the nearest tenth. Use a leading zero if it applies. Do not use a trailing zero.)

6. A nurse is preparing to administer dextrose 5% in water (D_5W) 1,000 mL IV to infuse over 10 hr. The nurse should set the IV infusion pump to deliver how many mL/hr? (Round the answer to the nearest whole number. Do not use a trailing zero.)

7. A nurse is preparing to administer acetaminophen 320 mg PO every 4 hr PRN for pain. The amount available is acetaminophen liquid 160 mg/5 mL. How many mL should the nurse administer per dose? (Round the answer to the nearest tenth. Use a leading zero if it applies. Do not use a trailing zero.)

8. A nurse is preparing to administer dextrose 5% in lactated Ringer's (D_5LR) 1,000 mL to infuse over 6 hr. The drop factor of the manual IV tubing is 15 gtt/mL. The nurse should adjust the manual IV infusion to deliver how many gtt/min? (Round the answer to the nearest whole number. Do not use a trailing zero.)

Application Exercises Key

1. 0.3 mL

Using Ratio and Proportion

STEP 1: What is the unit of measurement the nurse should calculate?   mL

STEP 2: What is the dose the nurse should administer? Dose to administer = Desired = 10 mg

STEP 3: What is the dose available? Dose available = Have = 40 mg

STEP 4: Should the nurse convert the units of measurement?   No

STEP 5: What is the quantity of the dose available? = Quantity = 1 mL

STEP 6: Set up the equation and solve for X.

$$\frac{Have}{Quantity} = \frac{Desired}{X} \qquad \frac{40\ mg}{1\ mL} \times \frac{10\ mg}{X\ mL}$$

$X = 0.25$

STEP 7: Round, if necessary.   0.25 = 0.3

STEP 8: Reassess to determine whether the amount to administer makes sense. If there are 40 mg/mL and the prescription reads 10 mg, it makes sense to administer 0.3 mL. The nurse should administer methylprednisolone injection 0.3 mL by IV bolus.

Using Desired Over Have

STEP 1: What is the unit of measurement the nurse should calculate?   mL

STEP 2: What is the dose the nurse should administer? Dose to administer = Desired = 10 mg

STEP 3: What is the dose available? Dose available = Have = 40 mg

STEP 4: Should the nurse convert the units of measurement?   No

STEP 5: What is the quantity of the dose available? = Quantity = 1 mL

STEP 6: Set up an equation and solve for X.

$$\frac{Desired \times Quantity}{Have} = \frac{10\ mg \times 1\ mL}{40\ mg} = X\ mL$$

$0.25 = X$

STEP 7: Round, if necessary.   0.25 = 0.3

STEP 8: Reassess to determine whether the amount to administer makes sense. If there are 40 mg/mL and the prescription reads 10 mg, it makes sense to administer 0.3 mL. The nurse should administer methylprednisolone injection 0.3 mL by IV bolus.

Using Dimensional Analysis

STEP 1: What is the unit of measurement the nurse should calculate?   mL

STEP 2: What is the quantity of the dose available? = Quantity = 1 mL

STEP 3: What is the dose available? Dose available = Have = 40 mg

STEP 4: What is the dose the nurse should administer? Dose to administer = Desired = 10 mg

STEP 5: Should the nurse convert the units of measurement? No

STEP 6: Set up an equation and solve for X.

$$X = \frac{Quantity}{Have} \times \frac{Conversion\ (Have)}{Conversion\ (Desired)} \times Desired$$

$$X\ mL = \frac{1\ mL}{40\ mg} \times 10\ mg$$

$X = 0.25$

STEP 7: Round, if necessary.   0.25 = 0.3

STEP 8: Reassess to determine whether the amount to administer makes sense. If there are 40 mg/mL and the prescription reads 10 mg, it makes sense to administer 0.3 mL. The nurse should administer methylprednisolone injection 0.3 mL by IV bolus.

Ⓝ NCLEX® Connection: Pharmacological and Parenteral Therapies, Dosage Calculation

---

2. 400 mL/hr

STEP 1: What is the unit of measurement the nurse should calculate?   mL/hr

STEP 2: What is the volume the nurse should infuse?   100 mL

STEP 3: What is the total infusion time?   15 min

STEP 4: Should the nurse convert the units of measurement?
No (mL = mL)
Yes (min ≠ hr)

$$\frac{60\ min}{15\ min} = \frac{1\ hr}{X\ hr}$$

$X = 0.25$

STEP 5: Set up an equation and solve for X.

$$\frac{Volume\ (mL)}{Time\ (hr)} = X\ mL/hr$$

$$\frac{100\ mL}{0.25\ hr} = X\ mL/hr$$

$400 = X$

STEP 6: Round, if necessary.

STEP 7: Reassess to determine whether the IV flow rate makes sense. If the prescription reads 100 mL to infuse over 15 min (0.25 hr), it makes sense to administer 400 mL/hr. The nurse should set the IV pump to deliver LR 100 mL IV at 400 mL/hr.

Ⓝ NCLEX® Connection: Pharmacological and Parenteral Therapies, Dosage Calculation

---

3. 83 gtt/min

Using Ratio and Proportion and Desired Over Have

STEP 1: What is the unit of measurement the nurse should calculate?   gtt/min

STEP 2: What is the quantity of the drop factor that is available?   10 gtt/mL

STEP 3: What is the volume the nurse should infuse?   250 mL

STEP 4: What is the total infusion time?   30 min

STEP 5: Should the nurse convert the units of measurement?   No

STEP 6: Set up an equation and solve for X.

$$\frac{Volume\ (mL)}{Time\ (min)} \times Drop\ factor\ (gtt/mL) = X$$

$$\frac{250\ mL}{30\ min} \times 10\ gtt/mL = X\ gtt/mL$$

$83.3333 = X$

STEP 7: Round, if necessary.   83.3333 = 83

STEP 8: Reassess to determine whether the IV flow rate makes sense. If the amount prescribed is 250 mL to infuse over 30 min, it makes sense to administer 83 gtt/min. The nurse should adjust the manual IV infusion to deliver 0.9% NaCl 250 mL at 83 gtt/min.

Ⓝ NCLEX® Connection: Pharmacological and Parenteral Therapies, Dosage Calculation

Using Dimensional Analysis

STEP 1: What is the unit of measurement to calculate?   gtt/min

STEP 2: What is the quantity of the drop factor that is available?   10 gtt/mL

STEP 3: What is the total infusion time?   30 min

STEP 4: What is the volume the nurse should infuse?   250 mL

STEP 5: Should the nurse convert the units of measurement?   No

STEP 6: Set up an equation and solve for X.

$$X = \frac{Quantity}{1\ mL} \times \frac{Conversion\ (Have)}{Conversion\ (Desired)} \times \frac{Volume}{Time}$$

$$X\ gtt/min = \frac{10\ gtt}{1\ mL} \times \frac{250\ mL}{30\ min}$$

$X = 83.3333$

STEP 7: Round, if necessary.   83.3333 = 83

STEP 8: Reassess to determine whether the IV flow rate makes sense. If the amount prescribed is 250 mL to infuse over 30 min, it makes sense to administer 83 gtt/min. The nurse should adjust the manual IV infusion to deliver 0.9% NaCl 250 mL at 83 gtt/min.

4. **2 tablets**

Using Ratio and Proportion	Using Desired Over Have	Using Dimensional Analysis

Using Ratio and Proportion

STEP 1: What is the unit of measurement the nurse should calculate? tablets

STEP 2: What is the dose the nurse should administer? Dose to administer = Desired = 200 mg

STEP 3: What is the dose available? Dose available = Have = 100 mg

STEP 4: Should the nurse convert the units of measurement? No

STEP 5: What is the quantity of the dose available? = Quantity = 1 tablet

STEP 6: Set up the equation and solve for X.

$$\frac{Have}{Quantity} = \frac{Desired}{X} \qquad \frac{100\ mg}{1\ tablet} \times \frac{200\ mg}{X\ tablets}$$

$X = 2$

STEP 7: Round, if necessary.

STEP 8: Reassess to determine whether the amount to administer makes sense. If there are 100 mg/tablet and the prescription reads 200 mg, it makes sense to administer 2 tablets. The nurse should administer metoprolol 2 tablets daily.

Using Desired Over Have

STEP 1: What is the unit of measurement the nurse should calculate? tablets

STEP 2: What is the dose the nurse should administer? Dose to administer = Desired = 200 mg

STEP 3: What is the dose available? Dose available = Have = 100 mg

STEP 4: Should the nurse convert the units of measurement? No

STEP 5: What is the quantity of the dose available? = Quantity = 1 tablet

STEP 6: Set up the equation and solve for X.

$$\frac{Desired \times Quantity}{Have} = X$$

$$\frac{200\ mg \times 1\ tablet}{100\ mg} = X\ tablets$$

$2 = X$

STEP 7: Round, if necessary.

STEP 8: Reassess to determine whether the amount to administer makes sense. If there are 100 mg/tablet and the prescription reads 200 mg, it makes sense to administer 2 tablets. The nurse should administer metoprolol 2 tablets daily.

Using Dimensional Analysis

STEP 1: What is the unit of measurement the nurse should calculate? tablets

STEP 2: What is the quantity of the dose available? = Quantity = 1 tablet

STEP 3: What is the dose available? Dose available = Have = 100 mg

STEP 4: What is the dose the nurse should administer? Dose to administer = Desired = 200 mg

STEP 5: Should the nurse convert the units of measurement? No

STEP 6: Set up the equation and solve for X.

$$X = \frac{Quantity}{Have} \times \frac{Conversion\ (Have)}{Conversion\ (Desired)} \times Desired$$

$$X\ tablets = \frac{1\ tablet}{100\ mg} \times 200\ mg$$

$X = 2$

STEP 7: Round, if necessary.

STEP 8: Reassess to determine whether the amount to administer makes sense. If there are 100 mg/tablet and the prescription reads 200 mg, it makes sense to administer 2 tablets. The nurse should administer metoprolol 2 tablets daily.

Ⓝ *NCLEX® Connection: Pharmacological and Parenteral Therapies, Dosage Calculation*

---

5. **0.5** mL

STEP 1: What is the unit of measurement the nurse should calculate? kg

STEP 2: Set up an equation and solve for X.

$$\frac{2.2\ lb}{1\ kg} = \frac{client's\ weight\ in\ lb}{X\ kg} \qquad \frac{2.2\ lb}{1\ kg} \times \frac{66\ lb}{X\ kg}$$

$X = 30$

STEP 3: Round, if necessary.

STEP 4: Reassess to determine whether the equivalent makes sense. If 1 kg = 2.2 lb, it makes sense that 66 lb = 30 kg.

STEP 5: What is the unit of measurement the nurse should calculate? mg

STEP 6: Set up an equation and solve for X.

$mg \times kg = X$

$0.5\ mg \times 30\ kg = 15\ mg$

$15 = X$

STEP 7: Round, if necessary.

STEP 8: Reassess to determine whether the amount makes sense. If the prescription reads 0.5 mg/kg every 6 hr and the school-age child weighs 30 kg, it makes sense to give 15 mg.

Using Ratio and Proportion

STEP 9: What is the unit of measurement the nurse should calculate? mL

STEP 10: What is the dose the nurse should administer? Dose to administer = Desired = 15 mg

STEP 11: What is the dose available? Dose available = Have = 30 mg

STEP 12: Should the nurse convert the units of measurement? No

STEP 13: What is the quantity of the dose available? = Quantity = 1 mL

STEP 14: Set up an equation and solve for X.

$$\frac{Have}{Quantity} = \frac{Desired}{X} \qquad \frac{30\ mg}{1\ mL} \times \frac{15\ mg}{X\ mL}$$

$X = 0.5$

STEP 15: Round, if necessary.

STEP 16: Reassess to determine whether the amount makes sense. If the prescription reads 0.5 mg/kg every 6 hr and the school-age child weighs 30 kg, it makes sense to give 15 mg. If there are 30 mg in 1 mL, it makes sense to give 0.5 mL. The nurse should give ketorolac 0.5 mL IV bolus every 6 hr.

Using Desired Over Have

STEP 9: What is the unit of measurement the nurse should calculate? mL

STEP 10: What is the dose the nurse should administer? Dose to administer = Desired = 15 mg

STEP 11: What is the dose available? Dose available = Have = 30 mg

STEP 12: Should the nurse convert the units of measurement? No

STEP 13: What is the quantity of the dose available? = Quantity = 1 mL

STEP 14: Set up an equation and solve for X.

$$\frac{Desired \times Quantity}{Have} = X \qquad \frac{15\ mg \times 1\ mL}{30\ mg} = X\ mL$$

$0.5 = X$

STEP 15: Round, if necessary.

STEP 16: Reassess to determine whether the amount makes sense. If the prescription reads 0.5 mg/kg every 6 hr and the school-age child weighs 30 kg, it makes sense to give 15 mg. If there are 30 mg in 1 mL, it makes sense to give 0.5 mL. The nurse should give ketorolac 0.5 mL IV bolus every 6 hr.

Using Dimensional Analysis

STEP 9: What is the unit of measurement the nurse should calculate? mL

STEP 10: What is the quantity of the dose available? = Quantity = 1 mL

STEP 11: What is the dose available? Dose available = Have = 30 mg

STEP 12: What is the dose the nurse should administer? Dose to administer = Desired = 15 mg

STEP 13: Should the nurse convert the units of measurement? No

STEP 14: Set up an equation and solve for X.

$$X = \frac{Quantity}{Have} \times \frac{Conversion\ (Have)}{Conversion\ (Desired)} \times Desired$$

$$X\ mL = \frac{1\ mL}{30\ mg} \times 15\ mg$$

$X = 0.5$

STEP 15: Round, if necessary.

STEP 16: Reassess to determine whether the amount makes sense. If the prescription reads 0.5 mg/kg every 6 hr and the school-age child weighs 30 kg, it makes sense to give 15 mg. If there are 30 mg in 1 mL, it makes sense to give 0.5 mL. The nurse should give ketorolac 0.5 mL IV bolus every 6 hr.

Ⓝ *NCLEX® Connection: Pharmacological and Parenteral Therapies, Dosage Calculation*

6. 100 mL/hr

STEP 1: What is the unit of measurement the nurse should calculate? mL/hr

STEP 2: What is the volume the nurse should infuse? 1,000 mL

STEP 3: What is the total infusion time? 10 hr

STEP 4: Should the nurse convert the units of measurement? No

STEP 5: Set up an equation and solve for X.

$$\frac{\text{Volume (mL)}}{\text{Time (hr)}} = X\,\text{mL/hr} \qquad \frac{1{,}000\ \text{mL}}{10\ \text{hr}} = X\,\text{mL/hr}$$

$$100 = X$$

STEP 6: Round, if necessary.

STEP 7: Reassess to determine whether the IV flow rate makes sense. If the prescription reads 1,000 mL to infuse over 10 hr, it makes sense to administer 100 mL/hr. The nurse should set the IV pump to deliver D₅W 1,000 mL IV at 100 mL/hr.

(N) *NCLEX® Connection: Pharmacological and Parenteral Therapies, Dosage Calculation*

---

7. 10 mL

Using Ratio and Proportion

STEP 1: What is the unit of measurement the nurse should calculate? mL

STEP 2: What is the dose the nurse should administer? Dose to administer = Desired = 320 mg

STEP 3: What is the dose available? Dose available = Have = 160 mg

STEP 4: Should the nurse convert the units of measurement? No

STEP 5: What is the quantity of the dose available? = Quantity = 5 mL

STEP 6: Set up the equation and solve for X.

$$\frac{\text{Have}}{\text{Quantity}} = \frac{\text{Desired}}{X}$$

$$\frac{160\ \text{mg}}{5\ \text{mL}} \times \frac{320\ \text{mg}}{X\ \text{mL}}$$

$$X = 10$$

STEP 7: Round, if necessary.

STEP 8: Reassess to determine whether the amount to administer makes sense. If there are 160 mg/5 mL and the prescription reads 320 mg, it makes sense to administer 10 mL. The nurse should administer acetaminophen liquid 10 mL PO every 4 hr PRN for pain.

Using Desired Over Have

STEP 1: What is the unit of measurement the nurse should calculate? mL

STEP 2: What is the dose the nurse should administer? Dose to administer = Desired = 320 mg

STEP 3: What is the dose available? Dose available = Have = 160 mg

STEP 4: Should the nurse convert the units of measurement? No

STEP 5: What is the quantity of the dose available? = Quantity = 5 mL

STEP 6: Set up the equation and solve for X.

$$\frac{\text{Desired} \times \text{Quantity}}{\text{Have}} = X$$

$$\frac{320\ \text{mg} \times 5\ \text{mL}}{160\ \text{mg}} = X\,\text{mL}$$

$$10 = X$$

STEP 7: Round, if necessary.

STEP 8: Reassess to determine whether the amount to administer makes sense. If there are 160 mg/5 mL and the prescription reads 320 mg, it makes sense to administer 10 mL. The nurse should administer acetaminophen liquid 10 mL PO every 4 hr PRN for pain.

Using Dimensional Analysis

STEP 1: What is the unit of measurement the nurse should calculate? mL

STEP 2: What is the quantity of the dose available? = Quantity = 5 mL

STEP 3: What is the dose available? Dose available = Have = 160 mg

STEP 4: What is the dose the nurse should administer? Dose to administer = Desired = 320 mg

STEP 5: Should the nurse convert the units of measurement? No

STEP 6: Set up the equation and solve for X.

$$X = \frac{\text{Quantity}}{\text{Have}} \times \frac{\text{Conversion (Have)}}{\text{Conversion (Desired)}} \times \text{Desired}$$

$$X\,\text{mL} = \frac{5\ \text{mL}}{160\ \text{mg}} \times 320\ \text{mg}$$

$$X = 10$$

STEP 7: Round, if necessary.

STEP 8: Reassess to determine whether the amount to administer makes sense. If there are 160 mg/5 mL and the prescription reads 320 mg, it makes sense to administer 10 mL. The nurse should administer acetaminophen liquid 10 mL PO every 4 hr PRN for pain.

(N) *NCLEX® Connection: Pharmacological and Parenteral Therapies, Dosage Calculation*

---

8. 42 gtt/min

Using Ratio and Proportion and Desired Over Have

STEP 1: What is the unit of measurement the nurse should calculate? gtt/min

STEP 2: What is the quantity of the drop factor that is available? 15 gtt/mL

STEP 3: What is the volume the nurse should infuse? 1,000 mL

STEP 4: What is the total infusion time? 6 hr

STEP 5: Should the nurse convert the units of measurement? No (mL = mL) Yes (hr ≠ min)

$$\frac{1\ \text{hr}}{60\ \text{min}} = \frac{6\ \text{hr}}{X\ \text{hr}}$$

$$X = 360\ \text{min}$$

STEP 6: Set up an equation and solve for X.

$$\frac{\text{Volume (mL)}}{\text{Time (min)}} \times \text{Drop factor (gtt/mL)} = X$$

$$\frac{1{,}000\ \text{mL}}{360\ \text{min}} \times 15\ \text{gtt/mL} = X\,\text{gtt/mL}$$

$$41.6666 = X$$

STEP 7: Round, if necessary. 41.6666 = 42

STEP 8: Reassess to determine whether the IV flow rate makes sense. If the amount prescribed is 1,000 mL to infuse over 6 hr (360 min), it makes sense to administer 42 gtt/min. The nurse should adjust the manual IV infusion to deliver D₅LR 1,000 mL at 42 gtt/min.

Using Dimensional Analysis

STEP 1: What is the unit of measurement to calculate? gtt/min

STEP 2: What is the quantity of the drop factor that is available? 15 gtt/mL

STEP 3: What is the total infusion time? 6 hr

STEP 4: What is the volume the nurse should infuse? 1,000 mL

STEP 5: Should the nurse convert the units of measurement? No (mL = mL) Yes (hr ≠ min)

$$\frac{1\ \text{hr}}{60\ \text{min}} = \frac{6\ \text{hr}}{X\ \text{hr}}$$

$$X = 360\ \text{min}$$

STEP 6: Set up an equation and solve for X.

$$X = \frac{\text{Quantity}}{1\ \text{mL}} \times \frac{\text{Conversion (Have)}}{\text{Conversion (Desired)}} \times \frac{\text{Volume}}{\text{Time}}$$

$$X\,\text{gtt/min} = \frac{15\ \text{gtt}}{1\ \text{mL}} \times \frac{1\ \text{hr}}{60\ \text{min}} \times \frac{1{,}000\ \text{mL}}{6\ \text{hr}}$$

$$X = 41.6666$$

STEP 7: Round, if necessary. 41.6666 = 42

STEP 8: Reassess to determine whether the IV flow rate makes sense. If the amount prescribed is 1,000 mL to infuse over 6 hr (360 min), it makes sense to administer 42 gtt/min. The nurse should adjust the manual IV infusion to deliver D₅LR 1,000 mL at 42 gtt/min.

(N) *NCLEX® Connection: Pharmacological and Parenteral Therapies, Dosage Calculation*

UNIT 4   PHYSIOLOGICAL INTEGRITY

SECTION: PHARMACOLOGICAL AND PARENTERAL THERAPIES

CHAPTER 49 *Intravenous Therapy*

Intravenous (IV) therapy involves infusing fluids via an IV catheter to administer medications, supplement fluid intake, or provide fluid replacement, electrolytes, or nutrients.

Nurses administer large-volume IV infusions, as well as IV boluses, usually in a small amount of fluid. Nurses or pharmacists mix IV medication in a large volume of fluid to give as a continuous IV infusion or intermittently in a small amount of fluid.

PROCEDURE

- The provider prescribes the type of IV fluid, the volume to infuse, and either the rate at which to infuse the IV fluid or the total amount of time it should take to infuse the fluid. The nurse regulates the IV infusion, either with an IV pump or manually, to be sure to deliver the right amount.
- Nurses administer large-volume IV infusions on a continuous basis, such as 0.9% sodium chloride IV to infuse at 100 mL/hr or 0.9% sodium chloride 500 mL to give IV over 3 hr.
- A fluid bolus is a large amount of IV fluid to give in a short time, usually less than 1 hr. A fluid bolus rapidly replaces fluid loss from dehydration, shock, hemorrhage, burns, or trauma. A large-gauge catheter (18-gauge or larger) is essential for maintaining the rapid rate necessary to give a fluid bolus to an adult.
- Nurses administer medications as an IV bolus, giving the medication in a small amount of solution, concentrated or diluted, and injecting it over a short time (1 to 2 min).

ADVANTAGES

- Rapid absorption and onset of action
- Constant therapeutic blood levels
- Less irritation to subcutaneous and muscle tissue

DISADVANTAGES

- Circulatory fluid overload is possible if the volume of solution is large or the infusion rate is rapid.
- Immediate absorption leaves little time to correct errors.
- Solutions and IV catheters can irritate the lining of the vein.
- Failure to maintain surgical asepsis can lead to local and systemic infection.

CONSIDERATIONS

NURSING ACTIONS

Nurses administer IV medication infusions in the following ways.

- Giving the medication the pharmacist mixed in a large volume of fluid (500 to 1,000 mL) as a continuous IV infusion, such as potassium chloride and vitamins
- Delivering the medication in premixed solution bags from the medication's manufacturer

Administering volume-controlled infusions

- Giving some medications, such as antibiotics, intermittently in a small amount of solution (25 to 250 mL) through a continuous IV fluid system or with saline or heparin lock systems
- Infusing the medications for short periods of time and on a schedule
- Using a secondary ("piggyback") IV bag or bottle or tandem setup, a volume-control administration set, or a mini-infusion pump

Giving an IV bolus dose

- Injecting the medications in small amounts of solution, concentrated or diluted, over a short time (1 to 2 min)
- Administering medications directly into the peripheral IV or access port to achieve an immediate medication level in the bloodstream, such as with pain medication
- Preparing medications in the correct concentration and at a safe rate (amount of medication per minute)
- Using extreme caution and observing for adverse reactions or complications such as redness, burning, or increasing pain

Older adult clients, clients taking anticoagulants, or clients who have fragile veins Ⓒ

- Avoid tourniquets.
- Use a blood pressure cuff instead.
- Do not slap the extremity to visualize veins.
- Avoid rigorous friction while cleaning the site.

Edema in extremities

- Apply digital pressure over the selected vein to displace edema.
- Apply pressure with a swab of cleaning solution.
- Cannulate the vein quickly.

Clients who are obese

Use anatomical landmarks to find veins.

PREPROCEDURE

EQUIPMENT

- IV start kit if available: Tourniquet, sterile drape, antiseptic swabs, transparent dressing, small roll of sterile tape, 2x2 or 4x4 gauze sponges, and safety positioning device.
- Correct size catheter
  - 16-gauge for clients who have trauma, rapid fluid volume
  - 18- to 20-gauge for clients who are having surgery, rapid blood administration
  - 22- to 24-gauge for other clients (children, adults)
- Tubing
- Prefilled syringe containing 1 to 3 mL of 0.9% sodium chloride solution
- Infusion pump
- Clean gloves
- Scissors or electric shaver for hair removal

NURSING ACTIONS

- Check the prescription (solution, rate).
- Identify allergies to latex or tape.
- Follow the rights of medication administration.
- Check compatibilities of IV solutions and medications.
- Perform hand hygiene.
- Examine the IV solution for clarity, leaks, and expiration date.
- Don clean gloves.
- Evaluate extremities and veins. Clip hair at and around the insertion site with scissors. Do not shave the area because an abrasion can occur, increasing the risk of infection.

CLIENT EDUCATION

- Identify the client and explain the procedure.
- Place the client in a comfortable position.

INTRAPROCEDURE

NURSING ACTIONS

- Apply a clean tourniquet or blood pressure cuff (especially for older adults) 10 to 15 cm (4 to 6 in) above the insertion site to compress only venous blood flow.
- Select the vein by using visualization, gravity, fist clenching, friction with the cleaning solution, or heat and choose
  - Distal veins first on the nondominant hand
  - A site that is not painful or bruised and will not interfere with activity
  - A vein that is resilient with a soft, bouncy sensation on palpation
  - Avoid the following.
    - Varicose veins that are permanently dilated and tortuous
    - Veins in the inner wrist with bifurcations, in flexion areas, near valves (appearing as bumps), in lower extremities, and in the antecubital fossa (except for emergency access)
    - Veins in the back of the hand
    - Veins that are sclerosed or hard
    - Veins in an extremity with impaired sensitivity (scar tissue, paralysis), lymph nodes removed, recent infiltration, a PICC line, or an arteriovenous fistula or graft
    - Veins that had previous venipunctures

- Untie the tourniquet or deflate the blood pressure cuff.
- Cleanse the area at the site using friction in a circular motion from the middle and outwardly with chlorhexidine or the cleaning agent the facility's protocol specifies. Allow it to air dry for 1 to 2 min.
- Remove the cover from the catheter, grasp the plastic hub, and examine the device for smooth edges.
- Retie the tourniquet or reinflate the blood pressure cuff.
- Anchor the vein below the site of insertion.
- Pull the skin taut and hold it.
- Warn the client of a sharp, quick stick.
- Use a steady, smooth motion to insert the catheter into the skin at an angle of 10° to 30° with the bevel up.
- Advance the catheter through the skin and into the vein, maintaining a 10° to 30° angle. A flashback of blood will confirm placement in the vein.
- Lower the hub of the catheter close to the skin to prepare for threading it into the vein approximately 0.6 cm (0.24 in).
- Loosen the needle from the catheter and pull back slightly on the needle so that it no longer extends past the tip of the catheter.
- Use the thumb and index finger to advance the catheter into the vein until the hub rests against the insertion site.
- Stabilize the IV catheter with one hand and release the tourniquet or blood pressure cuff with the other.
- Apply pressure approximately 3 cm (1.2 in) above the insertion site with the middle finger and stabilize the catheter with the index finger.
- Remove the needle and activate the safety device.
- Maintain pressure above the IV site and connect the appropriate equipment to the hub of the IV catheter.
- Apply a dressing and leave it in place until catheter removal, unless it becomes damp, loose, or soiled.
- Avoid encircling the entire extremity with tape and taping under the sterile dressing.
- For a continuous IV infusion, regulate the infusion rate according to the prescription.
- Dispose of used equipment and supplies.
- Document the following in the medical record.
  - The date and time of insertion
  - The insertion site and appearance
  - The catheter's size
  - The type of dressing
  - The IV fluid and rate
  - The number, locations, and conditions of previously attempted catheterizations
  - The client's response

Sample documentation: 6/1/20XX, 1635, Inserted #22-gauge IV catheter into left wrist cephalic vein (one attempt); applied sterile occlusive dressing. IV dextrose 5% in lactated Ringer's infusing at 100 mL/hr per infusion pump without redness or edema at the site. Tolerated without complications. S. Velez, RN

POSTPROCEDURE

NURSING ACTIONS

- **Maintaining the patency of IV access**
  - Do not stop a continuous infusion or allow blood to back up into the catheter for any length of time. Clots can form at the tip of the needle or catheter and lodge against the vein's wall, blocking the flow of fluid.
  - Instruct clients not to manipulate the flow rate device, change the settings on the IV pump, or lie on the tubing.
  - Make sure the IV insertion site's dressing is not too tight.
  - Flush intermittent IV catheters with the appropriate solution after every medication administration or every 8 to 12 hr when not in use, according to the facility's policy.
  - Monitor the site and infusion rate at least every hour.
- **Discontinuing IV therapy**
  - Check the prescription.
  - Prepare the equipment.
  - Perform hand hygiene.
  - Don clean gloves.
  - Clamp the IV tubing.
  - Remove the tape and dressing, stabilizing the IV catheter.
  - Apply a sterile gauze pad over the site without putting pressure on the vein. Do not use alcohol.
  - Using the other hand, withdraw the catheter by pulling it straight back from the site, keeping the hub parallel to the skin.
  - Elevate the extremity and apply pressure for 2 to 3 min and until bleeding stops.
  - Examine the site.
  - Apply tape over the gauze.
  - Use a pressure dressing, if necessary.
  - Check the catheter for intactness.
  - Dispose of the catheter in the designated puncture-resistant receptacle, and the IV solution and equipment in the appropriate location.
  - Document.

TYPES OF IV ACCESS

- Peripheral vein via a catheter
- Jugular or subclavian vein via a central venous access device

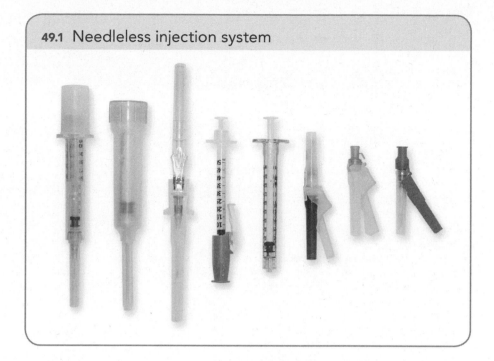

49.1 Needleless injection system

GUIDELINES FOR SAFE IV MEDICATION ADMINISTRATION

- Use an infusion pump to administer medications that can cause serious adverse reactions, such as potassium chloride. Never administer them by IV bolus.
- Never administer IV medications through tubing that is infusing blood, blood products, or parenteral nutrition solutions.
- Verify the compatibility of medications with IV solutions before infusing a medication through tubing that is infusing another medication or IV fluid.

NEEDLESTICK PREVENTION Qs

- Be familiar with IV insertion equipment.
- Do not use needles when needleless systems are available. **(49.1)**
- Use protective safety devices when available.
- Dispose of needles immediately in designated puncture-resistant receptacles.
- Do not break, bend, or recap needles.

PREVENTING IV INFECTIONS Q_s

- Perform hand hygiene before and after handling IV systems.
- Use standard precautions.
- Change IV sites according to the facility's policy (usually every 72 hr).
- Replacement of the administration set is dependent upon the type of infusion. Administration sets with a continuous infusion of fluids with or without secondary fluids should be changed every 96 hr. Intermittent infusions should be changed every 24 hr. Some products—such as blood or medications such as propofol—should be changed more frequently, according to facility policy.
- Remove catheters as soon as there is no clinical need for them.
- Replace catheters when suspecting any break in surgical aseptic technique, such as during emergency insertions.
- Use a sterile needle or catheter for each insertion attempt.
- Avoid writing on IV bags with pens or markers, because ink can contaminate the solution.
- Change tubing immediately for potential contamination.
- Do not allow fluids to hang for more than 24 hr unless it is a closed system (pressure bags for hemodynamic monitoring).
- Wipe all ports with alcohol or an antiseptic swab before connecting IV lines or inserting a syringe to prevent the introduction of micro-organisms into the system.
- Never disconnect tubing for convenience or to reposition the client.

COMPLICATIONS

Complications require notification of the provider and documentation. Use new tubing and catheters for restarting IV infusions after detecting complications.

Infiltration or extravasation

Pallor, local swelling at the site, decreased skin temperature around the site, damp dressing, slowed rate of infusion

TREATMENT
- Stop the infusion and remove the catheter.
- Elevate the extremity.
- Encourage active range of motion.
- Apply a warm or cold compress depending on the solution infusing.
- Restart the infusion proximal to the site or in another extremity.

PREVENTION
- Carefully select the site and catheter.
- Secure the catheter.

Phlebitis or thrombophlebitis

Edema; throbbing, burning, or pain at the site; increased skin temperature; erythema; a red line up the arm with a palpable band at the vein site; slowed rate of infusion

TREATMENT
- Promptly discontinue the infusion and remove the catheter.
- Elevate the extremity.
- Apply warm compresses three to four times/day.
- Restart the infusion in a different vein proximal to the site or in another extremity.
- Obtain a specimen for culture at the site and prepare the catheter for culture if drainage is present.

PREVENTION
- Rotate sites at least every 72 hr or sooner according to the facility's policy.
- Avoid the lower extremities.
- Use hand hygiene.
- Use surgical aseptic technique.

Hematoma

Ecchymosis at the site

TREATMENT
- Do not apply alcohol.
- Apply pressure after IV catheter removal.
- Use a warm compress and elevation after the bleeding stops.

PREVENTION
- Minimize tourniquet time.
- Remove the tourniquet before starting the IV infusion.
- Maintain pressure after IV catheter removal.

Fluid overload

Distended neck veins, increased blood pressure, tachycardia, shortness of breath, crackles in the lungs, edema, additional findings varying with the IV solution

TREATMENT
- Stop the infusion.
- Raise the head of the bed.
- Measure vital signs and oxygen saturation.
- Adjust the rate after correcting fluid overload.
- Administer diuretics.

PREVENTION
- Use an infusion pump.
- Monitor I&O.

Cellulitis

Pain, warmth, edema, induration, red streaking, fever, chills, malaise

TREATMENT
- Discontinue the infusion and remove the catheter.
- Elevate the extremity.
- Apply warm compresses three to four times/day.
- Obtain a specimen for culture at the site and prepare the catheter for culture if drainage is present.
- Administer the following.
  - Antibiotics
  - Analgesics
  - Antipyretics

PREVENTION
- Rotate sites at least every 72 hr.
- Avoid the lower extremities.
- Use hand hygiene.
- Use surgical aseptic technique.

Catheter embolus

Missing catheter tip on removal, severe pain at the site with migration, absence of findings if no migration

TREATMENT
- Place a tourniquet high on the extremity to limit venous flow.
- Prepare for removal under x-ray or via surgery.
- Save the catheter after removal to determine the cause.

PREVENTION: Do not reinsert the stylet into the catheter.

PRACTICE Active Learning Scenario

A nurse has inserted an IV catheter for a client who requires IV rehydration. What information should the nurse document in the client's medical record? Use the ATI Active Learning Template: Basic Concept to complete this item.

RELATED CONTENT: List the seven components of documentation following insertion of an IV catheter.

Application Exercises

1. A nurse is demonstrating how to insert an IV catheter. Which of the following statements by a nurse viewing the demonstration indicates understanding of the procedure?

   A. "I will thread the needle all the way into the vein until the hub rests against the insertion site after I see a flashback of blood."

   B. "I will insert the needle into the client's skin at an angle of 10 to 30 degrees with the bevel up."

   C. "I will apply pressure approximately 1.2 inches below the insertion site prior to removing the needle."

   D. "I will choose a vein in the antecubital fossa for IV insertion due to its size and easily accessible location."

2. A nurse is collecting data from a client who is receiving IV therapy and reports pain in his arm, chills, and "not feeling well." The nurse notes warmth, edema, induration, and red streaking on the client's arm close to the IV insertion site. Which of the following actions should the nurse plan to take first?

   A. Obtain a specimen for culture.

   B. Apply a warm compress.

   C. Administer analgesics.

   D. Discontinue the infusion.

3. During new employee orientation, a nurse is explaining how to prevent IV infections. Which of the following statements by an orientee indicates understanding of the preventive strategies?

   A. "I will leave the IV catheter in place after the client completes the course of IV antibiotics."

   B. "As long as I am working with the same client, I can use the same IV catheter for my second insertion attempt."

   C. "If my client needs to use the rest room, it would be safer to disconnect his IV infusion as long as I clean the injection port thoroughly with an antiseptic swab."

   D. "I will replace any IV catheter when I suspect contamination during insertion."

4. A nurse on the IV team is conducting an in-service education program about the complications of IV therapy. Which of the following statements by an attendee indicates an understanding of the manifestations of infiltration? (Select all that apply.)

   A. "The temperature around the IV site is cooler."

   B. "The rate of the infusion increases."

   C. "The skin at the IV site is red."

   D. "The IV dressing is damp."

   E. "The tissue around the venipuncture site is swollen."

5. A nurse is caring for a client receiving dextrose 5% in 0.9% sodium chloride IV at 120 mL/hr. Which of the following statements by the client should alert the nurse to suspect fluid overload? (Select all that apply.)

   A. "I feel lightheaded."

   B. "I feel as though my heart is racing."

   C. "I feel a little short of breath."

   D. "The nurse technician told me that my blood pressure was 150 over 90."

   E. "I think my ankles are less swollen."

Application Exercises Key

1. A. After seeing a flashback of blood, the nurse should lower the hub close to the skin to prepare for threading the needle into the vein, then loosen the needle from the catheter and pull back slightly on the needle so that it no longer extends past the tip of the catheter. The nurse should use the thumb and index finger to advance the catheter into the vein until the hub rests against the insertion site. Inserting the needle all the way into the vein could puncture the vein.

    B. **CORRECT:** The nurse should use a smooth, steady motion to insert the catheter through the skin at an angle of 10° to 30° with the bevel up. This is the optimal angle for preventing the puncture of the posterior wall of the vein.

    C. The nurse should apply pressure approximately 3 cm (1.2 in) above the insertion site to reduce the backflow of blood into the vein prior to removing the needle.

    D. The nurse should not use a vein in the antecubital fossa for IV insertion, except for emergency access, because it will limit the mobility of the client's arm.

    Ⓝ *NCLEX® Connection: Pharmacological and Parenteral Therapies, Parenteral/Intravenous Therapies*

2. A. The nurse should obtain a specimen for culture to identify pathogens causing infection. However, another action is the priority.

    B. The nurse should apply a warm compress to promote healing and comfort. However, another action is the priority.

    C. The nurse should administer analgesics to promote comfort. However, another action is the priority.

    D. **CORRECT:** The greatest risk to this client is injury from infection. The first action the nurse should take is to stop the infusion and remove the catheter because the catheter might be the source of infection.

    Ⓝ *NCLEX® Connection: Pharmacological and Parenteral Therapies, Medication Administration*

3. A. Nurses should remove catheters as soon as they are no longer clinically necessary to eliminate a portal of entry for pathogens.

    B. Nurses should use a sterile needle or catheter for each insertion attempt for safety and prevention of infection.

    C. Nurses should not disconnect tubing for convenience, because this increases the risk of bacteria entering the system.

    D. **CORRECT:** Nurses should replace IV catheters when suspecting any break in surgical aseptic technique, such as in emergency insertions.

    Ⓝ *NCLEX® Connection: Pharmacological and Parenteral Therapies, Medication Administration*

4. A. **CORRECT:** A decrease in skin temperature around the site is a manifestation of infiltration due to the IV solution entering the subcutaneous tissue around the venipuncture site.

    B. When infiltration occurs, the rate of infusion can slow or stop, not increase, as the solution is no longer infusing directly into the vein. This occurs due to dislodgement of the catheter or rupture of the vein.

    C. When infiltration occurs, the skin around the IV site is pale, not red, because the solution is no longer infusing directly into the vein and enters the subcutaneous tissue around the venipuncture site.

    D. **CORRECT:** A damp IV dressing is a common finding with infiltration due to the IV solution entering the subcutaneous tissue and leaking out through the venipuncture site.

    E. **CORRECT:** Swollen tissue around the venipuncture site is a manifestation of infiltration due to the IV solution entering the subcutaneous tissue and causing swelling, as the fluid is no longer infusing into the vein.

    Ⓝ *NCLEX® Connection: Pharmacological and Parenteral Therapies, Medication Administration*

5. A. A manifestation of fluid overload is hypertension. Lightheadedness is a manifestation of hypotension.

    B. **CORRECT:** A manifestation of fluid overload is tachycardia due to the increased blood volume, which causes the heart rate to increase.

    C. **CORRECT:** A manifestation of fluid overload is shortness of breath or dyspnea due to the increased amount of fluid entering the air spaces in the lungs, which reduces the amount of circulating oxygen.

    D. **CORRECT:** A manifestation of fluid overload is hypertension due to the increased blood volume, which causes the blood pressure to increase.

    E. A manifestation of fluid overload is edema. If the client's ankles are less swollen, this is an indication that the edema and the fluid overload are resolving.

    Ⓝ *NCLEX® Connection: Physiological Adaptation, Fluid and Electrolyte Imbalances*

PRACTICE Answer

Using the ATI Active Learning Template: Basic Concept

RELATED CONTENT

- Date and time of insertion
- Insertion site and appearance
- Catheter's size
- Type of dressing
- IV fluid and rate
- The number, locations, and conditions of previously attempted catheterizations
- Client's response

Ⓝ *NCLEX® Connection: Pharmacological and Parenteral Therapies, Parenteral/Intravenous Therapies*

CHAPTER 50   # Adverse Effects, Interactions, and Contraindications

To ensure safe medication administration and prevent errors, nurses must know the therapeutic effect, potential adverse effects, interactions, contraindications, and precautions for each medication they administer.

Every medication has the potential to cause adverse effects. These are undesired, inadvertent, and harmful effects of the medication. Adverse effects can range from mild to severe, and some can be life-threatening.

Medications are chemicals that affect the body. With concurrent use of medications, there is a potential for an interaction. Medications can also interact with foods and dietary supplements.

Contraindications and precautions for specific medications are conditions (diseases, age, pregnancy, lactation) that make it risky or completely unsafe for clients to take them.

Anticipation of adverse effects, interactions, contraindications, and precautions is an important component of client education. Both the nurse and the client should know the major adverse effects a medication can cause. Early identification of adverse effects allows for timely intervention to minimize harm.

ADVERSE EFFECTS

Central nervous system effects

From either central nervous system (CNS) stimulation (excitement) or CNS depression

NURSING CONSIDERATIONS
- Implement seizure precautions for CNS stimulation.
- For CNS depression, advise clients not to drive or participate in other dangerous activities.

Extrapyramidal symptoms

- Abnormal body movements: tremors, rigidity, restlessness, acute dystonia (spastic movements of the back, neck, tongue, and face), drooling, agitation, shuffling gait
- These can take a few hours or months to develop.

NURSING CONSIDERATIONS
- More common with medications affecting the CNS, such as those that treat mental health disorders.
- Keep clients safe when movements and balance are uncontrollable.

Anticholinergic effects

Result from muscarinic receptor blockade and affect the eye, smooth muscle tone, exocrine glands, and heart

NURSING CONSIDERATIONS
- Have clients sip fluids to relieve dry mouth.
- Tell clients to wear sunglasses outdoors to prevent photophobia.
- Suggest that clients urinate before taking the medication to lessen urinary retention.
- To prevent constipation, instruct clients to increase dietary fiber and fluids and to increase exercise.
- Remind clients to avoid activities that could lead to overheating, because adverse effects include a decrease in sweat.

Cardiovascular effects

- Involve blood vessels and the heart
- Antihypertensives can cause orthostatic hypotension.

NURSING CONSIDERATIONS: To relieve and prevent postural hypotension (lightheadedness, dizziness), instruct clients to sit or lie down and to get up and change positions slowly.

Gastrointestinal effects

From local irritation of the gastrointestinal (GI) tract, stimulation of the vomiting center, or stimulation or slowing of bowel motility

NURSING CONSIDERATIONS
- Many medications, such as NSAIDs, cause GI distress.
- Tell clients to try taking the medication with food and to notify the provider about consistent GI effects.

Hematologic effects

Relatively common and potentially life-threatening

NURSING CONSIDERATIONS
- Bone marrow depression can result from anticancer medications and hemorrhagic disorders from anticoagulants and thrombolytics.
- Instruct clients taking an anticoagulant to report bruising, discolored urine or stool, petechiae, and bleeding gums to the provider immediately.

Hepatotoxicity

Because metabolism of most medications takes place in the liver, the liver is particularly vulnerable to medication-induced injury. Damage to liver cells can impair medication metabolism and cause accumulation in the body or alter results of liver function tests with no obvious manifestations of liver dysfunction.

NURSING CONSIDERATIONS
- When combining two or more medications that are hepatotoxic, the risk for liver damage increases.
- Liver function tests are essential when a client starts taking a hepatotoxic medication and periodically thereafter.

Nephrotoxicity

- Primarily the result of antimicrobial agents and NSAIDs
- Impaired kidney function can interfere with medication excretion, leading to accumulation and adverse effects.

NURSING CONSIDERATIONS
- Aminoglycosides can cause kidney damage.
- Monitor serum creatinine and BUN levels of clients taking nephrotoxic medications.

Toxicity

Severe and potentially life-threatening effects from excessive dosing, but can also occur at therapeutic dose levels.

NURSING CONSIDERATIONS
- An overdose of acetaminophen can result in hepatotoxicity, which can lead to liver damage.
- The antidote acetylcysteine minimizes liver damage due to acetaminophen toxicity.
- There is a greater risk of toxicity and liver damage with chronic alcohol use.
- Liver damage from disease states can delay or prevent medication metabolism.

Allergic reaction

An immune response to a medication after previous exposure, causing antibody formation

NURSING CONSIDERATIONS
- Allergic reactions range from minor to serious. Diphenhydramine treats mild rashes and hives.
- Before administering any medications, obtain a complete medication and allergy history.

Anaphylactic reaction

A life-threatening immediate allergic reaction that causes respiratory distress, severe bronchospasm, and cardiovascular collapse

NURSING CONSIDERATIONS
- Treat anaphylaxis with epinephrine, bronchodilators, and antihistamines.
- Provide respiratory support and notify the provider.

Immunosuppression

A decreased or absent immune response

NURSING CONSIDERATIONS
- Glucocorticoids depress the immune response and increase the risk for infection.
- Monitor for indications of infection.

50.1 Over-the-counter medication interactions

Interactions	NURSING INTERVENTIONS
Ingredients in OTC medications can interact with other OTC or prescription medications.	Obtain a complete medication history that includes both prescription and OTC medications.
Inactive ingredients such as dyes, alcohol, and preservatives can cause adverse reactions.	Instruct clients to follow the manufacturer's recommendations for dosage.
The potential for overdose exists with the use of several preparations (including prescription medications) that have similar ingredients.	Obtain a history of herbal and other dietary supplements.

Interactions	NURSING INTERVENTIONS
Interactions of some prescription and OTC medications can interfere with therapeutic effects.	Advise clients to use caution and to check with their provider before using any OTC preparations such as antacids, laxatives, decongestants, and cough syrups. For example, antacids can interfere with the absorption of ranitidine and other medications. Tell clients to take antacids at least 1 hr apart from other medications

MEDICATION-MEDICATION INTERACTIONS

Increased therapeutic effects

NURSING CONSIDERATIONS: Taking some medications together can increase their therapeutic effect. For example, clients who have asthma inhale albuterol, a beta$_2$ adrenergic agonist, 5 min prior to inhaling fluticasone, a glucocorticoid, to increase the absorption of fluticasone.

Increased adverse effects

NURSING CONSIDERATIONS: Taking two medications that have the same adverse effects together increases the risk of or worsens these adverse effects. Diazepam and hydrocodone with acetaminophen both have CNS depressant effects. The risk increases when clients take both concurrently.

Decreased therapeutic effects

NURSING CONSIDERATIONS: One medication can increase the metabolism of another medication and therefore decrease the serum level and effectiveness of that medication. Phenytoin increases hepatic medication-metabolizing enzymes that affect warfarin and thereby decreases the serum level and the therapeutic effect of warfarin.

Decreased adverse effects

NURSING CONSIDERATIONS: One medication can counteract the adverse effects of another medication. Ondansetron, an antiemetic, counteracts the adverse effects of nausea and vomiting that result from chemotherapy.

Increased serum levels, leading to toxicity

NURSING CONSIDERATIONS: One medication can decrease the metabolism of a second medication and therefore increase the serum level of the second medication and lead to toxicity. Fluconazole, an antifungal, inhibits hepatic medication-metabolizing enzymes that affect aripiprazole, an antipsychotic, and thereby increases serum levels of aripiprazole.

MEDICATION-FOOD INTERACTIONS

Food can alter medication absorption and can contain substances that react with some medications.

Tyramine

Consuming foods that contain tyramine (avocados, figs, aged cheese, yeast extracts, beer, smoked meats) while taking monoamine oxidase inhibitors (MAOIs) can lead to hypertensive crisis.

NURSING CONSIDERATIONS: Tell clients taking an MAOI to avoid these foods. Q EBP

Vitamin K

Vitamin K can decrease the therapeutic effects of warfarin and put clients at risk for developing blood clots.

NURSING CONSIDERATIONS: Clients taking warfarin should maintain a consistent intake of dietary vitamin K to avoid sudden fluctuations that could affect the action of warfarin.

Dairy

Tetracycline can interact with a chelating agent such as milk to form an insoluble, unabsorbable compound.

NURSING CONSIDERATIONS: Instruct clients not to take tetracycline within 2 hr of consuming any dairy products.

Grapefruit juice

Grapefruit juice seems to act by inhibiting presystemic medication metabolism in the small bowel, thus increasing the absorption of some oral medications such as nifedipine, a calcium channel blocker. This combination can result in increased effects or intensified adverse reactions.

NURSING CONSIDERATIONS: Instruct clients not to drink grapefruit juice if they are taking a medication it affects.

Caffeine

Theophylline, a methylxanthine for asthma control, and caffeine can result in excessive CNS excitation.

NURSING CONSIDERATIONS: Instruct clients taking this medication to avoid beverages containing caffeine.

Antacids, vitamin C

Taking aluminum-containing antacids with citrus beverages can result in excessive absorption of aluminum.

NURSING CONSIDERATIONS: Tell clients taking antacids to avoid taking vitamin C supplements or drinking citrus juices.

CONTRAINDICATIONS AND PRECAUTIONS

- Take extra precautions for clients who are at greater risk for developing an adverse reaction to a medication. For example, morphine depresses respiratory function, so asthma and respiratory dysfunction require precautions with the use of morphine. Qs
- Contraindications for specific medications relate to clients' physical status, health, and allergy history. For example, an allergy to any medication is a contraindication for taking that medication. Pregnancy or health conditions such as kidney disease are also contraindications for many medications.

PREGNANCY RISK CATEGORIES

The U.S. Food and Drug Administration (FDA) places medications in categories according to the risks they pose to a fetus.

Category A: There is no evidence of risk to a fetus from taking the medication during pregnancy, according to adequate and well-controlled studies. Ferrous sulfate, an iron supplement, is a Category A medication.

Category B: There is no evidence of risk to an animal fetus according to studies, but there are no adequate and well-controlled studies of pregnant women. Or, there is evidence of risk to an animal fetus, but controlled studies of pregnant women show no evidence of risk to the fetus. Esomeprazole, an antiulcer medication, is in Category B.

Category C: Studies have demonstrated adverse effects on animal fetuses, but there are no adequate and well-controlled studies of pregnant women. Or, there have not been any studies of animals or pregnant women. Glipizide, an antidiabetic medication, is in Category C.

Category D: Studies have demonstrated adverse effects on human fetuses according to data from investigational or marketing experience, but potential benefits from the use of the medication during pregnancy might warrant its use. Sorafenib, an antineoplastic medication, is in Category D.

Category X: Studies have demonstrated adverse effects on animal and human fetuses, according to studies and data from investigational or marketing experience. Pregnancy is a contraindication for the use of the medication because the risks outweigh the potential benefits. Estradiol, an estrogen replacement, is a Category X medication.

Application Exercises

1. A nurse is collecting data from a client who takes haloperidol to treat schizophrenia. Which of the following findings should the nurse document as extrapyramidal symptoms (EPSs)? (Select all that apply.)

   A. Orthostatic hypotension

   B. Tremors

   C. Acute dystonia

   D. Decreased level of consciousness

   E. Restlessness

2. A nurse is teaching a client who has a new prescription for oxybutynin about managing the medication's anticholinergic effects. Which of the following instructions should the nurse include? (Select all that apply.)

   A. Take sips of water frequently.

   B. Wear sunglasses when outdoors in sunlight.

   C. Use a soft toothbrush when brushing teeth.

   D. Take the medication with an antacid.

   E. Urinate prior to taking the medication.

3. A nurse is reviewing a client's medications. They include cimetidine and imipramine. Knowing that cimetidine decreases the metabolism of imipramine, the nurse should identify that this combination is likely to result in which of the following effects?

   A. Decreased therapeutic effects of cimetidine

   B. Increased risk of imipramine toxicity

   C. Decreased risk of adverse effects of cimetidine

   D. Increased therapeutic effects of imipramine

4. A nurse in an outpatient clinic is caring for a client who has a new prescription for an antihypertensive medication. Which of the following instructions should the nurse give the client?

   A. "Get up and change positions slowly."

   B. "Avoid eating aged cheese and smoked meat."

   C. "Report any usual bruising or bleeding to the doctor immediately."

   D. "Eat the same amount of foods that contain vitamin K every day."

5. A nurse in an outpatient surgical center is admitting a client for a laparoscopic procedure. The client has a prescription for preoperative diazepam. Prior to administering the medication, which of the following actions is the nurse's priority?

   A. Teaching the client about the purpose of the medication

   B. Giving the medication at the administration time the provider prescribed

   C. Identifying the client's medication allergies

   D. Documenting the client's anxiety level

PRACTICE Active Learning Scenario

A nurse is reviewing the FDA's pregnancy risk categories in an in-service presentation. Use the ATI Active Learning Template: Basic Concept to complete this item.

RELATED CONTENT: Include the definition and an example of each of the five pregnancy risk categories.

1. A. Orthostatic hypotension is an adverse effect, but it is not an EPS.

    B. **CORRECT:** Tremors are an EPS. Others are rigidity, drooling, agitation, and a shuffling gait.

    C. **CORRECT:** Acute dystonia is an EPS. It includes spastic movements of the back, neck, tongue, and face.

    D. Decreased level of consciousness is an adverse effect, but it is not an EPS.

    E. **CORRECT:** Restlessness is an EPS. Others are rigidity, drooling, agitation, and a shuffling gait.

    Ⓝ *NCLEX® Connection: Pharmacological and Parenteral Therapies, Adverse Effects/Contraindications/Side Effects/Interactions*

2. A. **CORRECT:** Taking sips of water frequently will help relieve the anticholinergic effect of dry mouth.

    B. **CORRECT:** Wearing sunglasses will help relieve the anticholinergic effect of photophobia.

    C. Anticholinergic effects do not increase the client's risk for bleeding. Constipation is an example of an anticholinergic effect.

    D. Taking the medication with an antacid will not decrease anticholinergic effects. Constipation is an example of an anticholinergic effect.

    E. **CORRECT:** Urinating prior to taking the medication will help relieve the anticholinergic effect of urinary retention.

    Ⓝ *NCLEX® Connection: Pharmacological and Parenteral Therapies, Medication Administration*

3. A. A medication that increases the metabolism of another medication can decrease the effectiveness of that medication.

    B. **CORRECT:** A medication that decreases the metabolism of another medication increases the serum level of that medication, increasing the risk for toxicity.

    C. A medication that decreases the metabolism of another medication does not decrease the risk for adverse effects.

    D. A medication that decreases the metabolism of another medication does not increase that medication's therapeutic effects.

    Ⓝ *NCLEX® Connection: Pharmacological and Parenteral Therapies, Medication Administration*

4. A. **CORRECT:** Antihypertensive medications can cause orthostatic hypotension. The nurse should instruct the client to change positions slowly and to sit or lie down when feeling dizzy or lightheaded to prevent injury.

    B. Consuming foods that contain tyramine (avocados, figs, aged cheese, yeast extracts, beer, smoked meats) while taking monoamine oxidase inhibitors, not antihypertensives, can lead to hypertensive crisis.

    C. Clients taking an anticoagulant, not an antihypertensive, should report bruising, discolored urine or stool, petechiae, bleeding gums, and any other manifestations of bleeding to the provider immediately.

    D. Clients taking anticoagulants, not antihypertensives, should maintain a consistent intake of dietary vitamin K to avoid sudden fluctuations that could affect the action of the anticoagulant.

    Ⓝ *NCLEX® Connection: Pharmacological and Parenteral Therapies, Medication Administration*

5. A. The nurse should teach the client about the purpose of the medication to make sure the client understands why the provider prescribed it. However, another action is the priority.

    B. The nurse should administer the medication at the time the provider prescribed that the client receive it to help prepare the client for the surgical procedure. However, another action is the priority.

    C. **CORRECT:** The greatest risk to this client is injury from an allergic reaction. The priority action is to identify the client's allergies prior to medication administration.

    D. The nurse should document the client's anxiety level to have a baseline against which to measure the effectiveness of the medication. However, another action is the priority.

    Ⓝ *NCLEX® Connection: Pharmacological and Parenteral Therapies, Medication Administration*

PRACTICE Answer

Using the ATI Active Learning Template: Basic Concept

RELATED CONTENT

- Category A: There is no evidence of risk to a fetus from taking the medication during pregnancy, according to adequate and well-controlled studies. Ferrous sulfate, an iron supplement, is a Category A medication.
- Category B: There is no evidence of risk to an animal fetus according to studies, but there are no adequate and well-controlled studies of pregnant women. Or, there is evidence of risk to an animal fetus, but controlled studies of pregnant women show no evidence of risk to the fetus. Esomeprazole, an antiulcer medication, is in Category B.

- Category C: Studies have demonstrated adverse effects on animal fetuses, but there are no adequate and well-controlled studies of pregnant women. Or, there have not been any studies of animals or pregnant women. Glipizide, an antidiabetes medication, is in Category C.
- Category D: Studies have demonstrated adverse effects on human fetuses according to data from investigational or marketing experience, but potential benefits from the use of the medication during pregnancy might warrant its use. Sorafenib, an antineoplastic medication, is in Category D.

- Category X: Studies have demonstrated adverse effects on animal and human fetuses, according to studies and data from investigational or marketing experience. Pregnancy is a contraindication for the use of the medication because the risks outweigh the potential benefits. Estradiol, an estrogen replacement, is a Category X medication.

Ⓝ *NCLEX® Connection: Pharmacological and Parenteral Therapies, Medication Administration*

CHAPTER 51 *Individual Considerations of Medication Administration*

Various factors affect how clients respond to medications. It is important for nurses to identify these factors to help them individualize nursing care when administering medications.

FACTORS AFFECTING MEDICATION DOSAGES AND RESPONSES

Body weight: Because body tissues absorb medications, individuals with a greater body mass require larger doses. Because the percentage of body fat an individual has can alter the distribution of a medication, basing dosages on body surface area (BSA) can be a more precise method of regulating an individual's response to a medication.

Age: Liver and kidney function are immature in young children and often decreased in older adults, which can cause heightened sensitivities to medications and thus necessitate proportionately smaller medication doses. Ⓖ

Gender: Women respond differently to medications than men due to a higher proportion of body fat and the effects of female hormones.

Genetics: Genetic factors such as missing enzymes can alter the metabolism of certain medications, thus enhancing or reducing a medication's action. The usual effect is either fewer benefits from the medication or greater medication toxicity.

Biorhythmic cycles: Responses to some medications vary with the biologic rhythms of the body. For example, hypnotic medications work better when clients take them at their usual sleep time than at other times.

Tolerance: Reduced responsiveness to a medication clients take over time, such as morphine, is pharmacodynamic tolerance. Other medications, such as barbiturates, cause metabolic tolerance as metabolism of the medication increases over time and the effectiveness of the medication declines. Cross-tolerance can occur with other chemically similar medications.

Accumulation: Medication concentration in the body increases due to the inability to metabolize or excrete a medication rapidly enough, resulting in a toxic medication effect. For older adults, decreased kidney and liver function are the major causes of medication accumulation leading to toxicity. Ⓖ

Psychological factors: Emotional state and expectations can influence the effects of a medication. The placebo effect describes positive medication effects that psychological factors, not biochemical properties of the medication, influence.

Diet: Inadequate nutrition, such as starvation, can affect the protein-binding response of medications. It increases their response and thus increases the risk for medication toxicity.

Medical problems
- Inadequate gastric acid inhibits the absorption of medications that require an acid medium to dissolve.
- Diarrhea causes oral medications to pass through the gastrointestinal tract too quickly for adequate absorption.
- Vascular insufficiency prevents the distribution of a medication to affected tissue.
- Liver disease or failure impairs medication metabolism, which can cause toxicity.
- Kidney disease or failure prevents or delays medication excretion, which can cause toxicity.
- Prolonged gastric emptying time delays the absorption of medications in the intestines.

PHARMACOLOGY AND CHILDREN

Although most medications adults take are useful for children, the dosages are different. Providers base pediatric dosages on body weight or BSA.
- Newborns (younger than 1 month old) and infants (1 month to 1 year old) have immature liver and kidney function, alkaline gastric juices, and an immature blood-brain barrier, making them especially sensitive to medications that affect the CNS. Providers base some medication dosages on age due to a greater risk for decreased skeletal bone growth, acute cardiopulmonary failure, and hepatic toxicity.
- Be particularly alert when administering medications to children due to the risk for medication errors. Ⓠ**s**
  - Check that dosages are accurate for weight or BSA.
  - Initial pediatric dosages are an approximation.
  - Be aware that most medications do not undergo testing on children.
  - Some adult medication forms and concentrations require dilution, calculation, preparation, and administration of very small doses for children.
  - Limited sites exist for IV medication administration.
  - Give written and verbal instructions to parents to promote adherence to medication regimens.

Additional pharmacokinetic factors specific to children
- Decreased gastric acid production and slower gastric emptying time
- Decreased first-pass medication metabolism
- Increased absorption of topical medications (greater blood flow to the skin and thinner skin)
- Lower blood pressure (more blood flow to the liver and brain and less to the kidneys)
- Higher body water content (dilutes water-soluble medications)
- Decreased serum protein-binding sites (until age 1 year). This can result in an increase in the serum level of protein-binding medications.

PHARMACOLOGY AND OLDER ADULTS (65+ YEARS)

PHYSIOLOGIC CHANGES WITH AGING THAT AFFECT PHARMACOKINETICS

- Increased gastric pH (alkaline)
- Decreased gastrointestinal motility and gastric emptying time, resulting in a slower rate of absorption
- Decreased blood flow through the cardiovascular system, liver, and kidneys
- Decreased hepatic enzyme function
- Decreased kidney function and glomerular filtration rate
- Decreased protein-binding sites, resulting in lower serum albumin levels
- Decreased body water, increased body fat, and decreased lean body mass

OTHER FACTORS AFFECTING MEDICATION THERAPY

- Impaired memory or altered mental state
- Multiple or severe illnesses
- Changes in vision and hearing
- Decreased mobility and dexterity
- Poor adherence
- Inadequate supervision of long-term therapy
- Limited financial resources
- Polypharmacy: The practice of taking several medications simultaneously (prescription and over-the-counter [OTC]) with diminished bodily functions and some medical problems can contribute to the potential for medication toxicity.

NURSING INTERVENTIONS

Decreasing the risk of adverse medication effects
- Obtain a complete medication history and include all OTC medications.
- Make sure medication therapy starts at the lowest possible dose.
- Assess and monitor for therapeutic and adverse effects.
- Monitor plasma medication levels to provide a rational basis for dosage adjustment.
- Assess and monitor for medication-medication and medication-food interactions.
- Document findings.
- Notify the provider of adverse effects.

Promoting adherence
- Give clear and concise instructions, verbally and in writing.
- Ensure that the dosage form is appropriate. Administer liquid forms to clients who have difficulty swallowing. Qpcc
- Provide clearly marked containers that are easy to open.
- Assist the client with setting up a daily calendar with the use of pill containers.
- Discuss the availability of and access to local resources for obtaining and paying for medications.
- Suggest that the client obtain assistance from a friend, neighbor, or relative.

PHARMACOLOGY: PREGNANCY AND LACTATION

PREGNANCY

- Any medication women who are pregnant ingest will affect the fetus. The U.S. Food and Drug Administration (FDA) classifies medications in five categories that range from remote risk to proven risk of fetal harm.
- Most medications are potentially harmful to the fetus. Prescribers must weigh the benefits of maternal medication administration against possible fetal risk.
- Medications women take during pregnancy include nutritional supplements (iron, vitamins, minerals) and medications that treat nausea, vomiting, gastric acidity, and mild discomforts.
- Providers manage chronic medical disorders such as diabetes mellitus and hypertension in conjunction with careful maternal-fetal monitoring.
- Pregnancy is a contraindication for live-virus vaccines (measles, mumps, polio, rubella, yellow fever) due to possible teratogenic effects.

LACTATION

- Most medications women take during lactation enter breast milk. Women who are lactating should avoid medications that have an extended half-life, are sustained-released, or are harmful to infants.
- For medications that are safe, administer them immediately after breastfeeding to minimize the medication's concentration in the next feeding. Use the lowest effective dosage for the shortest possible time. Qs

Application Exercises

1. To promote adherence with medication self-administration, a nurse is making recommendations for an older adult client. Which of the following instructions should the nurse include? (Select all that apply.)

    A. Adjust dosages according to daily weight.

    B. Place pills in daily pill holders.

    C. Ask for liquid forms if the client has difficulty swallowing pills.

    D. Ask a relative to assist periodically.

    E. Request child-resistant caps on medication containers.

2. A young adult client in a provider's office tells the nurse that she uses fasting for several days each week to help control her weight. The client takes several medications for various chronic issues. The nurse should explain to the client that which of the following mechanisms that results from fasting puts her at risk for medication toxicity?

    A. Increasing the metabolism of the medications over time

    B. Increasing the protein-binding response

    C. Increasing medications' transit time through the intestines

    D. Decreasing the excretion of medications

3. A nurse is preparing medications for a preschooler. Which of the following factors should the nurse identify as altering how a medication affects children? (Select all that apply.)

    A. Increased gastric acid production

    B. Lower blood pressure

    C. Higher body water content

    D. Increased absorption of topical medications

    E. Increased gastric emptying time

4. A nurse is teaching a client who is lactating about taking medications. Which of the following actions should the nurse recommend to minimize in the entry of medication into breast milk?

    A. Drink 8 oz milk with each dose of medication.

    B. Use medications that have an extended half-life.

    C. Take each dose right after breastfeeding.

    D. Pump breast milk and freeze it prior to feeding to the newborn.

5. A nurse in an outpatient clinic is teaching a client who is in her first trimester of pregnancy. Which of the following statements should the nurse make?

    A. "You will need to get a rubella immunization if you haven't had one prior to pregnancy."

    B. "You can safely take over-the-counter medications."

    C. "You should avoid any vitamin preparations containing iron."

    D. "Your provider can prescribe medication for nausea if you need it."

PRACTICE Active Learning Scenario

A nurse is preparing to administer medications to an older adult client who has vascular insufficiency and impaired kidney function. Use the ATI Active Learning Template: Basic Concept to complete this item.

UNDERLYING PRINCIPLES
- Discuss medication considerations with vascular insufficiency.
- Discuss medication considerations with impaired kidney function.
- Identify at least four physiologic changes with aging that affect pharmacokinetics.

NURSING INTERVENTIONS: Identify at least three interventions for reducing the risk for adverse effects.

Application Exercises Key

1. A. The provider adjusts the client's dosages. Instructing the client to base dosages on daily weight increases the risk for error in medication self-administration.

   B. **CORRECT:** Organizing medications in daily pill holders promotes medication adherence.

   C. **CORRECT:** Providing a form of medication that is easier for the client to swallow promotes medication adherence.

   D. **CORRECT:** Including the client's support system promotes medication adherence.

   E. Some older adult clients have difficulty opening child-resistant caps. Request easy-open containers from the pharmacy.

   Ⓝ *NCLEX® Connection: Pharmacological and Parenteral Therapies, Medication Administration*

2. A. Some medications, not fasting, cause metabolic tolerance as metabolism of the medication increases over time and the effectiveness of the medication declines.

   B. **CORRECT:** Inadequate nutrition, such as starvation, can affect the protein-binding response of medications. It increases their response and thus increases the risk for medication toxicity.

   C. Disorders that cause diarrhea, not fasting, cause oral medications to pass through the gastrointestinal tract too quickly for adequate absorption. This mechanism does not cause toxicity.

   D. Kidney disease or failure, not fasting, prevents or delays medication excretion, which can cause toxicity.

   Ⓝ *NCLEX® Connection: Physiological Adaptation, Pathophysiology*

3. A. Children have decreased gastric acid production.

   B. **CORRECT:** Children have a lower blood pressure.

   C. **CORRECT:** Children have a higher body water content.

   D. **CORRECT:** Children have increased absorption of topical medications.

   E. Children have a slower gastric emptying time.

   Ⓝ *NCLEX® Connection: Health Promotion and Maintenance, Developmental Stages and Transitions*

4. A. The intake of food or fluid with medication does not affect entry of medications into breast milk.

   B. The client should avoid medications that have an extended half-life due to their increased entry into breast milk.

   C. **CORRECT:** Taking medication immediately after breastfeeding helps minimize medication concentration in the next feeding.

   D. Pumping and freezing breast milk does not affect entry of medications into breast milk.

   Ⓝ *NCLEX® Connection: Health Promotion and Maintenance, Developmental Stages and Transitions*

5. A. Pregnancy is a contraindication for live-virus vaccines, including rubella, due to possible teratogenic effects.

   B. Most medications, including over-the-counter, are potentially harmful to the fetus. The client should avoid any medications unless her provider prescribes them.

   C. Nutritional supplements that include iron are common recommendations during pregnancy to support the health of the mother and fetus.

   D. **CORRECT:** Providers can prescribe medications to treat nausea and other discomforts of pregnancy.

   Ⓝ *NCLEX® Connection: Health Promotion and Maintenance, Developmental Stages and Transitions*

PRACTICE Answer

Using the ATI Active Learning Template: Basic Concept

UNDERLYING PRINCIPLES

- Vascular insufficiency prevents distribution of a medication to affected tissue. The nurse should document and monitor for the medication's effectiveness and report concerns to the provider.
- Impaired kidney function prevents or delays medication excretion, which increases the risk for toxicity. Decreased kidney function is a major cause of medication accumulation leading to toxicity.
- Physiologic changes
  - Increased gastric pH (alkaline)
  - Decreased gastrointestinal motility and gastric emptying time, resulting in a slower rate of absorption
  - Decreased blood flow through the cardiovascular system, liver, and kidneys
  - Decreased hepatic enzyme function
  - Decreased kidney function and glomerular filtration rate
  - Decreased protein-binding sites, resulting in lower serum albumin levels
  - Decreased body water, increased body fat, and decreased lean body mass
  - Impaired memory or altered mental state
  - Multiple or severe illnesses
  - Changes in vision and hearing
  - Decreased mobility and dexterity

Ⓝ *NCLEX® Connection: Physiological Adaptation, Illness Management*

NURSING INTERVENTIONS

- Obtain a complete medication history, and include all OTC medications.
- Make sure medication therapy starts at the lowest possible dose.
- Assess and monitor for therapeutic and adverse effects.
- Monitor plasma medication levels to provide a rational basis for dosage adjustment.
- Assess and monitor for medication-medication and medication-food interactions.
- Document findings.
- Notify the provider of adverse effects.

ⓝ NCLEX® Connections

When reviewing the following chapters, keep in mind the relevant topics and tasks of the NCLEX outline, in particular:

Client Needs: Basic Care and Comfort

NUTRITION AND ORAL HYDRATION: Provide client nutrition through continuous or intermittent tube feedings.

Client Needs: Reduction of Risk Potential

DIAGNOSTIC TESTS: Perform diagnostic testing.

LABORATORY VALUES: Obtain specimens other than blood for diagnostic testing.

POTENTIAL FOR ALTERATIONS IN BODY SYSTEMS: Identify client potential for skin breakdown.

POTENTIAL FOR COMPLICATIONS OF DIAGNOSTIC TESTS/ TREATMENTS/PROCEDURES: Position the client to prevent complications following tests/treatments/procedures.

THERAPEUTIC PROCEDURES: Educate client about home management of care.

Client Needs: Physiological Adaptation

FLUID AND ELECTROLYTE IMBALANCES: Identify signs and symptoms of client fluid and/or electrolyte imbalance.

ILLNESS MANAGEMENT: Manage the care of a client with impaired ventilation/oxygenation.

CHAPTER 52 # Specimen Collection for Glucose Monitoring

Monitoring blood glucose levels is an essential component in the care of clients who have diabetes mellitus. Blood glucose testing is the preferred method of monitoring blood glucose levels. Q EBP

Urine testing is not an effective measure of glucose level because glucose levels must be greater than 220 mg/dL before glucose appears in the urine.

Clients who are able and willing to monitor independently can learn how to self-monitor blood glucose levels. Required abilities include alertness, the ability to comprehend and give a return demonstration of the process, adequate finger dexterity, and adequate visual acuity.

Blood glucose testing

For blood glucose testing, clients who have diabetes mellitus use a glucometer or a blood glucose meter with small test strips to "read" the blood sample. These systems require proper calibration, storage of supplies, and matching of lot numbers.

INDICATIONS

Regular testing is necessary for clients who have diabetes mellitus to manage the disease by maintaining safe blood glucose levels.

CONSIDERATIONS

PREPROCEDURE

NURSING ACTIONS
- Check the client's record and prescription.
  - Frequency and type of test: Testing times vary based on the goals of management and the complexity of the client's hypoglycemic medication schedule.
  - Results from previous tests: norms and ranges
  - Actions according to results
- Review the client's medication profile.
  - Note anticoagulant usage, history of bleeding disorders, and low platelet count.
  - Note the times and dose of hypoglycemic agents.
  - Note the use of corticosteroids, oral contraceptives, beta blockers, antipsychotics, and other medications that can elevate blood glucose levels.
- Gather materials, and prepare the equipment.
  - Blood glucose meter
  - Reagent strip compatible with the meter
  - Washcloth and soap or antiseptic swab
  - Clean gloves
  - Sterile lancet
  - Cotton ball
- Review the meter and the manufacturer's instructions.
- Check the strip solution's expiration date.
- Some meters require calibration; others require zeroing of the timer. No-code models require no calibration because the calibration is integrated into the test strips. Follow the manufacturer's directions.
- Explain the procedure to the client.
- Evaluate the selected puncture site.
  - Integrity of the skin (to avoid areas of bruising, open lesions)
  - Compromised circulation
- Perform hand hygiene and put on gloves.

INTRAPROCEDURE

NURSING ACTIONS

- Select a site from which to collect the blood sample. Q_{PCC}
  - Outer edge of a fingertip (most common site)
  - Alternate site (earlobe, heel, palm, arm, thigh)
- Rotate sites to avoid ongoing tenderness.
- Wrap the site in a warm, moist towel to enhance circulation, especially when it has been difficult to obtain an adequate sample.
- Cleanse the site with warm water and soap or an antiseptic swab (not alcohol), and allow it to dry. Alcohol can interfere with results. Q_{EBP}
- Hold the finger in a dependent position before puncturing to improve blood flow.
- Pierce the skin using a sterile lancet (or a lancet injector device) and holding it perpendicular to the skin.
- Wipe away the first drop of blood with a cotton ball.
- Place a drop of blood on the test strip.
  - Follow the manufacturer's procedure for applying blood to the strip.
  - If necessary, gently milk the finger to obtain a drop. (Forceful milking or squeezing can cause pain, bruising, and scarring.) Do not touch the site directly to stimulate bleeding.
  - Hold the test strip next to the blood on the fingertip.
  - Do not smear blood onto the strip because this can cause an inaccurate reading.
  - Allow the meter to process the reading. (Time varies with the meter.)
  - Apply a cotton ball over the puncture site.
  - Note the reading; turn off the meter; and dispose of the cotton ball, test strip, lancet, and gloves in proper receptacles.

POSTPROCEDURE

NURSING ACTIONS

- Perform hand hygiene.
- Document the meter's reading.
- Check the prescription for medication or treatment actions, and implement them.

INTERPRETATION OF FINDINGS

- Usually, a random blood glucose level greater than 200 mg/dL indicates hyperglycemia.
- Usually, a blood glucose level less than 70 mg/dL indicates hypoglycemia.
- Poor storage of glucose test strips can lead to falsely high or low readings. Typically, these test strips come in a vial to store at room temperature or as the manufacturer directs.

Urine glucose testing

INDICATIONS

Clients who have diabetes mellitus perform urine glucose testing at home at times of acute illness, stress, or a blood glucose greater than 240 mg/dL to identify the presence of ketones. Q_{EBP}

CONSIDERATIONS

PREPROCEDURE

NURSING ACTIONS

- Evaluate the client's ability to urinate.
- Verify the prescription for frequency and actions to take based on the results.
- Gather materials, and prepare the equipment.
  - Clean urine specimen cup
  - Chemical reagent strips, container with glucose reading scale
  - Clean gloves
  - Towelette or soap and washcloth
- Check the strip's expiration date.
- Explain the procedure.
- Perform hand hygiene, and put on clean gloves.

INTRAPROCEDURE

NURSING ACTIONS

- Assist the client with urine sample collection.
- Dip the reagent strip into the urine sample and gently shake off excess urine.
- Compare the strip's color change with the ranges on the container within the instructed time (usually 1 to 5 seconds).

POSTPROCEDURE

NURSING ACTIONS

- Dispose of the remaining urine sample, test strip, and gloves.
- Perform hand hygiene.
- Check the prescription for medication or treatment actions, and implement.

INTERPRETATION OF FINDINGS

If the test is positive for ketones, it indicates uncontrolled blood glucose.

Application Exercises

1. A nurse is determining a client's ability to learn self-monitoring of blood glucose using a glucometer. Which of the following abilities should the nurse confirm that the client has before proceeding with instruction? (Select all that apply.)

   A. Finger dexterity

   B. Visual acuity

   C. Color vision

   D. Basic literacy

   E. Demonstration ability

2. A nurse is reviewing a client's medication history. The client has an admission blood glucose of 260 mg/dL and no documented history of diabetes mellitus. Which of the following types of medications should alert the nurse to the possibility that the client has developed an adverse effect of pharmacological therapy? (Select all that apply.)

   A. Diuretics

   B. Corticosteroids

   C. Oral anticoagulants

   D. Opioid analgesics

   E. Antipsychotics

3. A nurse is providing education on how to check blood glucose levels to a client who has a new diagnosis of type 1 diabetes mellitus. The nurse should include which of the following instructions about transferring blood onto the reagent portion of the test strip?

   A. Smear the blood onto the strip.

   B. Squeeze the blood onto the strip.

   C. Touch the puncture to stimulate bleeding.

   D. Hold the test strip next to the blood on the fingertip.

4. A nurse attempts to collect a capillary blood specimen via finger stick for a blood glucose monitoring from a client who has diabetes mellitus. The nurse is unable to obtain an adequate drop of blood for the reagent strip. Which of the following actions should the nurse take first?

   A. Puncture another finger to obtain a capillary specimen.

   B. Test the urine with a urine reagent strip.

   C. Wrap the hand in a warm, moist cloth.

   D. Perform a venipuncture to obtain a venous sample.

5. A nurse is teaching self-monitoring of blood glucose (SMBG) to a client who has diabetes mellitus. Which of the following instructions should the nurse include? (Select all that apply.)

   A. Perform SMBG once daily at bedtime.

   B. Wipe the hand with an alcohol swab.

   C. Hold the hand in a dependent position prior to the puncture.

   D. Place the puncturing device perpendicular to the site.

   E. Prick the outer edge of the fingertip for the blood sample.

PRACTICE Active Learning Scenario

A nurse is teaching a group of nursing students how to perform urine glucose testing. Use the ATI Active Learning Template: Diagnostic Procedure to complete this item.

NURSING INTERVENTIONS: List the steps of the procedure in the three phases (pre-, intra-, post-procedure).

Application Exercises Key

1. A. **CORRECT:** The client should have the manual dexterity to cleanse and puncture his finger, collect the blood, and insert the strip into the meter, in order to use a glucometer to monitor blood glucose

   B. **CORRECT:** The client should have the visual acuity to see the digital reading of the results, in order to use a glucometer to monitor blood glucose.

   C. The client who has color blindness can have difficulty interpreting the colors on a reagent strip for urine glucose testing. However, the client should be able to perform blood glucose testing accurately.

   D. The client needs only to recognize numerals for basic use of a glucometer to monitor blood glucose. Reading skills are not necessary.

   E. **CORRECT:** The client should learn to use a glucometer accurately and safely, and therefore must perform for the nurse a return demonstration of the procedure in order to verify understanding.

   Ⓝ *NCLEX® Connection: Reduction of Risk Potential, Therapeutic Procedures*

2. A. **CORRECT:** Diuretics can cause hyperglycemia, especially in clients who have diabetes mellitus, and also can cause many electrolyte imbalances.

   B. **CORRECT:** Corticosteroids can cause hyperglycemia and glycosuria.

   C. Anticoagulants can cause excessive bleeding during blood sampling for glucose testing.

   D. Opioid analgesics cause many adverse effects, including respiratory depression, but they are unlikely to raise blood glucose levels.

   E. **CORRECT:** Antipsychotics, particularly atypical antipsychotics, can cause new-onset diabetes mellitus.

   Ⓝ *NCLEX® Connection: Pharmacological and Parenteral Therapies, Adverse Effects/Contraindications/Side Effects/Interactions*

3. A. Smearing the blood on the test strip can cause inaccurate results.

   B. The client should milk her finger gently to obtain a drop of blood. Forceful milking or squeezing can cause pain, bruising, and scarring.

   C. Touching the puncture site can cause transfer of micro-organisms to the site.

   D. **CORRECT:** Holding the pad of the strip next to the puncture allows the blood to flow until the amount on the strip is adequate. Too little blood can result in falsely low readings.

   Ⓝ *NCLEX® Connection: Reduction of Risk Potential, Therapeutic Procedures*

4. A. The nurse can puncture another finger to obtain a capillary specimen. However, the nurse should use a less restrictive intervention first.

   B. The nurse can obtain a urine glucose. However, the client's blood glucose level should be significantly elevated in order to detect glucose in the urine. The nurse should use a less restrictive intervention first.

   C. **CORRECT:** When providing client care, the nurse should first use the least restrictive intervention. The nurse should warm the client's finger with a warm, moist cloth to promote blood flow in preparation for the next finger stick.

   D. The nurse might need to request a venipuncture for checking the blood glucose level. However, the nurse should use a less restrictive intervention first.

   Ⓝ *NCLEX® Connection: Reduction of Risk Potential, Therapeutic Procedures*

5. A. The client can perform SMBG as often as before each meal and at bedtime. Generally, the timing and frequency of SMBG testing correlates with the client's medication schedule. Monitoring once a day at bedtime does not provide enough information to monitor blood glucose control effectively.

   B. The client should wash his hand with warm water and soap. Alcohol can alter the blood glucose reading.

   C. **CORRECT:** The client should hold the hand in a dependent position to increase blood flow to the fingers.

   D. **CORRECT:** The client should hold the lancet perpendicular to the skin to ensure the correct piercing depth.

   E. **CORRECT:** The client should use the outer edge of the fingertip for blood sampling. The client can also use a heel, palm, arm, or thigh.

   Ⓝ *NCLEX® Connection: Reduction of Risk Potential, Therapeutic Procedures*

PRACTICE Answer

Using ATI Active Learning Template: Diagnostic Procedure

NURSING INTERVENTIONS

Preprocedure
- Evaluate the client's ability to urinate.
- Verify the prescription for frequency and actions to take based on the results.
- Gather materials and prepare equipment: urine specimen cup, chemical reagent strips, container with the glucose reading scale, clean gloves, towelette or soap and washcloth.
- Check the strip's expiration date.
- Explain the procedure.
- Perform hand hygiene, and put on clean gloves.

Intraprocedure
- Assist the client with urine sample collection.
- Dip the reagent strip into the urine sample.
- Compare the strip's color change with the ranges on the container within the instructed time (usually 1 to 5 seconds).

Postprocedure
- Dispose of the remaining urine sample, test strip, and gloves.
- Perform hand hygiene.
- Check the prescription for medication or treatment actions, and implement.

Ⓝ *NCLEX® Connection: Reduction of Risk Potential, Therapeutic Procedures*

CHAPTER 53 Airway Management

Managing airway compromise includes respiratory assessment and measuring vital signs, including oxygen saturation via pulse oximetry and administration of oxygen.

Oxygen helps maintain adequate cellular oxygenation for clients who have many acute and chronic respiratory problems (hypoxemia, cystic fibrosis, asthma) or are at risk for developing hypoxia (respiratory illness, circulatory impairment).

Maintaining a patent airway is a nursing priority. It involves mobilizing secretions, suctioning the airway, and managing artificial airways (endotracheal tubes, tracheostomy tubes) to promote adequate gas exchange and lung expansion.

Pulse oximetry and oxygen therapy

- A pulse oximeter is a device with a sensor probe that attaches securely to the fingertip, toe, bridge of nose, earlobe, or forehead with a clip or band.
- A pulse oximeter measures pulse saturation (SpO_2) via a wave of infrared light that measures light absorption by oxygenated and deoxygenated hemoglobin in arterial blood. SpO_2 reliably reflects the percent of saturation of hemoglobin (SaO_2) when the SaO_2 is greater than 70%.
- Oxygen is a tasteless and colorless gas that accounts for 21% of atmospheric air.
- Oxygen flow rates vary to maintain an SpO_2 of 95% to 100% using the lowest amount of oxygen to achieve the goal without risking complications.
- The fraction of inspired oxygen (FiO_2) is the percentage of oxygen the client receives.

Pulse oximetry

Noninvasive measurement of the oxygen saturation of the blood for monitoring respiratory status when assessment findings include any of the following.
- Increased work of breathing
- Wheezing
- Coughing
- Cyanosis
- Changes in respiratory rate or rhythm
- Adventitious breath sounds
- Restlessness, irritability, confusion

CONSIDERATIONS

INTERVENTIONS FOR READINGS LESS THAN 90% (INDICATING HYPOXEMIA)
- Confirm probe placement.
- Confirm that the oxygen delivery system is functioning and that the client is receiving the prescribed oxygen levels.
- Place the client in semi-Fowler's or Fowler's position promote chest expansion and to maximize ventilation. Qpcc
- Encourage deep breathing.
- Remain with the client and provide emotional support to decrease anxiety.

INTERPRETATION OF FINDINGS

- The expected reference range is 95% to 100%. Acceptable levels range from 91% to 100%. Some illness states can allow for 85% to 89%. Readings less than 90% reflect hypoxemia.
- Values can be slightly lower for older adult clients and clients who have dark skin. Ⓖ
- Additional reasons for low readings include hypothermia, poor peripheral blood flow, too much light (sun, infrared lamps), low hemoglobin levels, jaundice, movement, edema, and nail polish.

Oxygen therapy

Oxygen is a therapeutic gas that treats hypoxemia (low levels of arterial oxygen). Administering and adjusting it requires a prescription.

INDICATIONS

MANIFESTATIONS OF HYPOXEMIA

EARLY
- Tachypnea
- Tachycardia
- Restlessness, anxiety, confusion
- Pale skin, mucous membranes
- Elevated blood pressure
- Use of accessory muscles, nasal flaring, tracheal tugging, adventitious lung sounds

LATE
- Stupor
- Cyanotic skin, mucous membranes
- Bradypnea
- Bradycardia
- Hypotension
- Cardiac dysrhythmias

CONSIDERATIONS

NURSING ACTIONS
- Monitor respiratory rate and pattern, level of consciousness, SpO_2, and arterial blood gases.
- Provide oxygen therapy at the lowest liter flow that will correct hypoxemia.
- Make sure the mask creates a secure seal over the nose and mouth.
- Assess/monitor hypoxemia and hypercarbia (elevated levels of CO_2): restlessness, hypertension, and headache.
- Auscultate the lungs for breath sounds and adventitious sounds, such as crackles and wheezes.
- Assess/monitor oxygenation status with pulse oximetry and arterial blood gases (ABGs).
- Promote oral hygiene.
- Encourage turning, coughing, deep breathing, and the use of incentive spirometry and suctioning.
- Promote rest and decrease environmental stimuli.
- Provide emotional support. Qpcc
- Assess nutritional status. Provide supplements.
- Assess skin integrity. Provide moisture and pressure-relief devices.
- Assess and document the response to oxygen therapy.
- Titrate oxygen to maintain the recommended oxygen saturation.
- Discontinue supplemental oxygen gradually.
- Monitor for respiratory depression (decreased respiratory rate and level of consciousness).
- Low-flow oxygen delivery systems deliver varying amounts of oxygen based on the delivery method and the client's breathing pattern.

LOW-FLOW OXYGEN DELIVERY SYSTEMS

Nasal cannula

Tubing with two small prongs for insertion into the nares

FRACTION OF INSPIRED OXYGEN: Delivers an FiO_2 of 24% to 44% at a flow rate of 1 to 6 L/min

ADVANTAGES
- Cannula is a safe, simple, and easy-to-apply method.
- Cannula is comfortable and well-tolerated.
- The client is able to eat, talk, and ambulate.

DISADVANTAGES
- The FiO_2 varies with the flow rate, and rate and depth of the client's breathing.
- Extended use can lead to skin breakdown and dry mucous membranes.
- Tubing is easily dislodged.

NURSING ACTIONS
- Assess the patency of the nares.
- Ensure that the prongs fit in the nares properly.
- Use water-soluble gel to prevent dry nares.
- Provide humidification for flow rates of 4 L/min and greater.

Simple face mask

Covers the client's nose and mouth

FRACTION OF INSPIRED OXYGEN
- It delivers an FiO_2 of 40% to 60% at flow rates of 5 to 8 L/min.
- The minimum flow rate is 5 L/min to ensure flushing of CO_2 from the mask.

ADVANTAGES
- A face mask is easy to apply and can be more comfortable than a nasal cannula.
- It is a simple delivery method.
- It is more comfortable than a nasal cannula.
- It provides humidified oxygen.

DISADVANTAGES
- Flow rates less than 5 L/min can result in rebreathing of CO_2.
- Clients who have anxiety or claustrophobia do not tolerate it well.
- Eating, drinking, and talking are impaired.
- Moisture and pressure can collect under the mask and cause skin breakdown.

NURSING ACTIONS
- Assess proper fit to ensure a secure seal over the nose and mouth.
- Make sure the client wears a nasal cannula during meals.
- Use with caution for clients who have a high risk of aspiration or airway obstruction.
- Monitor for skin breakdown.

Partial rebreather mask

Covers the client's nose and mouth

FRACTION OF INSPIRED OXYGEN: Delivers an FiO_2 of 40% to 70% at flow rates of 6 to 10 L/min.

ADVANTAGES: The mask has a reservoir bag attached with no valve, which allows the client to rebreathe up to ⅓ of exhaled air together with room air.

DISADVANTAGES
- Complete deflation of the reservoir bag during inspiration causes CO_2 buildup.
- The FiO_2 varies with the client's breathing pattern.
- Clients who have anxiety or claustrophobia do not tolerate it well.
- Eating, drinking, and talking are impaired.

NURSING ACTIONS
- Keep the reservoir bag from deflating by adjusting the oxygen flow rate to keep the reservoir bag ⅓ to ½ full on inspiration.
- Assess proper fit to ensure a secure seal over nose and mouth. Assess for skin breakdown beneath the edges of the mask and bridge of the nose.
- Make sure the client uses a nasal cannula during meals.
- Use with caution for clients who have a high risk of aspiration or airway obstruction.

Nonrebreather mask

Covers the client's nose and mouth

FRACTION OF INSPIRED OXYGEN: Delivers an FiO_2 of 60% to 100% at flow rates of 10 to 15 L/min to keep the reservoir bag ⅔ full during inspiration and expiration.

ADVANTAGES
- It delivers the highest O_2 concentration possible (except for intubation).
- A one-way valve situated between the mask and reservoir allows the client to inhale maximum O_2 from the reservoir bag. The two exhalation ports have flaps covering them that prevent room air from entering the mask.

DISADVANTAGES
- The valve and flap on the mask must be intact and functional during each breath.
- It is poorly tolerated by clients who have anxiety or claustrophobia.
- Eating, drinking, and talking are impaired.
- Use with caution for clients who have a high risk of aspiration or airway obstruction.

NURSING ACTIONS
- Perform an hourly assessment of the valve and flap.
- Assess proper fit to ensure a secure seal over the nose and mouth. Assess for skin breakdown beneath the edges of the mask and bridge of nose.
- Make sure the client uses a nasal cannula during meals.

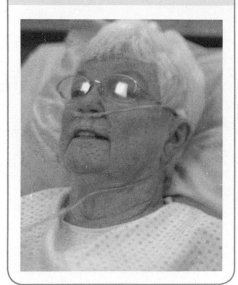

53.1 Nasal cannula

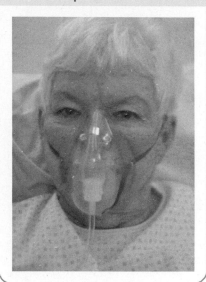

53.2 Simple face mask

HIGH-FLOW OXYGEN DELIVERY SYSTEMS

Venturi mask

Covers the client's nose and mouth

FRACTION OF INSPIRED OXYGEN: Delivers an FiO_2 of 24% to 60% at flow rates of 4 to 12 L/min via different size adapters, which allows specific amounts of air to mix with oxygen.

ADVANTAGES
- It delivers the most precise oxygen concentration.
- Humidification is not required.
- Best for clients who have chronic lung disease.

DISADVANTAGES
- Use is expensive.
- Eating, drinking, and talking are impaired.

NURSING ACTIONS
- Assess frequently to ensure an accurate flow rate.
- Assess proper fit to ensure a secure seal over the nose and mouth. Assess for skin breakdown beneath the edges of the mask particularly on the nares.
- Make sure the tubing is free of kinks.
- Ensure that the client wears a nasal cannula during meals.

Aerosol mask

Face tent: fits loosely around the face and neck

Tracheostomy collar: a small mask that covers the surgically created opening of the trachea

FRACTION OF INSPIRED OXYGEN
- Delivers an FiO_2 of 24% to 100% at flow rates of at least 10 L/min.
- Provides high humidification with oxygen delivery.

ADVANTAGES

- Use with clients who do not tolerate masks well.
- Useful for clients who have facial trauma, burns, and thick secretions.

DISADVANTAGES: High humidification requires frequent monitoring.

NURSING ACTIONS

- Empty condensation from the tubing often.
- Ensure adequate water in the humidification canister.
- Ensure that the aerosol mist leaves from the vents during inspiration and expiration
- Make sure the tubing does not pull on the tracheostomy.

COMPLICATIONS

Oxygen toxicity

Oxygen toxicity can result from high concentrations of oxygen (typically greater than 50%), long durations of oxygen therapy (typically more than 24 to 48 hr), and the severity of lung disease. Q EBP

MANIFESTATIONS: Nonproductive cough, substernal pain, nasal stuffiness, nausea, vomiting, fatigue, headache, sore throat, and hypoventilation

NURSING ACTIONS

- Use the lowest level of oxygen necessary to maintain an adequate SpO_2.
- Monitor ABGs and notify the provider if SpO_2 levels are outside the expected reference range.
- Decrease the FiO_2 as the client's SpO_2 improves.

Oxygen-induced hypoventilation

Clients who have conditions that cause alveolar hypoventilation can be sensitive to the administration of oxygen.

NURSING ACTIONS

- Monitor respiratory rate and pattern, level of consciousness, and SpO_2.
- Provide oxygen therapy at the lowest liter flow rate that manages hypoxemia.
- If the client tolerates it, use a Venturi mask to deliver precise oxygen levels.
- Notify the provider of impending respiratory depression such as a decreased respiratory rate and a decreased level of consciousness.

Combustion Qs

Oxygen is combustible.

NURSING ACTIONS

- Post "No Smoking" or "Oxygen in Use" signs to alert others of the fire hazard.
- Know where to find the closest fire extinguisher.
- Educate about the fire hazard of smoking with oxygen use.
- Have clients wear a cotton gown because synthetic or wool fabrics can generate static electricity.
- Ensure that all electric devices (razors, hearing aids, radios) are working well.
- Make sure all electric machinery (monitors, suction machines) is grounded.
- Do not use volatile, flammable materials (alcohol, acetone) near clients receiving oxygen.

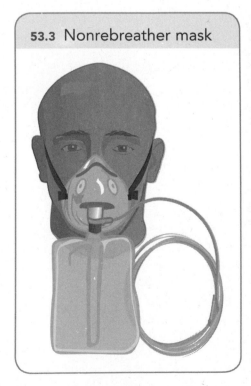

53.3 Nonrebreather mask

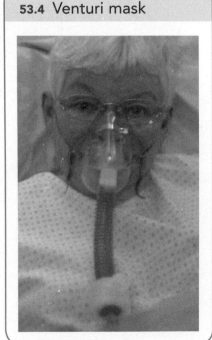

53.4 Venturi mask

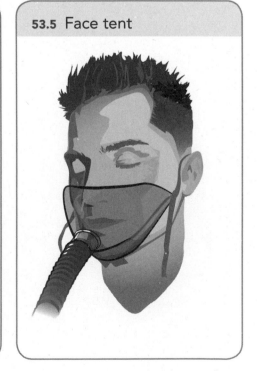

53.5 Face tent

Specimen collection and airway clearance

Mucosal secretion buildup or aspiration of emesis can obstruct a client's airway.

- Adequate hydration and coughing help the client maintain airway patency.
- Nursing interventions that mobilize secretions and maintain airway patency include assistance with coughing, hydration, positioning, humidification, nebulizer therapy, chest physiotherapy, and suctioning.
- These interventions promote adequate gas exchange and lung expansion.

INDICATIONS

CLIENTS AT RISK FOR DEVELOPING AIRWAY COMPROMISE: infants, clients who have neuromuscular disorders, clients who are quadriplegic, clients who have cystic fibrosis

INDICATIONS THAT CLIENTS NEED HELP MAINTAINING AIRWAY CLEARANCE: hypoxemia (restlessness, irritability, tachypnea, tachycardia, cyanosis, decreased level of consciousness, decreased SpO_2 levels), adventitious breath sounds, visible secretions, absence of spontaneous cough

CONSIDERATIONS

- Humidification of oxygen moistens the airways, which loosens and mobilizes pulmonary secretions.
- Nebulization breaks up medications (bronchodilators, mucolytic agents) into minute particles that disperse throughout the respiratory tract and improves clearance of pulmonary secretions.
- Chest physiotherapy involves the use of chest percussion, vibration, and postural drainage to help mobilize secretions. Chest percussion and vibration facilitate movement of secretions into the central airways. For postural drainage, one or more positions allow gravity to assist with the removal of secretions from specific areas of the lung. Qpcc
- Early-morning postural drainage mobilizes secretions that have accumulated through the night.

NURSING ACTIONS

- Collect sputum specimens by suctioning during coughing.
- Whenever possible, encourage coughing. Coughing is more effective than artificial suctioning at moving secretions into the upper trachea and laryngopharynx.
- Suction orally, nasally, or endotracheally, not routinely but only when clients need it.
- Maintain surgical asepsis when performing any form of tracheal suctioning to avoid bacterial contamination of the airway.

Sputum specimen collection

Collection of sputum for analysis

INDICATIONS

- For cytology to identify aberrant cells or cancer
- For culture and sensitivity to grow and identify micro-organisms and the antibiotics effective against them
- To identify acid-fast bacillus (AFB) to diagnose tuberculosis (requires three consecutive morning samples)

CONSIDERATIONS

NURSING ACTIONS

- Obtain specimens early in the morning.
- Wait 1 to 2 hr after the client eats to obtain a specimen to decrease the likelihood of emesis or aspiration.
- Perform chest physiotherapy to help mobilize secretions.
- Use a sterile specimen container, a label, a laboratory requisition slip, a biohazard bag for delivery of the specimen to the laboratory, clean gloves, and a mask and goggles if necessary.
- Use a container with a preservative to obtain a specimen for cytology.
- Use a sterile container for routine cultures and AFB testing.
- If a client cannot cough effectively and expectorate sputum into the container, collect the specimen by endotracheal suctioning.
- Older adult clients have a weak cough reflex and decreased muscle strength, making it difficult for them to expectorate. They can require suctioning for sputum specimen collection. Ⓖ

INTERPRETATION OF FINDINGS

- Presence of micro-organisms indicating infection
- Presence of cancer cells

Chest physiotherapy

- The use of a set of techniques that loosen respiratory secretions and move them into the central airways where coughing or suctioning can remove them
- For clients who have thick secretions and are unable to clear their airways
- Contraindicated for clients who are pregnant; have a rib, chest, head, or neck injury; have increased intracranial pressure; have had recent abdominal surgery; have a pulmonary embolism; or have bleeding disorders or osteoporosis

Percussion: the use of cupped hands to clap rhythmically on the chest to break up secretions

Vibration: the use of a shaking movement during exhalation to help remove secretions

Postural drainage: the use of various positions to allow secretions to drain by gravity

CONSIDERATIONS

NURSING ACTIONS

- Schedule treatments 1 hr before or 2 hr after meals, and at bedtime to decrease the likelihood of vomiting or aspirating.
- Administer a bronchodilator medication or nebulizer treatment 30 min to 1 hr prior to postural drainage.
- Offer the client an emesis basin and facial tissues.
- Apply manual percussion to the chest wall using cupped hands or a specific device.
- Place hands on the affected area, tense hand and arm muscles, and move the heel of the hands to create vibrations as the client exhales. Have the client cough after each set of vibrations.
- Have the client remain in each position for 10 to 15 min to allow time for percussion, vibration, and postural drainage.
- Discontinue the procedure if the client reports faintness or dizziness.
- Note that older adult clients have decreased respiratory muscle strength and chest wall compliance, which puts them at risk for aspiration. They require more frequent position changes and other interventions to promote mobility of secretions. ⓒ

Positioning: Ensure proper positioning to promote drainage of specific areas of the lungs.
- Both lobes in general: high Fowler's
- Apical segments of both lobes: sitting on the side of the bed
- Right upper lobe, anterior segment: supine with head elevation
- Right upper lobe, posterior segment: on the left side with a pillow under the right side of the chest
- Right middle lobe, anterior segment: three-quarters supine with dependent lung in Trendelenburg
- Right middle lobe, posterior segment: prone with thorax and abdomen elevation
- Right lower lobe, lateral segment: on the left side in Trendelenburg
- Left upper lobe, anterior segment: supine with head elevation
- Left upper lobe, posterior segment: on the right side with a pillow under the left side of the chest
- Left lower lobe, lateral segment: on the right side in Trendelenburg
- Both lower lobes, anterior segments: supine in Trendelenburg
- Both lower lobes, posterior segments: prone in Trendelenburg

Suctioning

Suction orally, nasally, or endotracheally when clients have early signs of hypoxemia, such as restlessness, confusion, tachypnea, tachycardia, decreased SpO_2 levels, adventitious breath sounds, audible or visible secretions, cyanosis, and absence of spontaneous cough.

CONSIDERATIONS

NURSING ACTIONS

- Don the required personal protective equipment.
- Assist the client to high-Fowler's or Fowler's position for suctioning if possible.
- Encourage the client to breathe deeply and cough in an attempt to clear the secretions without artificial suction.
- Obtain baseline breath sounds and vital signs, including SaO_2 by pulse oximeter. Can monitor SaO_2 continually during the procedure.
- For oropharyngeal suctioning, use a Yankauer or tonsil-tipped rigid suction catheter and move the catheter around the mouth, gum line, and pharynx.
- For nasopharyngeal and nasotracheal suctioning, use a flexible catheter and lubricate the distal 6 to 8 cm (2 to 3 in) with water-soluble lubricant.
- For endotracheal suctioning, use a suction catheter. The catheter should not exceed one half of the internal diameter of the endotracheal tube to prevent hypoxia. The nurse should use no larger than a 16 French suction catheter when suctioning an 8 mm endotracheal tube or tracheostomy tube. Hyperoxygenate the client using a bag-valve-mask (BVM) or specialized ventilator function with an FiO_2 of 100%.
- Use medical asepsis for suctioning the mouth.
- Use surgical asepsis for all other types of suctioning.
- Use suction pressure no higher than 120 to 150 mm Hg.
- Limit each suction attempt to no longer than 10 to 15 seconds to avoid hypoxia and the vagal response. Repeat suctioning if needed. Limit total suctioning time to 5 minutes. Ⓠ EBP

Additional guidelines for nasopharyngeal and nasotracheal suctioning

- Insert the catheter into the naris during inhalation.
- Do not apply suction while inserting the catheter.
- Follow the natural course of the naris and slightly slant the catheter downward while advancing it.
- Advance the catheter the approximate distance from the tip of the nose to the base of the earlobe.
- Apply suction intermittently by covering and releasing the suction port with the thumb for 10 to 15 seconds.
- Apply suction only while withdrawing the catheter and rotating it with the thumb and forefinger.
- Do not perform more than two passes with the catheter. Allow at least 1 min between passes for ventilation and oxygenation.

Additional guidelines for endotracheal suctioning

- Remove the bag or ventilator from the tracheostomy or endotracheal tube and insert the catheter into the lumen of the airway. Advance the catheter until resistance is met. The catheter should reach the level of the carina (location of bifurcation into the mainstem bronchi).
- Pull the catheter back 1 cm (0.4 in) prior to applying suction to prevent mucosal damage.
- Apply suction intermittently by covering and releasing the suction port with the thumb for 10 to 15 seconds.
- Apply suction only while withdrawing the catheter and rotating it with the thumb and forefinger.
- Reattach the BVM or ventilator and administer 100% oxygen.
- Rinse catheter and suction tubing with sterile saline until clear.
- Do not reuse the suction catheter for subsequent suctioning sessions.

Artificial airways and tracheostomy care

A tracheotomy is a sterile surgical incision into the trachea through the skin and muscles for the purpose of establishing an airway.

- A tracheotomy can be an emergency or a scheduled surgical procedure; it can be temporary or permanent.
- A tracheostomy is the stoma/opening that results from a tracheotomy to provide and secure a patent airway.
- Artificial airways can be placed orotracheally, nasotracheally, or through a tracheostomy to assist with respiration.
- Tracheostomy tubes vary in their composition (plastic, steel, silicone), number of parts, size (long vs. short), and shape (50° to 90° angles).
- There is no standard tracheostomy sizing system. However, the diameter of the tracheostomy tube must be smaller than the trachea.
- The outside cannula has a flange or neck plate that sits against the skin of the neck and has holes on each side for attaching ties around the neck to stabilize the tracheostomy tube.
- Airflow in and out of a tracheostomy without air leakage (a cuffed tracheostomy tube) bypasses the vocal cords, resulting in an inability to produce sound or speech.
- Uncuffed tubes and fenestrated tubes, in place or capped, allow speech. Clients who have a cuffed tube can be off mechanical ventilation, can breathe around the tube, and can use a specific valve to allow for speech. The cuff is deflated and the valve occludes the opening.
- Indications for a tracheostomy include acute or chronic upper airway obstruction, edema, anaphylaxis, burns, trauma, head/neck surgery, copious secretions, obstructive sleep apnea refractory to conventional therapy, and the need for long-term mechanical ventilation or reconstruction after laryngeal trauma or laryngeal cancer surgery.

ARTIFICIAL AIRWAY TUBE TYPES

Single-lumen (cannula)

- Long, single-cannula tube
- For clients who have long or thick necks

NURSING CONSIDERATIONS: Do not use with clients who have excessive secretions.

Double-lumen (cannula)

- An outer cannula fits into the stoma and keeps the airway open.
- An inner cannula fits snugly into the outer cannula and locks into place.
- An obturator is a thin, solid tube the provider places inside the tracheostomy and uses as a guide for inserting the outer cannula, and removes immediately after outer cannula insertion.

NURSING CONSIDERATIONS

- This device allows removing, cleaning, reusing, discarding, and replacing the inner cannula with a disposable inner cannula.
- It is useful for clients who have excessive secretions.

Cuffed tube

It has a balloon that inflates around the outside of the distal segment of the tube to protect the lower airway by producing a seal between the upper and lower airway.

NURSING CONSIDERATIONS
- A cuffed tube permits mechanical ventilation.
- A cuffed tube prevents aspiration of oropharyngeal secretions.
- Cuffs do not hold the tube in place.
- Cuff pressures must be monitored to prevent tracheal tissue necrosis.
- The client is unable to speak.
- Children do not require a cuffed tube.

Cuffless tube

It has no balloon and is for clients who have long-term airway-management needs.

NURSING CONSIDERATIONS
- The client must be at low risk for aspiration.
- Cuffless tubes are not for clients on mechanical ventilation.
- This device allows the client to speak.

Fenestrated tube with cuff

- It has one large or multiple openings (fenestrations) in the posterior wall of the outer cannula with a balloon around the outside of the distal segment of the tube.
- It also has an inner cannula.

NURSING CONSIDERATIONS
- This device allows for mechanical ventilation.
- Removing the inner cannula allows the fenestrations to permit air to flow through the openings.
- This device allows the client to speak.

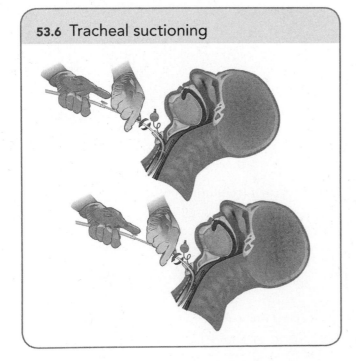

53.6 Tracheal suctioning

Fenestrated tube without cuff

- It has one larger or multiple openings (fenestrations) in the posterior wall of the outer cannula with no balloon.
- It also has an inner cannula.

NURSING CONSIDERATIONS
- The holes in the tube help wean the client from the tracheostomy.
- Removing the inner cannula allows the fenestrations to permit air to flow through the openings.
- This device allows the client to speak.

CONSIDERATIONS

NURSING ACTIONS
- Keep the following at the bedside: two extra tracheostomy tubes (one the client's size and one size smaller, in case of accidental decannulation), the obturator for the existing tube, an oxygen source, suction catheters and a suction source, and a BVM.
- Provide methods to communicate with staff (paper and pen, dry-erase board).
- Provide an emergency call system and a call light. Qs
- Provide adequate humidification and hydration to thin secretions and reduce the risk of mucous plugs.
- Give oral care every 2 hr.
- Provide tracheostomy care every 8 hr to reduce the risk of infection and skin breakdown.
  - Suction the tracheostomy tube, if necessary, using sterile suctioning supplies.
  - Remove soiled dressings and excess secretions.
  - Apply the oxygen source loosely if the client's SpO_2 decreases during the procedure.
  - Use cotton-tipped applicators and gauze pads to clean exposed outer cannula surfaces. Use the facility-approved solution. Clean in a circular motion from the stoma site outward.
  - Use surgical asepsis to remove and clean the inner cannula (with the facility-approved solution). Use a new inner cannula if it is disposable.
  - Clean the stoma site and then the tracheostomy plate.
  - Place a fresh split-gauze tracheostomy dressing of nonraveling material under and around the tracheostomy holder and plate.
  - Replace tracheostomy ties if they are wet or soiled. Secure the new ties before removing the soiled ones to prevent accidental decannulation.
  - If a knot is needed, tie a square knot that is visible on the side of the neck. Check that one or two fingers fit between the tie and the neck.
- Change nondisposable tracheostomy tubes every 6 to 8 weeks or per protocol.
- Reposition the client every 2 hr to prevent atelectasis and pneumonia.
- Minimize dust in the room. Do not shake bedding.
- If the client is permitted to eat, position him upright and tip his chin to his chest to enable swallowing. Assess for aspiration.

COMPLICATIONS

Accidental decannulation

Accidental decannulation in the first 72 hr after surgery is an emergency because the tracheostomy tract has not matured, and replacement can be difficult.

> **!** Ventilate the client with a BVM. Call for assistance.

NURSING ACTIONS
- Always keep the tracheostomy obturator and two spare tracheostomy tubes at the bedside.
- If unable to replace the tracheostomy tube, administer oxygen through the stoma. If unable to administer oxygen through the stoma, occlude the stoma and administer oxygen through the nose and mouth.

If accidental decannulation occurs after the first 72 hr
- Immediately hyperextend the neck and with the obturator inserted into the tracheostomy tube, quickly and gently replace the tube and remove the obturator. Qpcc
- Secure the tube.
- Assess tube placement by auscultating for bilateral breath sounds.

Damage to the trachea

Tracheal stenosis: Narrowing of the tracheal lumen due to scar formation resulting from irritation of the tracheal mucosa from the tracheal tube cuff.

NURSING CONSIDERATIONS
- Keep the cuff pressure between 14 and 20 mm Hg.
- Check the cuff pressure at least once every 8 hr.
- Keep the tube in the midline position and prevent pulling or traction on the tracheostomy tube.

Tracheal wall necrosis: Tissue damage that results when the pressure of the inflated cuff impairs blood flow to the tracheal wall.

PRACTICE Active Learning Scenario

A nurse is reviewing with a group of nursing students how to perform postural drainage. Use the ATI Active Learning Template: Nursing Skill to complete this item.

DESCRIPTION OF SKILL: List the specific positions that facilitate secretion drainage from at least eight specific lung areas.

Application Exercises

1. A nurse is assessing a client who has an acute respiratory infection that puts her at risk for hypoxemia. Which of the following findings are early indications that should alert the nurse that the client is developing hypoxemia? (Select all that apply.)
   - A. Restlessness
   - B. Tachypnea
   - C. Bradycardia
   - D. Confusion
   - E. Pallor

2. A provider is discharging a client who has a prescription for home oxygen therapy via nasal cannula. Client and family teaching by the nurse should include which of the following instructions? (Select all that apply.)
   - A. Apply petroleum jelly around and inside the nares.
   - B. Remove the nasal cannula during mealtimes.
   - C. Check the position of the cannula frequently.
   - D. Report any nasal stuffiness, nausea, or fatigue.
   - E. Post "No Smoking" signs in a prominent location.

3. A nurse is caring for a client who is having difficulty breathing. The client is lying in bed and is already receiving oxygen therapy via nasal cannula. Which of the following interventions is the nurse's priority?
   - A. Increase the oxygen flow.
   - B. Assist the client to Fowler's position.
   - C. Promote removal of pulmonary secretions.
   - D. Obtain a specimen for arterial blood gases.

4. A nurse is preparing to perform endotracheal suctioning for a client. The nurse should follow which of the following guidelines? (Select all that apply.)
   - A. Apply suction while withdrawing the catheter.
   - B. Perform suctioning on a routine basis, every 2 to 3 hr.
   - C. Maintain medical asepsis during suctioning.
   - D. Use a new catheter for each suctioning attempt.
   - E. Limit total suctioning time to 5 minutes.

5. A nurse is caring for a client who has a tracheostomy. Which of the following actions should the nurse take when providing tracheostomy care? (Select all that apply.)
   - A. Apply the oxygen source loosely if the SpO_2 decreases during the procedure.
   - B. Use surgical asepsis to remove and clean the inner cannula.
   - C. Clean the outer surfaces in a circular motion from the stoma site outward.
   - D. Replace the tracheostomy ties with new ties.
   - E. Cut a slit in gauze squares to place beneath the tube holder.

1. A. CORRECT: The nurse should monitor for restlessness, which is an early manifestation of hypoxemia, along with tachycardia, elevated blood pressure, use of accessory muscles, nasal flaring, tracheal tugging, and adventitious lung sounds.

   B. CORRECT: The nurse should monitor for tachypnea, which is an early manifestation of hypoxemia.

   C. Bradycardia is a late manifestation of hypoxemia, along with stupor, cyanotic skin and mucous membranes, bradypnea, hypotension, and cardiac dysrhythmias.

   D. CORRECT: The nurse should monitor for confusion, which is an early manifestation of hypoxemia.

   E. CORRECT: The nurse should monitor for pallor, which is an early manifestation of hypoxemia.

   (N) NCLEX® Connection: Physiological Adaptation, Illness Management

2. A. The nurse should teach the client to apply a water-based lubricant to protect the nares from drying during oxygen therapy.

   B. The nurse should teach the client to leave the nasal cannula on while eating because it does not interfere with eating.

   C. CORRECT: The nurse should teach the client that a disadvantage of the nasal cannula is that it dislodges easily. The client should form the habit of checking its position periodically and readjusting it as necessary.

   D. CORRECT: The nurse should teach the client about oxygen toxicity, which is a complication of oxygen therapy, usually from high concentrations or long durations. Manifestations include a nonproductive cough, substernal pain, nasal stuffiness, nausea, vomiting, fatigue, headache, sore throat, and hypoventilation. The client should report any of these promptly.

   E. CORRECT: The nurse should teach the client that oxygen is combustible and thus increases the risk of fire injuries. No one in the house should smoke or use any device that might generate sparks in the area where the oxygen is in use.

   (N) NCLEX® Connection: Reduction of Risk Potential, Therapeutic Procedures

3. A. The nurse might need to increase the client's oxygen flow, as hypoxemia can be the cause of his difficulty breathing. However, another action is the priority.

   B. CORRECT: The priority action the nurse should take when using the airway, breathing, circulation (ABC) approach to care delivery is to relieve dyspnea (difficulty breathing). Fowler's position facilitates maximal lung expansion and thus optimizes breathing. With the client in this position, the nurse can better assess and determine the cause of the client's dyspnea.

   C. The nurse might need to suction the client or encourage expectoration of pulmonary secretions. However, another action is the priority,

   D. The nurse should check the client's oxygenation status. However, another action is the priority.

   (N) NCLEX® Connection: Physiological Adaptation, Illness Management

4. A. CORRECT: The nurse should apply suction pressure only while withdrawing the catheter to prevent damaging the tracheal tissue.

   B. The nurse should suction the client only as needed, because suctioning is not without risk. It can cause mucosal damage, bleeding, and bronchospasm.

   C. The nurse should use surgical asepsis when performing endotracheal suctioning to prevent contamination with microorganism that can cause an infection.

   D. CORRECT: The nurse should use a new suction catheter, unless an in-line suctioning system is in place, to prevent contamination with microorganism that can cause an infection.

   E. CORRECT: To prevent hypoxemia, the nurse should limit total suctioning time to 5 minutes and allow at least 1 min between passes for ventilation and oxygenation.

   (N) NCLEX® Connection: Physiological Adaptation, Alterations in Body Systems

5. A. CORRECT: The nurse should provide supplemental oxygen in response to any decline in oxygen saturation while performing tracheostomy care.

   B. CORRECT: The nurse should use a sterile disposable tracheostomy cleaning kit or sterile supplies and maintain surgical asepsis throughout this part of the procedure.

   C. CORRECT: The nurse should cleanse the surface around the stoma in a circular motion from the stoma site outward. Cleansing in this manner helps move mucus and contaminated material away from the stoma for easy removal.

   D. The nurse should replace the tracheostomy ties if they are wet or soiled. There is a risk of tube dislodgement with replacing the ties, so he should not replace them routinely.

   E. The nurse should use a commercially prepared tracheostomy dressing with a slit in it. Cutting gauze squares can loosen lint or gauze fibers the client could aspirate.

   (N) NCLEX Connection: Reduction of Risk Potential, Potential for Complications of Diagnostic Tests/Treatments/Procedures

PRACTICE Answer

Using the ATI Active Learning Template: Nursing Skill

DESCRIPTION OF SKILL

- Both lobes in general: high-Fowler's
- Apical segments of both lobes: sitting on the side of the bed
- Right upper lobe, anterior segment: supine with head elevation
- Right upper lobe, posterior segment: on the left side with a pillow under the right side of the chest
- Right middle lobe, anterior segment: three-quarters supine with dependent lung in Trendelenburg
- Right middle lobe, posterior segment: prone with thorax and abdomen elevation
- Right lower lobe, lateral segment: on the left side in Trendelenburg
- Left upper lobe, anterior segment: supine with head elevation
- Left upper lobe, posterior segment: on the right side with a pillow under the left side of the chest
- Left lower lobe, lateral segment: on the right side in Trendelenburg
- Both lower lobes, anterior segments: supine in Trendelenburg
- Both lower lobes, posterior segments: prone in Trendelenburg

(N) NCLEX® Connection: Physiological Adaptation, Alterations in Body Systems

UNIT 4   PHYSIOLOGICAL INTEGRITY

SECTION: REDUCTION OF RISK POTENTIAL

CHAPTER 54 *Nasogastric Intubation and Enteral Feedings*

Nasogastric intubation is the insertion of a nasogastric (NG) tube to manage gastrointestinal (GI) dysfunction and provide enteral nutrition via NG. Nurses also give enteral feedings through jejunal and gastric tubes.

Nasogastric intubation

An NG tube is a hollow, flexible, cylindrical device the nurse inserts through the nasopharynx into the stomach.

INDICATIONS

Decompression
- Removal of gases or stomach contents to relieve distention, nausea, or vomiting
- Tube types: Salem sump, Miller–Abbott, Levin

Feeding
- Alternative to the oral route for administering nutritional supplements
- Tube types: Duo, Levin, Dobhoff

Lavage
- Washing out the stomach to treat active bleeding, ingestion of poison, or for gastric dilation
- Tube types: Ewald, Levin, Salem sump

Compression
- Using an internal balloon to apply pressure for preventing hemorrhage
- Tube type: Sengstaken–Blakemore

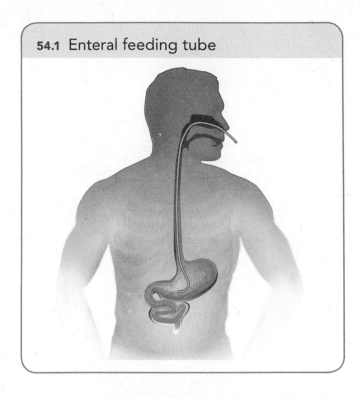

54.1 Enteral feeding tube

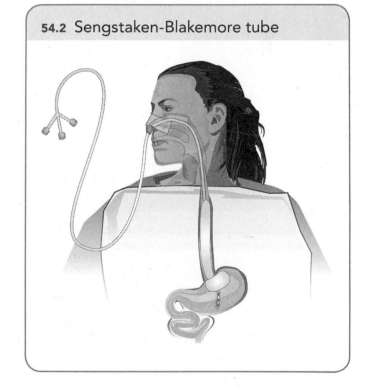

54.2 Sengstaken-Blakemore tube

CONSIDERATIONS

PREPROCEDURE

NURSING ACTIONS

- Review the prescription and purpose, plan for drainage or suction, and understand the need for placement for diagnostic purposes.
- Identify the client, and explain the procedure.
- Review the client's history (nasal problems, anticoagulants, previous trauma, past history of aspiration).
- Evaluate the client's ability to assist and cooperate.
- Establish a means of communication to signal distress, such as the client raising a hand. Qᴘᴄᴄ
- Perform hand hygiene.
- Set up the equipment.
  - NG tube: selected according to the indication
  - Tape or use a commercial fixation device to secure the dressing
  - Clean gloves
  - Water-soluble lubricant
  - Topical anesthetic
  - Cup of water and straw
  - Catheter-tipped syringe, usually 30 to 60 mL
  - Basin to prepare for gag-induced nausea
  - pH test strip or meter to measure gastric secretions for acidity
  - Stethoscope
  - Disposable towel to maintain a clean environment
  - Clamp or plug to close the tubing after insertion
  - Suction apparatus if attaching the tube to continuous or intermittent suction
  - Gauze square to cleanse the outside of the tubing after insertion
  - Safety pin and elastic band or commercial device to secure the tubing and prevent accidental removal
- Position a disposable towel and basin.
- Provide privacy.

INTRAPROCEDURE

NURSING ACTIONS

- Auscultate for bowel sounds, and palpate the abdomen for distention, pain, and rigidity.
- Raise the bed to a level comfortable for the nurse.
- Assist the client to high-Fowler's position (if possible).
- Assess the nares for the best route to determine how to avoid a septal deviation or other obstruction during the insertion process.
- Use the correct procedure for tube insertion, wearing clean gloves, and evaluate the outcome.
- If the client vomits, clear the airway, and provide comfort prior to continuing. Qs
- Check placement. Aspirate gently to collect gastric contents, testing pH (4 or less is expected), and assess odor, color, and consistency.

- After placement verification, secure the NG tube on the nose, avoiding pressure on the nares.
  - Confirm placement with an x-ray. Qᴇʙᴘ
  - Injecting air into the tube and then listening over the abdomen is not an acceptable practice.
- If the tube is not in the stomach, advance it 5 cm (2 in), and repeat the placement check.
- Clamp the NG tube, or connect it to the suction device.
- Salem sump tubing has a blue pigtail for negative air release. Do not insert any substance into the blue pigtail because it will break the seal and the tubing will leak.

POSTPROCEDURE

NURSING ACTIONS

- The insertion and maintenance of an NG tube is a nursing responsibility, but nurses may delegate measuring output, providing comfort, and giving oral care.
- For removal, wear clean gloves.
  - Inform the client of the prescription and process, emphasizing that removal is less stressful than placement.
  - Measure and record any drainage, assessing it for color, consistency, and odor.
  - Ensure comfort. Qᴘᴄᴄ
  - Document all relevant information.
    - Tubing removal and condition of the tube
    - Volume and description of the drainage
    - Abdominal assessment, including inspection, auscultation, percussion, and palpation
    - Last and next bowel movement and urine output

COMPLICATIONS

Excoriation of nares and stomach

- Apply water-soluble lubricant to the nares as necessary.
- Assess the color of the drainage. Report dark, coffee-ground, or blood-streaked drainage immediately.
- Consider switching the tube to the other naris.

Discomfort

- Rinse the mouth with water for dryness.
- Throat lozenges can help.
- Provide oral hygiene frequently.

Occlusion of the NG tube leading to distention

- Irrigate the tube per the facility's protocol to unclog blockages. Use tap water with enteral feedings. Have the client change position in case the tip of the tube is against the stomach wall.
- Verify that suction equipment functions properly.

Enteral feedings

Enteral feeding is a method of providing nutrients to clients who cannot consume foods orally.

ENTERAL FORMULAS

Polymeric: 1 to 2 kcal/mL
- Milk-based, blenderized foods
- Whole-nutrient formulas, either commercial or from the dietary department
- Only for clients whose GI tract can absorb whole nutrients

Modular formulas: 3.8 to 4 kcal/mL
- Single-macronutrient preparation
- Not nutritionally complete
- Supplement to other foods

Elemental formulas: 1 to 3 kcal/mL
- Predigested nutrients
- Not nutritionally complete
- Easier for a partially dysfunctional GI tract to absorb

Specialty formulas: 1 to 2 kcal/mL
- For meeting specific nutritional needs
- Not nutritionally complete
- Primarily for clients who have hepatic failure, respiratory disease, or HIV infection

ENTERAL ACCESS TUBES

Gastroparesis, esophageal reflux, or a history of aspiration pneumonia generally requires intestinal placement.

Nasogastric or nasointestinal
- Therapy duration less than 4 weeks
- Inserted via the nose

Gastrostomy or jejunostomy
- Therapy duration longer than 4 weeks
- Inserted surgically

Percutaneous endoscopic gastrostomy or jejunostomy
- Therapy duration longer than 4 weeks
- Inserted endoscopically

INDICATIONS

- Critical illness/trauma
- Neurological and muscular disorders: brain neoplasm, stroke, dementia, myopathy, Parkinson's disease
- Cancer that affects the head and neck, upper GI tract
- GI disorders: enterocutaneous fistula, inflammatory bowel disease, mild pancreatitis
- Respiratory failure with prolonged intubation
- Inadequate oral intake

CONSIDERATIONS

PREPARATION OF THE CLIENT

NURSING ACTIONS
- Review the prescription. Generally, the provider and dietary staff consult to determine the type of tube feeding formula. Qpcc
- Set up the equipment.
  - Feeding bag
  - Tubing
  - 30- to 60-mL syringe (compatible with the tubing)
  - Stethoscope
  - pH indicator strip
  - Infusion pump (if not a gravity drip)
  - Appropriate enteral formula
  - Irrigant solution: sterile or tap water, according to the facility's policy
  - Clean gloves
  - Supplies for blood glucose (if protocol or prescription indicates)
  - Suction equipment to use in case of aspiration

ONGOING CARE

NURSING ACTIONS
- Prepare the formula, tubing, and infusion device.
  - Check expiration dates, and note the content of the formula.
  - Ensure that the formula is at room temperature.
  - Set up the feeding system via gravity or pump.
  - Mix or shake the formula, fill the container, prime the tubing, and clamp it.
- Assist the client to Fowler's position, or elevate the head of the bed to a minimum of 30°.
- Auscultate for bowel sounds.
- Monitor tube placement.
  - Check gastric contents for pH. A good indication of appropriate placement is obtaining gastric contents with a pH between 0 and 4.
  - Aspirate for residual volume. Qs
  - Note the appearance of the aspirate.
  - Return aspirated contents, or follow the facility's protocol.
- Flush the tubing with at least 30 mL tap water.
- Administer the formula.
  - **Intermittent feeding**
    - Prepare the formula and a 60-mL syringe.
    - Remove the plunger from the syringe.
    - Hold the tubing above the instillation site.
    - Open the stopcock on the tubing, and insert the barrel of the syringe with the end up.
    - Fill the syringe with 40 to 50 mL formula.
    - If using a feeding bag, fill the bag with the total amount of formula for one feeding, and hang it to drain via gravity until empty (about 30 to 45 min).
    - If using a syringe, hold it high enough for the formula to empty gradually via gravity.
    - Continue to refill the syringe until the amount for the feeding is instilled. Follow with at least 30 mL tap water to flush the tube and prevent clogging.

- **Continuous-drip feeding**
  - Connect the feeding bag system to the feeding tube.
  - If using a pump, program the instillation rate, and set the total volume to instill.
  - Start the pump.
  - Flush the enteral tubing with at least 30 mL irrigant, usually tap water, every 4 to 6 hr, and check tube placement again.
  - Monitor intake and output, and include 24-hr totals.
  - Monitor capillary blood glucose every 6 hr until the client tolerates the maximum administration rate for 24 hr.
  - Use an infusion pump for intestinal tube feedings.
  - Follow the manufacturer's recommendations for formula hang time. Refrigerate unused formula, and discard after 24 hr.
  - Check gastric residual every 4 to 8 hr. Each facility's protocol specifies the actions to take for the amount of residual. **Qs**
  - Do not delegate this skill to assistive personnel.

COMPLICATIONS

Gastric residual exceeds 250 mL for each of two consecutive assessments

NURSING ACTIONS
- Withhold the feeding.
- Notify the provider.
- Keep the client in semi-Fowler's position.
- Recheck residual in 1 hr.

Diarrhea three times or more in a 24-hr period

NURSING ACTIONS
- Slow the instillation rate.
- Notify the provider.
- Confer with the dietitian.
- Provide skin care and protection.

Nausea or vomiting

NURSING ACTIONS
- Slow the instillation rate.
- Keep the head of the bed at 30°.
- Make sure the formula is at room temperature.
- Turn the client to the side.
- Notify the provider.
- Check the tube's patency.
- Aspirate for residual.
- Auscultate for bowel sounds.
- Obtain a chest x-ray.

Aspiration of formula **Qs**

NURSING ACTIONS
- Withhold the feeding.
- Turn the client to the side.
- Suction the airway.
- Provide oxygen if indicated.
- Monitor vital signs for elevated temperature.
- Monitor for decreased oxygen saturation or increased respiratory rate.
- Auscultate breath sounds for increased congestion.
- Notify the provider.
- Obtain a chest x-ray.

Skin irritation around the tubing site

NURSING ACTIONS
- Provide a skin barrier for any drainage at the site.
- Monitor the tube's placement.

Application Exercises

1. A nurse is delivering an enteral feeding to a client who has an NG tube in place for intermittent feedings. When the nurse pours water into the syringe after the formula drains from the syringe, the client asks the nurse why the water is necessary. Which of the following responses should the nurse make?

   A. "Water helps clear the tube so it doesn't get clogged."

   B. "Flushing helps make sure the tube stays in place."

   C. "This will help you get enough fluids."

   D. "Adding water makes the formula less concentrated."

2. A nurse is caring for a client who is receiving continuous enteral feedings. Which of the following nursing interventions is the highest priority when the nurse suspects aspiration of the feeding?

   A. Auscultate breath sounds.

   B. Stop the feeding.

   C. Obtain a chest x-ray.

   D. Initiate oxygen therapy.

3. A nurse is preparing to instill an enteral feeding for a client who has an NG tube in place. Which of the following actions is the nurse's highest assessment priority before performing this procedure?

   A. Check how long the feeding container has been open.

   B. Verify the placement of the NG tube.

   C. Confirm that the client does not have diarrhea.

   D. Make sure the client is alert and oriented.

4. A nurse is caring for a client in a long-term care facility who is receiving enteral feedings via an NG tube. Which of the following actions should the nurse complete prior to administering the tube feeding? (Select all that apply.)

   A. Auscultate bowel sounds.

   B. Assist the client to an upright position.

   C. Test the pH of gastric aspirate.

   D. Warm the formula to body temperature.

   E. Discard any residual gastric contents.

5. A nurse is preparing to insert an NG tube for a client who requires gastric decompression. Which of the following actions should the nurse perform before beginning the procedure? (Select all that apply.)

   A. Review a signal the client can use if feeling any distress.

   B. Lay a towel across the client's chest.

   C. Administer oral pain medication.

   D. Obtain a Dobhoff tube for insertion.

   E. Have a petroleum-based lubricant available.

PRACTICE Active Learning Scenario

A nurse is teaching a group of nursing students about administering enteral feedings. Use the ATI Active Learning Template: Nursing Skill to complete this item.

INDICATIONS: List at least four indications for enteral feedings.

NURSING INTERVENTIONS (INTRAPROCEDURE): List the steps of administering an enteral feeding.

Application Exercises Key

1. A. **CORRECT:** The nurse should flush the tube after instilling the feeding to help keep the NG tube patent by clearing any excess formula from the tube so that it doesn't clump and clog the tube.

   B. The nurse should tape a securing device, not flush the tube with water, to help maintain the position of the NG tube.

   C. The nurse should administer additional fluids. The small amount used for flushing the NG tube will not be adequate.

   D. The nurse should contact the dietary staff to prepare formula according to the prescription before the nurse instills it.

   Ⓝ *NCLEX® Connection: Reduction of Risk Potential, Potential for Alterations in Body Systems*

2. A. The nurse should listen to breath sounds whenever there is suspicion of the client aspirating. However, another assessment is the priority.

   B. **CORRECT:** The greatest risk to the client is aspiration pneumonia. The first action the nurse should take is to stop the feeding so that no more formula can enter the lungs.

   C. The nurse should obtain a chest x-ray whenever there is suspicion of the client aspirating. However, another assessment is the priority.

   D. The nurse should initiate oxygen therapy whenever there is suspicion of the client aspirating. However, another assessment is the priority.

   Ⓝ *NCLEX® Connection: Reduction of Risk Potential, Potential for Complications of Diagnostic Tests/Treatments/Procedures*

3. A. Checking that the container has not exceeded its expiration date, either for having it open or for opening it, is important. However, there is a higher assessment priority among these options.

   B. **CORRECT:** The greatest risk to the client receiving enteral feedings is injury from aspiration. The priority nursing assessment before initiating an enteral feeding is to verify proper placement of the NG tube.

   C. The nurse should assess the client for any possible complications of enteral feedings, such as diarrhea. However, there is another assessment that is the priority.

   D. The nurse should determine the client's level of consciousness as an assessment parameter that is ongoing and should precede any procedure. However, another assessment is the priority.

   Ⓝ *NCLEX® Connection: Reduction of Risk Potential, Potential for Complications of Diagnostic Tests/Treatments/Procedures*

4. A. **CORRECT:** The nurse should auscultate for bowel sounds, because the client's gastrointestinal tract might not be able to absorb nutrients. The nurse should then withhold feedings and notify the provider.

   B. **CORRECT:** The nurse should place the client in an upright position, with at least a 30° elevation of the head of the bed. Upright positioning helps prevent aspiration.

   C. **CORRECT:** Before administering enteral feedings, the nurse should verify the placement of the NG tube. The only reliable method is x-ray confirmation, which is impractical prior to every feeding. Testing the pH of gastric aspirate is an acceptable method between x-ray confirmations.

   D. The nurse should have the enteral formula at room temperature before administering the enteral feeding.

   E. The nurse should return the residual to the client's stomach, unless the volume of gastric contents is more than 250 mL or the facility has other guidelines in place.

   Ⓝ *NCLEX® Connection: Reduction of Risk Potential, Potential for Complications of Diagnostic Tests/Treatments/Procedures*

5. A. **CORRECT:** The nurse should establish a means for the client to communicate that she wants to stop the procedure, before inserting an NG tube.

   B. **CORRECT:** The nurse should place a disposable towel across the client's chest to provide for a clean environment and protect the client's gown from becoming soiled.

   C. Because the purpose of the procedure is to remove stomach contents, the procedure would also remove the oral pain medication.

   D. The nurse should plan to use the prescribed type of tube for gastric decompression, which is a Salem sump, Miller-Abbott, or Levin. A Dobhoff tube is for feeding.

   E. The nurse should plan to use a water-based lubricant to reduce complications from aspiration.

   Ⓝ *NCLEX® Connection: Reduction of Risk Potential, Potential for Complications of Diagnostic Tests/Treatments/Procedures*

PRACTICE Answer

Using the ATI Active Learning Template: Nursing Skill

INDICATIONS

- Critical illness, trauma
- Neurological and muscular disorders: brain neoplasm, cerebrovascular accident, dementia, myopathy, Parkinson's disease
- GI disorders: enterocutaneous fistula, inflammatory bowel disease, mild pancreatitis
- Respiratory failure with prolonged intubation
- Inadequate oral intake

NURSING INTERVENTIONS (INTRAPROCEDURE)

- Prepare the formula and a 60 mL syringe.
- Remove the plunger from the syringe.
- Hold the tubing above the instillation site.
- Open the stopcock on the tubing, and insert the barrel of the syringe with the end up.
- Fill the syringe with 40 to 50 mL formula.
- If using a feeding bag, fill the bag with the total amount of formula for one feeding, and hang it to drain via gravity until empty (about 30 to 45 min).
- If using a syringe, hold it high enough for the formula to empty gradually via gravity.
- Continue to refill the syringe until the amount for the feeding is instilled.
- Follow with at least 30 mL tap water to flush the tube and prevent clogging.

Ⓝ *NCLEX® Connection: Reduction of Risk Potential, Potential for Complications of Diagnostic Tests/Treatments/Procedures*

When reviewing the following chapters, keep in mind the relevant topics and tasks of the NCLEX outline, in particular:

Client Needs: Reduction of Risk Potential

CHANGES/ABNORMALITIES IN VITAL SIGNS: Assess and respond to changes in client vital signs.

POTENTIAL FOR COMPLICATIONS OF DIAGNOSTIC TESTS/ TREATMENTS/PROCEDURES: Apply knowledge of nursing procedures and psychomotor skills when caring for a client with potential for complications.

SYSTEM SPECIFIC ASSESSMENTS
Assess the client for peripheral edema.

Identify factors that result in delayed wound healing.

Client Needs: Physiological Adaptation

ALTERATIONS IN BODY SYSTEMS
Monitor wounds for signs and symptoms of infection.

Perform wound care or dressing change.

FLUID AND ELECTROLYTE IMBALANCES: Identify signs and symptoms of client fluid and/or electrolyte imbalance.

MEDICAL EMERGENCIES: Perform emergency care procedures.

PATHOPHYSIOLOGY: Understand general principles of pathophysiology.

Client Needs: Basic Care and Comfort

MOBILITY/IMMOBILITY: Perform skin assessment and implement measures to maintain skin integrity and prevent skin breakdown.

CHAPTER 55 *Pressure Ulcers, Wounds, and Wound Management*

Wounds are a result of injury to the skin. Although there are many different methods and degrees of injury, the basic phases of healing are essentially the same for most wounds.

A pressure ulcer (formerly called a decubitus ulcer) is a specific type of tissue injury from unrelieved pressure or friction over bony prominences that results in ischemia and damage to the underlying tissue.

WOUND HEALING AND MANAGEMENT

STAGES OF WOUND HEALING

Inflammatory stage

Begins with the injury and lasts 3 to 6 days.

EFFECTS TO THE WOUND
- Controlling bleeding with vasoconstriction and retraction of blood vessels, and with clot formation.
- Delivering oxygen, white blood cells, and nutrients to the area via the blood supply. Hemostasis occurs along with fibrin formation. Macrophages engulf microorganisms and cellular debris (phagocytosis).

Proliferative stage

Lasts the next 3 to 24 days.

EFFECTS TO THE WOUND
- Replacing lost tissue with connective or granulated tissue or collagen.
- Contracting the wound's edges.
- Resurfacing of new epithelial cells.

Maturation or remodeling stage

Occurs after day 21 and involves the strengthening of the collagen scar and the restoration of a more normal appearance. It can take more than 1 year to complete, depending on the extent of the original wound.

HEALING PROCESSES

Primary intention

- Little or no tissue loss
- Edges approximated, as with a surgical incision
- Heals rapidly
- Low risk of infection
- No or minimal scarring

  Example: Closed surgical incision with staples or sutures or liquid glue to seal laceration

Secondary intention

- Loss of tissue
- Wound edges widely separated, unapproximated (pressure ulcers, open burn areas)
- Longer healing time
- Increase for risk of infection
- Scarring
- Heals by granulation

  Example: Pressure ulcer left open to heal

Tertiary intention

- Widely separated
- Deep
- Spontaneous opening of a previously closed wound
- Closure of wound occurs when free of infection
- Risk of infection
- Extensive drainage and tissue debris
- Closed later
- Long healing time

  Example: Abdominal wound initially left open until infection is resolved and then closed

FACTORS AFFECTING WOUND HEALING

Age: Increased age delays healing. Ⓒ
- Loss of skin turgor
- Skin fragility
- Decrease in peripheral circulation and oxygenation
- Slower tissue regeneration
- Decrease in absorption of nutrients
- Decrease in collagen
- Impaired immune system function
- Dehydration due to decreased thirst sensation

Overall wellness: A wound in a young, healthy client will heal faster than a wound in an older adult who has a chronic illness.

Decreased leukocyte count: Delays wound healing because the immune system function is to fight infection by destroying invading pathogens.

Some medications (anti-inflammatory and antineoplastic) interfere with the body's ability to respond to and prevent infection.

Malnourished clients: Nutrition provides energy and elements for wound healing.

Tissue perfusion provides circulation that delivers nutrients for tissue repair and infection control.

Low Hgb levels: Hgb is essential for oxygen delivery to healing tissues.

Obesity: Fatty tissue lacks blood supply.

Chronic diseases, such as diabetes mellitus and cardiovascular disorders, place additional stress on the body's healing mechanisms.

Smoking impairs oxygenation and clotting.

Wound stress, such as from vomiting or coughing, puts pressure on the suture line and disrupts the wound healing process.

General principles of wound management

- Wounds impair skin integrity.
- Inflammation is a localized protective response to injury or destruction of tissue.
- Wounds heal by various processes and in stages.
- Wound infections result from the invasion of pathogenic micro-organisms.
- Principles of wound care include assessment, cleansing, and protection.

ASSESSMENT/DATA COLLECTION

APPEARANCE
- Note the color of open wounds.
  - **Red:** Healthy regeneration of tissue
  - **Yellow:** Presence of purulent drainage and slough
  - **Black:** Presence of eschar that hinders healing and requires removal
- Assess the length, width, and depth, and any undermining, sinus tracts or tunnels, and redness or swelling. Use a clock face with 12:00 toward the client's head to document the location of sinus tracts.
- Use the RYB color code guide for wound care: red (cover), yellow (clean), black (debride, removal of necrotic tissue). Q EBP
- **Closed wounds:** Skin edges should be well-approximated.

DRAINAGE (EXUDATE) is a result of the healing process and occurs during the inflammatory and proliferative phases of healing.
- Note the amount, odor, consistency and color of drainage from a drain or on a dressing.
- Note the integrity of the surrounding skin.
- With each cleansing, observe the skin around a drain for irritation and breakdown.
- For accurate measurement of drainage, weigh dressing.

1 g = 1 mL drainage

- Note and document the number of dressings and frequency of dressing changes.
  - **Serous drainage:** The portion of the blood (serum) that is watery and clear or slightly yellow in appearance (e.g., fluid in blisters).
  - **Sanguineous drainage:** Contains serum and red blood cells. It is thick and appears reddish. Brighter drainage indicates fresh bleeding; darker drainage indicates older bleeding/drainage.
  - **Serosanguineous drainage:** Contains both serum and blood. It is watery and appears blood-streaked or blood-tinged.
  - **Purulent drainage:** The result of infection. It is thick and contains white blood cells, tissue debris, and bacteria. It may have a foul odor, and its color such as yellow, tan, brown reflects the type of organism present (green for a *Pseudomonas aeruginosa* infection).
  - **Purosanguineous:** A mixed drainage of pus and blood (e.g., newly infected wound).

WOUND CLOSURE: Staples, sutures, wound-closure strips

STATUS of any drains or tubes

PAIN: Note the location, quality, intensity, timing, setting, associated manifestations, and aggravating/relieving factors.

NURSING INTERVENTIONS

- Provide adequate hydration and meet protein and calorie needs.
  - Encourage an intake of 2,000 to 3,000 mL of fluid/day, from food and beverage sources if not contraindicated (heart and chronic kidney disease).
  - Provide education about good sources of protein (meat, fish, poultry, eggs, dairy products, beans, nuts, whole grains). Q PCC
  - Note if serum albumin levels are low (below 3.5 g/dL), because a lack of protein increases the risk for a delay in wound healing and infection.
  - Provide nutritional support (vitamin and mineral supplements, nutritional supplements, and enteral and parenteral nutrition). Most adult clients need at least 1,500 kcal/day for nutritional support.
- Perform wound cleansing.
  - For clean wounds, such as a surgical incision, cleanse from the least contaminated (the incision) toward the most contaminated (the surrounding skin). Q s
  - Use gentle friction when cleansing or applying solutions to the skin to avoid bleeding or further injury to the wound.
  - Although the provider might prescribe other mild cleansing agents, isotonic solutions remain the preferred cleansing agents.
  - Never use the same gauze to cleanse across an incision or wound more than once.
  - Do not use cotton balls and other products that shed fibers.
  - If irrigating, use a piston syringe or a sterile straight catheter for deep wounds with small openings. Apply 5 to 8 psi of pressure. A 30 to 60 mL syringe with a 19-gauge needle provides approximately 8 psi. Use normal saline, lactated Ringer's, or an antibiotic/antimicrobial solution.

- Remove sutures and staples.
- Administer analgesics and monitor for effective pain management.
- Administer antimicrobials (topical, systemic) and monitor for effectiveness (reduced fever, increase in comfort, decreasing WBC count).
- Document the location and type of wound and incision, the status of the wound and type of drainage, the type of dressing and materials, client teaching, and how the client tolerated the procedure.

WOUND DRESSINGS

Protects the wound from microbes

Woven gauze (sponges): Absorbs exudate from the wound

Nonadherent material: Does not stick to the wound bed

Damp to damp 4-inch by 4-inch dressings: Used to mechanically debride a wound until granulation tissue starts to form in the wound bed. Must keep moist at all times to prevent pain and disruption of wound healing.

Self-adhesive, transparent film: A temporary "second skin" ideal for small, superficial wounds

Hydrocolloid: An occlusive dressing that swells in the presence of exudate; composed of gelatin and pectin, it forms a seal at the wound's surface to prevent evaporation of moisture from the skin.
- Maintains a granulating wound bed
- Can stay in place up to 7 days

Hydrogel: Composition is mostly water. Gels after contact with exudate, promoting autolytic debridement and cooling. Rehydrates and fills dead space.
- For infected, deep wounds, or necrotic tissue
- Not for moderately to heavily draining wounds
- Provides a moist wound bed
- Can stay in place for 3 days

VACUUM-ASSISTED CLOSURE SYSTEM

- Use of foam strips laid into the wound bed with an occlusive sealed drape applied and suction tubing is placed for negative pressure (suction) to occur once the tubing is connected to the systems therapy unit.
  ○ Speed tissue generation
  ○ Decrease swelling
  ○ Enhance healing in a moist protected environment

COMPLICATIONS AND NURSING IMPLICATIONS

Dehiscence and evisceration

Dehiscence: A partial or total rupture (separation) of a sutured wound, usually with separation of underlying skin layers.

Evisceration: A dehiscence that involves the protrusion of visceral organs through a wound opening.

MANIFESTATIONS
- A significant increase in the flow of serosanguineous fluid on the wound dressings
- Immediate history of sudden straining (coughing, sneezing, vomiting)
- Client report of a change or "popping" or "giving way" in the wound area
- Visualization of viscera

PREVENTION: Thin, folded blanket or small pillow over surgical wounds when client coughs in order to support the wound Qs

RISK FACTORS
- Chronic disease
- Advanced age
- Obesity
- Invasive abdominal cancer
- Vomiting
- Excessive straining, coughing, sneezing
- Dehydration, malnutrition
- Ineffective suturing
- Abdominal surgery
- Infection

NURSING INTERVENTIONS

> Evisceration and dehiscence require emergency treatment.

- Call for help. Notify the provider immediately due to the need for surgical intervention.
- Stay with the client.
- Cover the wound and any protruding organs with sterile towels or dressings soaked with sterile normal saline solution to decrease the chance of bacteria invasion and drying of the tissues. Do not attempt to reinsert the organs. QEBP
- Position the client supine with the hips and knees bent.
- Observe for indications of shock.
- Maintain a calm environment.
- Keep the client NPO in preparation for returning to surgery.

Hemorrhage

- Can be caused by clot dislodgement, broken stitch, or blood vessel damage.
- Internal bleeding will present with swelling or distension in the area and sanguineous drainage.
- Hematoma is a local area of blood that appears as a red/blue bruise.
- Wound hemorrhage is an emergency. Pressure dressing should be applied, with notification of the provider and monitoring of vital signs.

Infection

RISK FACTORS

- Extremes in age (immature immune system, decrease in immune function)
- Impaired circulation and oxygenation (COPD, peripheral vascular disease)
- Wound condition and nature (gunshot wound vs. surgical incision)
- Impaired or suppressed immune system
- Malnutrition, such as with alcohol use disorder
- Chronic disease, such as diabetes mellitus or hypertension
- Poor wound care, such as breaches in aseptic technique

MANIFESTATIONS: 3 to 11 days after injury or surgery

- Purulent drainage
- Pain
- Redness, edema (in and around the wound)
- Fever
- Chills
- Odor
- Increased pulse, respiratory rate
- Increase in WBC count

NURSING INTERVENTIONS

- Prevent infection by using aseptic technique when performing dressing changes.
- Provide optimal nutrition to promote the immune response.
- Provide for adequate rest to promote healing.
- Administer antibiotic therapy after collecting specimens for culture and sensitivity testing. **Q**EBP

Pressure ulcers

The National Pressure Ulcer Advisory Panel (NPUAP) classifies pressure ulcers in six stages/categories (visit www.npuap.org for additional information). **(55.1)**

Suspected deep tissue injury, depth unknown: Discoloration but intact skin from damage to underlying tissue.

Stage I, nonblanchable erythema: Intact skin with an area of persistent, nonblanchable redness, typically over a bony prominence, that can feel warmer or cooler than the adjacent tissue. The tissue is swollen and has congestion, with possible discomfort at the site. With darker skin tones, the ulcer can appear blue or purple.

Stage II, partial thickness: Involves the epidermis and the dermis. The ulcer is visible with reddish-pinkish bed without slough or bruising, superficial, and can appear as an abrasion, blister, or shallow crater. Edema persists. The ulcer can become infected, possibly with pain and scant drainage.

Stage III, full-thickness skin loss: Damage to or necrosis of subcutaneous tissue. The ulcer can extend down to, but not through, underlying fascia. The ulcer appears as a deep crater with or without undermining or tunneling of adjacent tissue and without exposed muscle or bone. Drainage and infection are common.

Stage IV, full-thickness tissue loss: Destruction, tissue necrosis, or damage to muscle, bone, or supporting structures. There can be sinus tracts, deep pockets of infection, tunneling, undermining, eschar (black scab-like material), or slough (tan, yellow, or green scab-like material).

Unstageable/unclassified, full-thickness skin or tissue loss, depth unknown: No determination of stage because eschar or slough obscures the wound. The actual depth of injury is unknown.

ASSESSMENT/DATA COLLECTION

The primary focus of prevention and treatment of pressure ulcers is to relieve the pressure and provide optimal nutrition and hydration.

- Monitor all clients regularly for skin-integrity status and for risk factors that contribute to impaired skin integrity.
- Use a risk assessment tool (Braden, Norton scales) for periodic systemic monitoring for skin breakdown risk.
- Pressure ulcers are a significant source of morbidity and mortality among older adults and those who have limited mobility. **©**

55.1 Stages of pressure ulcers

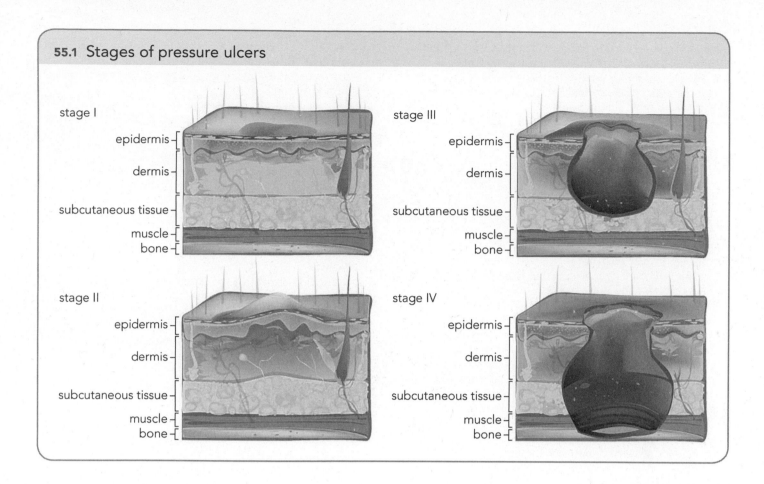

RISK FACTORS

- Aging skin (older adult clients)
- Immobility
- Incontinence, excessive moisture
- Skin friction, shearing
- Vascular disorders
- Obesity
- Inadequate nutrition, hydration
- Anemia
- Fever, dehydration Q𝐄𝐁𝐏
- Impaired circulation
- Edema
- Sensory deficits
- Impaired cognitive functioning, neurological disorders
- Chronic diseases (diabetes mellitus, chronic kidney disease, heart failure, chronic lung disease)
- Sedation that impairs spontaneous repositioning

NURSING INTERVENTIONS

PREVENTION

Avoid skin trauma.
- Keep skin clean, dry, and intact. Provide a firm, wrinkle-free foundation with wrinkle-free linens.
- Reposition the client in bed at least every 2 hr and every 1 hr in a chair. Document position changes.
- Keep the head of the bed at or below a 30° angle (or flat), unless contraindicated, to relieve pressure on the sacrum, buttocks, and heels. Q𝐄𝐁𝐏
- Raise heels off of the bed to prevent pressure.
- Ambulate clients as soon and as often as possible.
- Instruct clients who are mobile to shift their weight every 15 min when sitting.
- Keep clients from sliding down in bed, as this increases shearing forces that pull tissue layers apart and cause damage. Lift, rather than pull, clients up in bed or in a chair, because pulling creates friction that can damage the outer layer of skin (epidermis).

Provide supportive devices.
- Use pressure-reducing surfaces and devices (overlays; replacement mattresses; specialty beds; kinetic therapy; foam, gel, or air cushions).

Maintain skin hygiene.

- Inspect the skin frequently and document the client's risk using a tool such as the Braden scale. $\bigcirc$EBP
- Clean the skin with a mild cleansing agent, and pat it dry immediately following urine or stool incontinence.
- Bathe with tepid (not hot) water and avoid scrubbing.
- Apply dimethicone-based moisture barrier creams or alcohol-free barrier films to the skin of clients who have incontinence.
- Do not use powder or cornstarch to prevent friction or repel moisture due to their abrasive grit and aspiration potential.
- Implement active and passive exercises for clients who are immobile.
- Do not massage bony prominences. $\bigcirc$s

Encourage proper nutrition.

- Provide adequate hydration (2,000 to 3,000 mL/day) and meet protein and calorie needs.
- Note if serum albumin levels are low (less than 3.5 g/dL), because a lack of protein puts the client at greater risk for skin breakdown, slowed healing, and infection.
- Provide nutritional support as indicated, such as vitamin and mineral supplements (especially A, C, zinc, copper), nutritional supplements, and enteral and parenteral nutrition.
- Monitor lymphocyte count.
- Lift, rather than pull, clients up in bed or in a chair, because pulling creates friction that can damage the outer layer of skin (epidermis). $\bigcirc$PCC

TREATMENT

SUSPECTED DEEP TISSUE INJURY AND STAGE I

- Relieve pressure.
- Encourage frequent turning and repositioning.
- Use pressure-relieving devices, such as an air-fluidized bed.
- Implement pressure-reduction surfaces (air mattress, foam mattress). **(55.2)**
- Keep the client dry, clean, well-nourished, and hydrated.

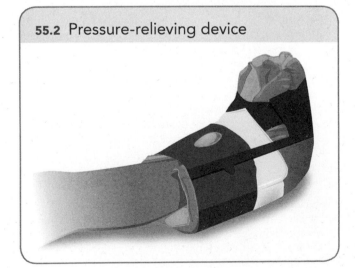

55.2 Pressure-relieving device

STAGE II

- Maintain a moist healing environment (saline or occlusive dressing). Apply hydrocolloid dressing
- Promote natural healing while preventing the formation of scar tissue.
- Provide nutritional supplements.
- Administer analgesics.

STAGE III

- Clean and/or debride the following.
  - Prescribed dressing
  - Surgical intervention
  - Proteolytic enzymes
- Provide nutritional supplements.
- Administer analgesics.
- Administer antimicrobials (topical and/or systemic).

STAGE IV

- Clean and/or debride the following.
  - Prescribed dressing
  - Surgical intervention
  - Proteolytic enzymes
- Perform nonadherent dressing changes every 12 hr.
- Treatment can include skin grafts or specialized therapy such as hyperbaric oxygen.
- Provide nutritional supplements.
- Administer analgesics.
- Administer antimicrobials (topical and/or systemic).

UNSTAGEABLE: Debride until staging is possible.

> Note: Do not use alcohol, Dakin's solution, acetic acid, povidone-iodine, hydrogen peroxide, or any other cytotoxic cleansers on a pressure ulcer wound.

COMPLICATIONS AND NURSING IMPLICATIONS

Deterioration to higher-stage ulceration or infection

- Check the ulcer frequently and report an increase in the size or depth of the lesion, changes in granulation tissue (color, texture), and changes in exudates (color, quantity, odor).
- Follow the facility's protocol for ulcer treatment.
- Might need to confer with wound care specialist. $\bigcirc$TC

Systemic infection

- Monitor for indications of sepsis (changes in level of consciousness, persistent recurrent fever, tachycardia, tachypnea, hypotension, oliguria, or an increase in WBC count).
- Prevent infection by using asepsis when performing ulcer treatment and dressing changes.
- Provide optimal nutrition to promote the immune response.
- Provide for adequate rest to promote healing.
- Administer antibiotic therapy after collecting specimens for culture and sensitivity testing.

Application Exercises

1. A nurse is caring for an adolescent client who is 2 days postoperative following an appendectomy and has type I diabetes mellitus. The client is tolerating a regular diet. He has ambulated successfully around the unit with assistance. He requests pain medication every 6 to 8 hr while reporting pain at a 2 on a scale of 0 to 10 after receiving the medication. His incision is approximated and free of redness, with scant serous drainage on the dressing. The nurse should recognize that the client has which of the following risk factors for impaired wound healing? (Select all that apply.)

   A. Extremes in age

   B. Impaired circulation

   C. Impaired/suppressed immune system

   D. Malnutrition

   E. Poor wound care

2. A nurse is collecting data from a client who is 5 days postoperative following abdominal surgery. The surgeon suspects an incisional wound infection and has prescribed antibiotic therapy for the nurse to initiate after collecting wound and blood specimens for culture and sensitivity. Which of the following findings should the nurse expect? (Select all that apply.)

   A. Increase in incisional pain

   B. Fever and chills

   C. Reddened wound edges

   D. Increase in serosanguineous drainage

   E. Decrease in thirst

3. A nurse educator is reviewing the wound healing process with a group of nurses. The nurse educator should include in the information which of the following alterations for wound healing by secondary intention? (Select all that apply.)

   A. Stage III pressure ulcer

   B. Sutured surgical incision

   C. Casted bone fracture

   D. Laceration sealed with adhesive

   E. Open burn area

4. A client who had abdominal surgery 24 hr ago suddenly reports a pulling sensation and pain in his surgical incision. The nurse checks the surgical wound and finds it separated with viscera protruding. Which of the following actions should the nurse take? (Select all that apply.)

   A. Cover the area with saline-soaked sterile dressings.

   B. Apply an abdominal binder snugly around the abdomen.

   C. Use sterile gauze to apply gentle pressure to the exposed tissues.

   D. Position the client supine with his hips and knees bent.

   E. Offer the client a warm beverage, such as herbal tea.

5. A nurse is caring for an older adult client who is at risk for developing pressure ulcers. Which of the following interventions should the nurse use to help maintain the integrity of the client's skin? (Select all that apply.)

   A. Keep the head of the bed elevated 30°.

   B. Massage the client's bony prominences frequently.

   C. Apply cornstarch liberally to the skin after bathing.

   D. Have the client sit on a gel cushion when in a chair.

   E. Reposition the client at least every 3 hr while in bed.

PRACTICE Active Learning Scenario

A nurse is teaching a group of nursing students about the National Pressure Ulcer Advisory Panel's classification system for pressure ulcers. Use the ATI Active Learning Template: Basic Concept to complete this item.

RELATED CONTENT: List the six pressure ulcer stages along with a brief description of the assessment findings typical for ulcers at each stage.

Application Exercises Key

1. A. The client is not at either extreme of the age spectrum.

    B. **CORRECT:** The client who has type I diabetes mellitus is at risk for impaired circulation.

    C. **CORRECT:** The client who has type I diabetes mellitus is at risk for impaired immune system function.

    D. There is no indication that the client is malnourished.

    E. That there is no indication that there have been any breaches in aseptic technique during wound care.

    Ⓝ *NCLEX® Connection: Health Promotion and Maintenance, Health Screening*

2. A. **CORRECT:** The nurse should expect the client to have pain and tenderness at the wound site with an incisional infection.

    B. **CORRECT:** The nurse should expect the client to have fever and chills with an incisional infection.

    C. **CORRECT:** The nurse should expect the client to have reddened or inflamed wound edges with an incisional infection.

    D. The nurse should expect the client to have purulent drainage with an incisional infection.

    E. The nurse should not expect changes in thirst as an indication of an incisional infection.

    Ⓝ *NCLEX® Connection: Physiological Adaptation, Alterations in Body Systems*

3. A. **CORRECT:** Open pressure ulcers heal by secondary intention, which is the process for wounds that have tissue loss and widely separated edges.

    B. Sutured surgical incisions heal by primary intention, which is the process for wounds that have little or no tissue loss and well-approximated edges.

    C. Unless the bone edges have pierced the skin, a casted bone fracture is an injury to underlying structures and does not require healing of the skin.

    D. Lacerations sealed with tissue adhesive heal by primary intention, which is the process for wounds that have little or no tissue loss and well-approximated edges.

    E. **CORRECT:** Open burn areas heal by secondary intention, which is the process for wounds that have tissue loss and widely separated edges.

    Ⓝ *NCLEX® Connection: Reduction of Risk Potential, System Specific Assessments*

4. A. **CORRECT:** The nurse should cover the wound with a sterile dressing soaked with sterile normal saline solution to keep the exposed organs and tissues moist until the surgeon can assess and intervene.

    B. An abdominal binder can help prevent, not treat, a wound evisceration.

    C. The nurse should not handle or apply pressure to any exposed organs or tissues because these actions increase the risks of trauma and perforation.

    D. **CORRECT:** This position minimizes pressure on the abdominal area.

    E. The nurse must keep the client NPO in anticipation of the surgical team taking him back to the surgical suite for repair of the evisceration.

    Ⓝ *NCLEX® Connection: Basic Care and Comfort, Mobility/Immobility*

5. A. **CORRECT:** The nurse should slightly elevate the client head of bed reduce shearing forces that could tear sensitive skin on the sacrum, buttocks, and heels.

    B. The nurse can traumatize deep tissues if she massages the skin over bony prominences.

    C. The nurse can abrade the client's sensitive skin and increase the risk for aspiration if cornstarch or powders are used.

    D. **CORRECT:** The nurse should have the client sit on a gel, air, or foam cushion to redistribute weight away from ischial areas.

    E. The nurse should reposition the client at least every 2 hr. Frequent position changes are important for preventing skin breakdown, but every 3 hr is not frequent enough.

    Ⓝ *NCLEX® Connection: Basic Care and Comfort, Mobility/Immobility*

PRACTICE Answer

Using the ATI Active Learning Template: Basic Concept

RELATED CONTENT

- Suspected deep tissue injury, depth unknown: Discoloration but intact skin from damage to underlying tissue.
- Stage I, nonblanchable erythema: Intact skin with an area of persistent, nonblanchable redness, typically over a bony prominence, that can feel warmer or cooler than the adjacent tissue. The tissue is swollen and has congestion, with possible discomfort at the site. With darker skin tones, the ulcer can appear blue or purple.

- Stage II, partial thickness: Involves the epidermis and the dermis. The ulcer is visible with reddish-pinkish bed without slough or bruising, superficial, and can appear as an abrasion, blister, or shallow crater. Edema persists. The ulcer can become infected, possibly with pain and scant drainage.
- Stage III, full-thickness skin loss: Damage to or necrosis of subcutaneous tissue. The ulcer can extend down to, but not through, underlying fascia. The ulcer appears as a deep crater with or without undermining or tunneling of adjacent tissue and without exposed muscle or bone. Drainage and infection are common.

- Stage IV, full-thickness tissue loss: Destruction, tissue necrosis, or damage to muscle, bone, or supporting structures. There can be sinus tracts, deep pockets of infection, tunneling, undermining, eschar (black scab-like material), or slough (tan, yellow, or green scab-like material).
- Unstageable/unclassified, full-thickness skin or tissue loss, depth unknown: No determination of stage because eschar or slough obscures the wound. The actual depth of injury is unknown.

Ⓝ *NCLEX® Connection: Physiological Adaptation, Pathophysiology*

CHAPTER 56

CHAPTER 56 Bacterial, Viral, Fungal, and Parasitic Infections

Pathogens are the micro-organisms or microbes that cause infections. Virulence is the ability of a pathogen to invade the host and cause disease. Herpes zoster is a common viral infection that erupts years after exposure to chickenpox and invades a specific nerve tract.

PATHOGENS

Bacteria: Most common type of pathogen (*Staphylococcus aureus, Escherichia coli, Mycobacterium tuberculosis*)

Viruses: Organisms that use the host's genetic machinery to reproduce (rhinovirus, HIV, hepatitis, herpes zoster, herpes simplex)

Fungi: Molds and yeasts (*Candida albicans*, Aspergillus)

Prions: Protein particles that have the ability to cause infections (Creutzfeldt–Jakob disease)

Parasites: Organisms that live on and often cause harm to a host organism
- **Protozoa** (malaria, toxoplasmosis)
- **Helminths** (worms: flatworms, roundworms)
- **Flukes** (schistosomes)
- **Arthropods** (lice, mites, ticks)

INFECTION PROCESS

The infection process (chain of infection) includes the following.

Causative agent

Bacteria, virus, fungus, prion, parasite

Reservoir

Human, animal, food, water, soil, insects, fomites

Portal of exit from (means for leaving) the host

Respiratory tract (droplet, airborne): *Mycobacterium tuberculosis* and Parainfluenza virus

Gastrointestinal tract: Shigella, *Salmonella enteritidis, Salmonella typhi*, hepatitis A, *Clostridium difficile*

Genitourinary tract: *Escherichia coli*, herpes simplex virus (type 1), HIV

Skin/mucous membranes: Herpes simplex virus and varicella

Blood/body fluids: HIV and hepatitis B and C

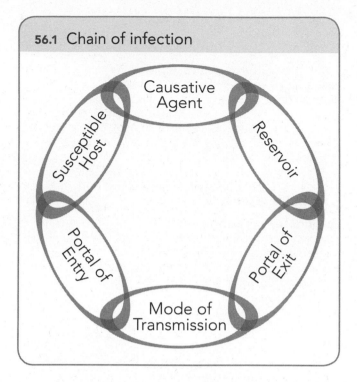

56.1 Chain of infection

Mode of transmission

CONTACT
- **Direct physical contact:** Person to person
- **Indirect contact with a vehicle of transmission:** Inanimate object, water, food, blood
- **Fecal–oral transmission:** Handling food after using a restroom and failing to wash hands

DROPLET: Large droplets travel through the air up to 3 to 6 feet (sneezing, coughing, and talking)

AIRBORNE: Small droplets remain in the air and can travel extended distances depending on airflow (sneezing and coughing)

VECTOR-BORNE: Animals or insects as intermediaries (ticks transmit Lyme disease; mosquitoes transmit West Nile virus and malaria)

Portal of entry to the host

Often the same as the portal of exit

Susceptible host

Compromised defense mechanisms (immunosuppression, breaks in skin) leave the host more susceptible to infections.

IMMUNE DEFENSES

Nonspecific innate-native immunity

Allows the body to restrict entry or immediately respond to a foreign organism (antigen) through the activation of phagocytic cells, complement, and inflammation

- Nonspecific innate-native immunity provides temporary immunity but does not have memory of past exposures.
- Intact skin is the body's first line of defense against microbial invasion.
- The skin, mucous membranes, secretions, enzymes, phagocytic cells, and protective proteins work in concert to prevent infections.

Inflammatory response

- Phagocytic cells (neutrophils, eosinophils, macrophages), the complement system, and interferons are involved.
- An inflammatory response localizes the area of microbial invasion and prevents its spread.

Specific adaptive immunity

Allows the body to make antibodies in response to a foreign organism (antigen)

- Requires time to react to antigens
- Provides permanent immunity due to memory of past exposures
- Involves B and T lymphocytes
- Produces specific antibodies against specific antigens (immunoglobulins: IgA, IgD, IgE, IgG, IgM).

ASSESSMENT/DATA COLLECTION

RISK FACTORS

ENVIRONMENTAL FACTORS
- Excessive alcohol consumption
- Nicotine use: smoking, smokeless tobacco
- Malnutrition

MEDICATION THERAPY (IMMUNOSUPPRESSIVE AGENTS)
- Glucocorticosteroids
- Antineoplastics

CHRONIC DISEASES
- Diabetes mellitus
- Cancer
- HIV, AIDS
- Peripheral vascular disease
- Chronic pulmonary disease
- Heart failure

AGE
Older adults are at increased risk for infections due to the following. ©
- Slowed response to antibiotic therapy
- Slowed immune response: indicators of infection more difficult to identify, resulting in possible delays in diagnosis and treatment
- Loss of subcutaneous tissue and thinning of the skin
- Decreased vascularity and slowed wound healing
- Decreased cough and gag reflexes
- Chronic illnesses (diabetes mellitus, COPD, neurological or musculoskeletal impairments)
- Decreased gastric acid production
- Decreased mobility
- Bowel/bladder incontinence
- Dementia
- Greater incidence of invasive devices (urinary catheters, feeding tubes, tracheostomies, intravenous lines)

> Common indications of infection are not always present in the older adult client. Altered mental status, agitation, or incontinence can be present instead. ©

EXPECTED FINDINGS

- Chills
- Sore throat
- Fatigue and malaise
- Change in level of consciousness, nuchal rigidity, photophobia, headache
- Nausea, vomiting, anorexia, abdominal cramping, and diarrhea
- Localized pain or discomfort

PHYSICAL ASSESSMENT FINDINGS
- Fever
- Increased pulse and respiratory rate, decreased blood pressure
- Localized redness and edema
- Enlarged lymph nodes
- Dyspnea, cough, purulent sputum, and crackles in lung fields
- Dysuria, urinary frequency, hematuria, and pyuria
- Rash, skin lesions, purulent wound drainage, and erythema
- Dysphagia, hyperemia, and enlarged tonsils

LABORATORY TESTS

White blood cell (WBC) count with differential
- An elevated WBC count is an indicator of infection (expected reference range is 5,000 to 10,000/mm^3).
- The differential identifies specific types of WBCs that can assist in diagnosis of the severity of infection or the specific type of pathogen.

Erythrocyte sedimentation rate (ESR)
- The rate at which red blood cells settle out of plasma
- An elevated ESR is an indicator of an active inflammatory process or infection (expected reference range is 15 to 20 mm/hr).
- An increase indicates an active inflammatory process or infection.

Immunoglobulin electrophoresis
- Determines the presence and quantity of specific immunoglobulins (IgG, IgA, IgM).
- Used to detect hypersensitivity disorders, autoimmune disorders, chronic viral infections, immunodeficiency, multiple myeloma, and intrauterine infections.

Antibody screening tests
- Detect the presence of antibodies against specific causative agents (bacteria, fungi, viruses, parasites).
- A positive antibody test indicates that the client has been exposed to and developed antibodies to a specific pathogen, but it does not provide information about whether or not the client is currently infected (HIV antibodies).

Auto-antibody screening tests
- Detect the presence of antibodies against a person's own DNA (self-cells).
- The presence of antibodies against self cells is associated with autoimmune conditions (systemic lupus erythematosus, rheumatoid arthritis).

Antigen tests
- Detect the presence of a specific pathogen (HIV).
- Used to identify certain infections or disorders.

Stool for ova and parasites
- Detects presence of ova and parasites, such as hookworm ova in stool.
- Three separate stool specimens usually collected.
- Each specimen must be transported to the laboratory while it is still warm.

Culture and sensitivity
- A culture is a microscopic examination to identify an infecting organism.
- Cultures can be obtained from blood, sputum, urine, wound, and soft tissue.
- Cultures should be obtained before any antibiotic therapy is initiated.
- The sensitivity report indicates which antibiotics are effective against the identified organism.

DIAGNOSTIC PROCEDURES

X-rays, **computed tomography (CT) scan**, **magnetic resonance imaging (MRI)**, and **biopsies** are used to determine the presence of infection, abscesses, and lesions.

Gallium scan
- A nuclear scan that uses a radioactive substance to identify hot spots of WBCs within the client's body.
- Radioactive gallium citrate is injected intravenously and accumulates in areas where inflammation is present.

PATIENT-CENTERED CARE

NURSING CARE
- Assess the following.
  - Presence of risk factors for infection
  - Recent travel or exposure to an infectious disease
  - Behaviors that can put the client at increased risk
  - Increased temperature, heart and respiratory rate, thirst, anorexia
  - Presence of chills, which occur when temperature is rising, and diaphoresis, which occurs when temperature is decreasing
  - Presence of hyperpyrexia (greater than 105.8° F), which can cause brain and organ damage
- Implement infection control measures.
  - Perform frequent hand hygiene to prevent transmission of infection to other clients.
  - Maintain a clean environment.
  - Perform wound care measures, such as sterile dressing changes.
  - Use personal protective equipment/barriers (gloves, masks, gowns, goggles).
  - Encourage recommended immunizations.
  - Implement protective precautions as needed.
    - **Standard:** Implemented for all clients
    - **Contact:** *Clostridium difficile*, herpes simplex virus, impetigo, methicillin-resistant *Staphylococcus aureus* (MRSA), vancomycin-resistant *Staphylococcus aureus* (VRSA)
    - **Droplet:** *Haemophilus influenzae* type B (Hib), pertussis, mumps, rubella, plague, streptococcal pneumonia, meningococcal pneumonia
    - **Airborne:** Measles, varicella, tuberculosis
- Encourage adequate rest and nutrition.
- Provide diversional activities if needed.
- Encourage increased fluid intake or maintain intravenous fluid replacement to prevent dehydration.
- Protect and maintain the client's protective barriers (skin, mucous membranes).

MEDICATIONS

Antipyretics

Acetaminophen and aspirin are used for fever and discomfort as prescribed.

NURSING CONSIDERATIONS
- Monitor fever to determine effectiveness of medication.
- Document temperature fluctuations on the medical record for trending.

Antimicrobial therapy

Antimicrobial medications kill pathogens or prevent their growth. Anthelmintics are given for worm infestations. There are currently no treatments for prions.

NURSING CONSIDERATIONS
- Administer antimicrobial therapy as prescribed.
- Monitor for medication effectiveness (reduced fever, increased level of comfort, decreasing WBC count).
- Maintain a medication schedule to assure consistent therapeutic blood levels of the antibiotic.

CLIENT EDUCATION

- Teach the client regarding the following.
  - Any infection control measures needed at home
  - Self-administration of medication therapy
  - Complications that need to be reported immediately
- Infants should receive the *H. influenzae* type b (Hib) vaccine.
- Adults and older adults at risk should receive the pneumococcal polysaccharide vaccine (PPSV). ⓒ
- Adolescents should receive the meningococcal vaccine on schedule and prior to living in a residential or communal setting.

COMPLICATIONS

Medication-resistant infections

Antimicrobials are becoming less effective for some strains of pathogens, due to the pathogen's ability to adapt and become resistant to previously sensitive antibiotics. This significantly limits the number of antibiotics that are effective against the pathogen. Use of antibiotics, especially broad-spectrum antibiotics, has significantly decreased to prevent new strains from evolving. Taking the measures below can ensure an antimicrobial is warranted and increase the effectiveness of treatment.

- MRSA is a strain of *S. aureus* that is resistant to all antibiotics, except vancomycin
- VRSA is a strain of *S. aureus* that is resistant to vancomycin but so far is sensitive to other antibiotics specific to the strain.

NURSING ACTIONS

- Obtain specimens for culture and sensitivity prior to initiation of antimicrobial therapy. ⓆEBP
- Monitor antimicrobial levels and ensure that therapeutic levels are maintained.
- Implement precautions to prevent the spread of the infection.

CLIENT EDUCATION

- Complete the full course of antimicrobial therapy.
- Avoid overuse of antimicrobials.

Sepsis

A systemic inflammatory response syndrome resulting from the body's response to a serious infection, usually bacterial (peritonitis, meningitis, pneumonia, wound infections, urinary tract infections)

- Sepsis is a potentially life-threatening complication that can lead to widespread inflammation, blood clotting, organ failure, and shock.
- Blood cultures definitively diagnose sepsis. Systemic antimicrobials are prescribed accordingly. Vasopressors and anticoagulants may be prescribed for shock and blood clotting manifestations. Mechanical ventilation, dialysis, and other interventions can be needed for treatment of specific organ failure.

RISK FACTORS: Very young age, very old age, weakened immune system, and severe injuries (trauma).

Herpes zoster (shingles)

Herpes zoster is a viral infection. It initially produces chickenpox, after which the virus lies dormant in the dorsal root ganglia of the sensory cranial and spinal nerves. It is then reactivated as shingles later in life.

- Shingles is usually preceded by a prodromal period of several days, during which pain, itching, tingling, or burning can occur along the involved dermatome.
- Shingles can be very painful and debilitating.

ASSESSMENT/DATA COLLECTION

RISK FACTORS

- Concurrent illness
- Stress
- Compromise to the immune system
- Fatigue
- Poor nutritional status

Possible immunocompromise makes older adult clients more susceptible to herpes zoster infection. Assess the client carefully for typical and atypical indications of infection. ⓒ

EXPECTED FINDINGS

- Paresthesia
- Pain that is unilateral and extends horizontally along a dermatome

PHYSICAL ASSESSMENT FINDINGS

- Vesicular, unilateral rash (the rash and lesions occur on the skin area innervated by the infected nerve)
- Changes in or loss of vision if the eye is affected
- Rash that is erythematous, vesicular, pustular, or crusting (depending on the stage)
- Rash that usually lasts several weeks
- Low-grade fever

LABORATORY TESTS

- Cultures provide a definitive diagnosis (but the virus grows so slowly that cultures are often of minimal diagnostic use).
- Occasionally, an immunofluorescence assay can be done.

PATIENT-CENTERED CARE

NURSING CARE

- Assess/monitor the following.
  - Pain
  - Condition of lesions
  - Presence of fever
  - Neurologic complications
  - Indications of infection
- Use an air mattress or bed cradle for pain prevention/control of affected areas.
- Isolate the client until the vesicles have crusted over.
- Maintain strict wound care precautions.
- The virus can be transmitted through direct contact, causing chickenpox. Avoid exposing the client to infants, pregnant women who have not had chickenpox, and clients who are immunocompromised. Qs
- Moisten dressings with cool tap water or 5% aluminum acetate (Burow's solution) and apply to the affected skin for 30 to 60 min, four to six times per day as prescribed.
- Use lotions, such as calamine lotion, or recommend oatmeal baths to help relieve itching and discomfort.
- Administer medications as prescribed.

MEDICATIONS

- Analgesics (NSAIDs, narcotics) enhance client comfort.
- If started soon after the rash appears, antiviral agents, such as acyclovir, can decrease the severity of the infection and shorten the clinical course.
- Recommend zoster vaccine live for clients 60 and older to prevent shingles. This vaccine does not treat active shingles infections. QEBP

COMPLICATIONS

Postherpetic neuralgia

- Characterized by pain that persists for longer than 1 month following resolution of the vesicular rash.
- Tricyclic antidepressants may be prescribed.
- Postherpetic neuralgia is common in adults older than 60 years of age. Ⓖ

Application Exercises

1. A nurse is discussing direct and indirect contact modes of transmission of infection at a staff education session. Which of the following incidents are examples of direct mode of transmission? (Select all that apply.)
   - A. A client vomits on a nurse's uniform.
   - B. A nurse has a needle stick injury.
   - C. A mosquito bites a hiker in the woods.
   - D. A nurse finds a hole in his glove while handling a soiled dressing.
   - E. A person fails to wash her hands after using the bathroom.

2. A nurse in a residential care facility is assessing an older adult client. Which of the following findings should the nurse identify as atypical indications of infection? (Select all that apply.)
   - A. Urinary incontinence
   - B. Malaise
   - C. Acute confusion
   - D. Fever
   - E. Agitation

3. A nurse is preparing to admit a client who is suspected to have pulmonary tuberculosis. Which of the following actions should the nurse plan to perform first?
   - A. Implement airborne precautions.
   - B. Obtain a sputum culture.
   - C. Administer prescribed antituberculosis medications.
   - D. Recommend a screening test for family members.

4. A nurse in a primary care clinic is assessing a client who has a history of herpes zoster. Which of the following findings suggests the client is experiencing postherpetic neuralgia?
   - A. Linear clusters of vesicles present on the right shoulder
   - B. Purulent drainage from both eyes
   - C. Decreased white blood cell count
   - D. Report of continued pain following resolution of rash

5. A charge nurse is teaching about the care of a client who has methicillin-resistant Staphylococcus aureus (MRSA) with a newly licensed nurse. Which of the following statements by the newly licensed nurse indicates an understanding of the teaching?
   - A. "I should obtain a specimen for culture and sensitivity after the first dose of an antimicrobial."
   - B. "MRSA is usually resistant to vancomycin, so another antimicrobial will be prescribed."
   - C. "I will need to monitor the client's serum antimicrobial levels during the course of therapy."
   - D. "To decrease resistance, antimicrobial therapy is discontinued when the client is no longer febrile."

Application Exercises Key

1. A. **CORRECT:** Transmission from emesis is person-to-person or direct contact.

   B. Transmission from a needle or other inanimate object is indirect contact.

   C. Transmission from an insect is vector-borne.

   D. Transmission from a soiled dressing or other inanimate object is indirect contact.

   E. **CORRECT:** Transmission from contaminated hands is person-to-person or direct contact.

   Ⓝ *NCLEX® Connection: Safety and Infection Control, Standard Precautions/Transmission-Based Precautions/Surgical Asepsis*

2. A. **CORRECT:** Urinary incontinence is an atypical indication of infection in an older adult client.

   B. Malaise is a typical indication of infection.

   C. **CORRECT:** Acute confusion is an atypical indication of infection in an older adult client.

   D. Fever is a typical indication of infection.

   E. **CORRECT:** Agitation is an atypical indication of infection in an older adult client.

   Ⓝ *NCLEX® Connection: Safety and Infection Control, Standard Precautions/Transmission-Based Precautions/Surgical Asepsis*

3. A. **CORRECT:** The greatest safety risk to the nurse and others is transmission of the infection from airborne exposure to tuberculosis. The priority intervention the nurse should take is to place the client on airborne precautions.

   B. The nurse should obtain a sputum culture, but another action is the priority.

   C. The nurse should administer prescribed medications to treat tuberculosis, but another action is the priority.

   D. The nurse should recommend screening tests for those in close contact with the client to determine if antibiotic therapy is needed, but another action is the priority.

   Ⓝ *NCLEX® Connection: Safety and Infection Control, Standard Precautions/Transmission-Based Precautions/Surgical Asepsis*

4. A. Localized linear clusters of vesicles are an expected finding of herpes zoster rather than postherpetic neuralgia.

   B. Eye infection is a potential complication of herpes zoster but does not suggest postherpetic neuralgia.

   C. Immunosuppression increases the risk for herpes zoster but does not suggest postherpetic neuralgia.

   D. **CORRECT:** Pain that persists following resolution of the vesicular rash is an indication of postherpetic neuralgia.

   Ⓝ *NCLEX® Connection: Physiological Adaptation, Illness Management*

5. A. The nurse should obtain a specimen for culture and sensitivity prior to the initiation of antimicrobial therapy.

   B. MRSA is resistant to all antibiotics except vancomycin.

   C. **CORRECT:** The nurse should monitor antimicrobial levels to ensure that therapeutic levels are maintained.

   D. Discontinuing antimicrobial therapy prior to completing a full course of treatment increases the risk of producing resistant pathogens.

   Ⓝ *NCLEX® Connection: Safety and Infection Control, Standard Precautions/Transmission-Based Precautions/Surgical Asepsis*

PRACTICE Active Learning Scenario

A nurse is admitting a client who has a new diagnosis of herpes zoster. Use the ATI Active Learning Template: System Disorder and the Medical-Surgical Nursing Review Module to complete this item.

PATHOPHYSIOLOGY RELATED TO CLIENT PROBLEM: Identify the mode of transmission.

RISK FACTORS: Identify at least three risk factors for acquiring herpes zoster.

EXPECTED FINDINGS: Identify at least three indications of infection with herpes zoster

NURSING CARE: Identify information the nurse should provide the client and family about acquiring adaptive immunity for herpes zoster.

CLIENT EDUCATION: Identify one preventative measure to prevent the transmission of herpes zoster.

PRACTICE Answer

Using the ATI Active Learning Template: System Disorder

PATHOPHYSIOLOGY RELATED TO CLIENT PROBLEM: Contact transmission

RISK FACTORS
- Concurrent illness
- Stress
- Compromise to the immune system
- Fatigue
- Poor nutritional status

EXPECTED FINDINGS
- Paresthesia
- Pain that is unilateral and extends horizontally along a dermatome
- Vesicular, unilateral rash (the rash and lesions occur on the skin area innervated by the infected nerve)
- Changes in or loss of vision if the eye is affected
- Rash that is erythematous, vesicular, pustular, or crusting (depending on the stage)
- Rash that usually lasts several weeks
- Low-grade fever

NURSING CARE
- Assess/monitor the following.
  - Pain
  - Condition of lesions
  - Presence of fever
  - Neurologic complications
  - Indications of infection
- Use an air mattress or bed cradle for pain prevention/control of affected areas.
- Isolate the client until the vesicles have crusted over.
- Maintain strict wound care precautions.
- Moisten dressings with cool tap water or 5% aluminum acetate (Burow's solution) and apply to the affected skin for 30 to 60 min, four to six times per day as prescribed.
- Use lotions, such as calamine lotion, or recommend oatmeal baths to help relieve itching and discomfort.
- Administer medications as prescribed

CLIENT EDUCATION
- The virus can be transmitted through direct contact, causing chickenpox. Avoid exposing the client to infants, pregnant women who have not had chickenpox, and clients who are immunocompromised.
- Recommend zoster vaccine live for clients 60 and over to prevent shingles. This vaccine does not treat active shingles infections.

Ⓝ *NCLEX® Connection: Safety and Infection Control, Standard Precautions/Transmission-Based Precautions/Surgical Asepsis*

CHAPTER 57 *Fluid Imbalances*

Body fluids are distributed between intracellular fluid (ICF) and extracellular fluid (ECF) compartments. ECF is comprised of intravascular (plasma), interstitial (fluid that surrounds the cells), lymph, and transcellular fluids (cerebrospinal, pericardial, pancreatic, pleural, intraocular, biliary, peritoneal, and synovial fluids).

Fluid can move between compartments (through selectively permeable membranes) by a variety of methods (diffusion, active transport, filtration, osmosis) in order to maintain homeostasis. Fluid imbalances that the nurse should be familiar with are fluid volume deficit and fluid volume excess.

Fluid volume deficit

- Fluid volume deficit (FVD) includes the following.
  - **Isotonic FVD** is the loss of water and electrolytes from the ECF. Isotonic FVD is often referred to as hypovolemia because intravascular fluid is also lost.
  - **Dehydration** is the loss of water from the body without the loss of electrolytes. This hemoconcentration results in increases in Hct, serum electrolytes, and urine specific gravity.
- Compensatory mechanisms include sympathetic nervous system responses of increased thirst, antidiuretic hormone (ADH) release, and aldosterone release.
- FVD can lead to hypovolemic shock.
- Older adults have an increased risk for dehydration due to multiple physiological factors including a decrease in total body mass, which includes total body water content, and a decrease in the ability to detect thirst. ⊙

ASSESSMENT/DATA COLLECTION

RISK FACTORS

CAUSES OF ISOTONIC FVD (HYPOVOLEMIA)
- Excessive gastrointestinal (GI) loss: vomiting, nasogastric suctioning, diarrhea
- Excessive skin loss: diaphoresis
- Excessive renal system losses: diuretic therapy, diabetes insipidus, kidney disease, adrenal insufficiency, osmotic diuresis
- Third spacing: peritonitis, intestinal obstruction, ascites, burns
- Excessive loss of fluids from a wound
- Hemorrhage
- Altered intake: anorexia, nausea, impaired swallowing, confusion, nothing by mouth (NPO)

CAUSES OF DEHYDRATION
- Hyperventilation
- Prolonged fever
- Diabetic ketoacidosis
- Enteral feeding without sufficient water intake

EXPECTED FINDINGS

VITAL SIGNS: Hypothermia or hyperthermia, tachycardia, thready pulse, hypotension, orthostatic hypotension, decreased central venous pressure, tachypnea (increased respirations), hypoxia

NEUROMUSCULOSKELETAL: Dizziness, syncope, confusion, weakness, fatigue

GI: Thirst, dry mucous membranes, dry furrowed tongue, nausea, vomiting, anorexia, acute weight loss

RENAL: Oliguria (decreased production of urine)

OTHER FINDINGS: Diminished capillary refill, cool clammy skin, diaphoresis, sunken eyeballs, flattened neck veins, absence of tears, decreased skin turgor

> Assessment of skin turgor in the older adult might not provide reliable findings due to a natural loss of skin elasticity. ⊙

LABORATORY TESTS

Hct: Increased in both hypovolemia and dehydration unless the fluid volume deficit is due to hemorrhage

Serum osmolarity
Dehydration: Increased hemoconcentration osmolarity (greater than 295 mOsm/kg); increased protein, BUN, electrolytes, glucose

Urine specific gravity
Dehydration: Increased concentration (urine specific gravity greater than 1.030)

Serum sodium
Dehydration: Increased hemoconcentration (greater than 145 mEq/L)

PATIENT-CENTERED CARE

NURSING CARE

- Observe respiratory rate, symmetry, and effort.
- Monitor for shortness of breath and dyspnea.
- Check urinalysis, oxygen saturation (SaO₂), CBC, and electrolytes.
- Administer supplemental oxygen as prescribed.
- Measure the client's weight daily at same time of day using the same scale.
- Observe for nausea and vomiting.
- Monitor vital signs. (Check for hypotension and orthostatic hypotension.)
- Check neurological status to determine level of consciousness. Qs
- Assess heart rhythm (can be irregular or tachycardic).
- Initiate and maintain IV access.
- For fluid replacement, administer IV fluids as prescribed (isotonic solutions such as lactated Ringer's or 0.9% sodium chloride; blood transfusions).
- Monitor I&O. Encourage fluids as tolerated. Alert the provider to a urine output less than 30 mL/hr.
- Monitor level of consciousness and ensure client safety.
- Observe level of gait stability.
- Encourage the client to use the call light and ask for assistance.
- Encourage the client to change positions slowly (rolling from side to side or standing up).
- Check capillary refill (expected reference range 3 seconds or less).
- Provide frequent oral care.
- Prevent skin breakdown.

Fluid volume excesses

- Fluid volume excesses include the following.
  - **Fluid volume excess** (FVE) is the isotonic retention of water and sodium in high proportions. FVE is often referred to as hypervolemia because of the resulting increased blood volume.
  - **Overhydration**, or hypoosmolar fluid imbalance, is the retention of more water than electrolytes. This hemodilution results in decreases in Hct, serum electrolytes, and protein.
- Severe FVE can lead to pulmonary edema and heart failure.
- Compensatory mechanisms include an increased release of natriuretic peptides, resulting in increased excretion of sodium and water by the kidneys, and a decreased release of aldosterone.

ASSESSMENT/DATA COLLECTION

RISK FACTORS

CAUSES OF HYPERVOLEMIA
- Chronic stimulus to the kidney to conserve sodium and water (heart failure, cirrhosis, increased glucocorticosteroids)
- Altered kidney function with reduced excretion of sodium and water (kidney failure)
- Interstitial to plasma fluid shifts (hypertonic fluids, burns)
- Age-related changes in cardiovascular and kidney function Ⓒ
- Excessive sodium intake from IV fluids, diet, or medications (sodium bicarbonate antacids, hypertonic enema solutions)

CAUSES OF OVERHYDRATION
- Water replacement without electrolyte replacement (strenuous exercise with profuse diaphoresis)
- Syndrome of inappropriate antidiuretic hormone (SIADH), which is the excess secretion of ADH
- Head injuries
- Barbiturates
- Anesthetics

EXPECTED FINDINGS

VITAL SIGNS: Tachycardia, bounding pulse, hypertension, tachypnea, increased central venous pressure

NEUROMUSCULOSKELETAL: Confusion, muscle weakness

GI: Weight gain, ascites

RESPIRATORY: Dyspnea, orthopnea, crackles

OTHER FINDINGS: Edema, distended neck veins

LABORATORY TESTS

Hct
- Hypervolemia: Decreased Hct
- Overhydration: Decreased Hct = hemodilution

Serum osmolarity
Overhydration: Osmolarity less than 280 mOsm/kg

Serum sodium
Hypervolemia: Sodium within expected reference range

Electrolytes, BUN, and creatinine
Overhydration/hypervolemia: Decreased electrolytes, BUN, and creatinine

Arterial blood gases
- Respiratory alkalosis: Decreased $PaCO_2$ (less than 35 mm Hg), increased pH (greater than 7.45)
- Urine specific gravity: Less than 1.010 (if not due to SIADH)

DIAGNOSTIC PROCEDURES

Chest x-rays can indicate pulmonary congestion.

PATIENT-CENTERED CARE

NURSING CARE

- Observe respiratory rate, symmetry, and effort.
- Auscultate breath sounds in all lung fields. Lung sounds can be diminished with crackles.
- Monitor for shortness of breath and dyspnea.
- Check ABGs, SaO_2, CBC, and chest x-ray results.
- Position the client in semi-Fowler's position.
- Measure the client's weight daily at same time of day using the same scale.
- Monitor and document edema (pretibial, sacral, periorbital).
- Monitor I&O.
- Implement prescribed restrictions for fluid and sodium intake.
  - Provide fluids in small glass to promote the perception of a full glass of fluid.
  - Set 1- to 2-hr short-term goals for the fluid restriction to promote client control and understanding. Qpcc
- Administer supplemental oxygen as needed. Reduce IV flow rates.
- Administer diuretics (osmotic, loop) as prescribed.
- Monitor and document circulation to the extremities.
- Reposition the client at least every 2 hr.
- Support arms and legs to decrease dependent edema.

Application Exercises

1. A nurse is performing an admission assessment on a client who has hypovolemia due to vomiting and diarrhea. The nurse should expect which of the following findings? (Select all that apply.)

   A. Distended neck veins

   B. Hyperthermia

   C. Tachycardia

   D. Syncope

   E. Decreased skin turgor

2. A nurse on a medical-surgical unit is caring for a group of clients. The nurse should identify that which of the following clients is at risk for hypovolemia?

   A. A client who has nasogastric suctioning.

   B. A client who has chronic constipation.

   C. A client who has syndrome of inappropriate antidiuretic hormone

   D. A client who took an overdose of sodium bicarbonate antacids

3. A nurse is reviewing the laboratory test results for a client who has an elevated temperature. The nurse should recognize which of the following findings is a manifestation of dehydration? (Select all that apply.)

   A. Hct 55%

   B. Serum osmolarity 260 mOsm/kg

   C. Serum sodium 150 mEq/L

   D. Urine specific gravity 1.035

   E. Serum creatinine 0.6 mg/dL

4. A nurse on a medical-surgical unit is caring for a group of clients. For which of the following clients should the nurse anticipate a prescription for fluid restriction?

   A. A client who has a new diagnosis of adrenal insufficiency

   B. A client who has heart failure

   C. A client who is receiving treatment for diabetic ketoacidosis

   D. A client who has abdominal ascites

5. A nurse is planning care for a client who has dehydration. Which of the following actions should the nurse include?

   A. Administer antihypertensive on schedule.

   B. Check the client's weight each morning.

   C. Notify the provider of a urine output greater than 30 mL/hr.

   D. Encourage independent ambulation four times a day.

Application Exercises Key

1. A. Distended neck veins is an expected finding of hypervolemia.

   B. Hypothermia is an expected finding of hypovolemia.

   C. **CORRECT:** Tachycardia is an expected finding of hypovolemia.

   D. **CORRECT:** Syncope is an expected finding of hypovolemia.

   E. **CORRECT:** Decreased skin turgor is an expected finding of hypovolemia.

   Ⓝ *NCLEX® Connection: Physiological Adaptation, Fluid and Electrolyte Imbalances*

2. A. **CORRECT:** The nurse should identify that a client who has nasogastric suctioning is at risk for hypovolemia due to excessive gastrointestinal losses.

   B. Diarrhea, rather than constipation, places the client at risk for hypovolemia due to excessive gastrointestinal losses.

   C. Syndrome of inappropriate antidiuretic hormone places the client at risk for hypervolemia due to overhydration.

   D. An overdose of sodium bicarbonate antacids places the client at risk for hypervolemia due to excessive sodium intake.

   Ⓝ *NCLEX® Connection: Physiological Adaptation, Fluid and Electrolyte Imbalances*

3. A. **CORRECT:** This Hct is greater than the expected reference range of 42-52% for men and 37-47% for women and is an indication of dehydration due to hemoconcentration.

   B. This serum osmolarity is within the expected reference range of 285-295 mOsm/kg. A serum osmolarity greater than 295 mOsm/kg is an indication of dehydration.

   C. **CORRECT:** This serum sodium level is greater than the expected reference range of 136-145 mEq/L and is an indication of dehydration due to hemoconcentration.

   D. **CORRECT:** This urine specific gravity is greater than the expected reference range of 1.005-1.030. An increased urine specific gravity is an indication of dehydration.

   E. This serum creatinine is within the expected reference range of 0.6 to 1.3 mg/dL. An elevated serum creatinine level is an indication of dehydration.

   Ⓝ *NCLEX® Connection: Basic Care and Comfort, Nutrition and Oral Hydration*

4. A. A client who has adrenal insufficiency is at risk for isotonic fluid volume deficit (hypovolemia) because of a decrease in aldosterone secretion and an increase in sodium and water excretion .

   B. **CORRECT:** The nurse should anticipate a client who has heart failure to require fluid and sodium restriction to reduce the workload on the heart.

   C. A client who has diabetic ketoacidosis is at risk for dehydration because hyperglycemia can cause osmotic dieresis which leads to dehydration and electrolyte loss.

   D. A client who has ascites is at risk for hypovolemia because of a fluid shift from the intravascular space to the abdomen.

   Ⓝ *NCLEX® Connection: Physiological Adaptation, Illness Management*

5. A. Hypotension is a manifestation of dehydration therefore the administration of antihypertensive medication would further lower the client's blood pressure and increase the risk for injury.

   B. **CORRECT:** The nurse should include obtaining the client's weight each day in the plan of care. To ensure accuracy the client's weight should be obtained at the same time each day using the same scale. By determining the client's weight gain or loss each day the nurse can evaluate the client's response to treatment.

   C. A urine output greater than 30 mL/hr is an expected finding and is an indicator of adequate fluid balance. The nurse should plan to monitor the client's urine output and notify the provider if it is less than 30 mL/hr.

   D. The client who has dehydration is at risk for falls due to orthostatic hypotension, possible decrease in level of consciousness, and possible gait instability. The nurse should encourage the client to use the call light and ask for assistance when getting out of bed or ambulating.

   Ⓝ *NCLEX® Connection: Physiological Adaptation, Fluid and Electrolyte Imbalances*

PRACTICE Answer

Using the ATI Active Learning Template: System Disorder

DESCRIPTION OF DISORDER/DISEASE PROCESS:
Fluid volume excess (FVE) is the isotonic retention of water and sodium in high proportions.

COMPLICATIONS

- FVE is often referred to as hypervolemia because of the resulting increased blood volume.
- Severe FVE can lead to pulmonary edema and heart failure.

EXPECTED FINDINGS

Assessment findings
- Vital signs: Tachycardia, bounding pulse, hypertension, tachypnea, increased central venous pressure
- Neuromusculoskeletal: Confusion, muscle weakness
- GI: Weight gain, ascites
- Respiratory: Dyspnea, orthopnea, crackles
- Other findings: Edema, distended neck veins

Laboratory findings
- Decreased Hct
- Serum sodium within the expected reference range
- Decreased Electrolytes
- Decreased BUN, and creatinine
- Arterial blood gases
- Respiratory alkalosis: decreased $PaCO_2$ (less than 35 mm Hg), increased pH (greater than 7.45)
- Urine specific gravity less than 1.010

PATIENT-CENTERED CARE

- Observe respiratory rate, symmetry, and effort.
- Auscultate breath sounds in all lung fields. Lung sounds can be diminished with crackles.
- Monitor for shortness of breath and dyspnea.
- Check ABGs, SaO_2, CBC, and chest x-ray results.
- Position the client in semi-Fowler's position.
- Measure the client's weight daily at same time of day using the same scale.
- Monitor and document edema (pretibial, sacral, periorbital).
- Monitor I&O.
- Implement prescribed restrictions for fluid and sodium intake.
- Provide fluids in a small glass to promote the perception of a full glass of fluid.
- Set 1- to 2-hr short-term goals for the fluid restriction to promote client control and understanding.
- Administer supplemental oxygen as needed. Reduce IV flow rates.
- Administer diuretics (osmotic, loop) as prescribed.
- Monitor and document circulation to the extremities.
- Reposition the client at least every 2 hr.
- Support arms and legs to decrease dependent edema.

Ⓝ *NCLEX® Connection: Physiological Adaptation, Fluid and Electrolyte Imbalances*

UNIT 4   PHYSIOLOGICAL INTEGRITY
SECTION: PHYSIOLOGICAL ADAPTATION

CHAPTER 58 # Electrolyte Imbalances

Electrolytes are minerals (sometimes called salts) that are present in all body fluids. They regulate fluid balance and hormone production, strengthen skeletal structures, and act as catalysts in nerve response, muscle contraction, and the metabolism of nutrients.

When dissolved in water or another solvent, electrolytes separate into ions and then conduct either a positive (cations: magnesium, potassium, sodium, calcium) or negative (anions: phosphate, sulfate, chloride, bicarbonate) electrical current.

Major electrolytes in the body include sodium, potassium, chloride, magnesium, phosphorus, and calcium. Nurses monitor laboratory values to identify any electrolyte imbalances. Electrolytes are distributed between intracellular fluid (ICF) and extracellular fluid (ECF) compartments. While laboratory tests can accurately reflect the electrolyte concentrations in plasma, it is not possible to directly measure electrolyte concentrations within cells.

It is important to recognize the manifestations of electrolyte imbalance. Clients at greatest risk for electrolyte imbalance are infants, children, older adults, clients who have cognitive disorders, and clients who have chronic illnesses.

Sodium imbalances

- Sodium (Na^+) is the major electrolyte found in ECF and is present in most body fluids or secretions.
- Sodium is essential for maintenance of acid–base and fluid balance, active and passive transport mechanisms, and irritability and conduction of nerve and muscle tissue.
- Expected serum sodium levels are between 136 and 145 mEq/L.

Hyponatremia

- Hyponatremia is a serum sodium level less than 136 mEq/L.
- Hyponatremia results from an excess of water in the plasma or loss of sodium-rich fluids.
- Hyponatremia delays and slows the depolarization of membranes.
- Water moves from the ECF into the ICF, which causes cells to swell (cerebral edema).
- Serious complications can result from untreated acute hyponatremia (coma, seizures, respiratory arrest).

ASSESSMENT/DATA COLLECTION

RISK FACTORS

- Deficient ECF volume
- Excessive GI losses: vomiting, nasogastric suctioning, diarrhea, tap water enemas
- Renal losses: diuretics, kidney disease, adrenal insufficiency, excessive sweating
- Skin losses: burns, wound drainage, gastrointestinal obstruction, peripheral edema, ascites
- Increased or normal ECF volume: excessive oral water intake, syndrome of inappropriate antidiuretic hormone secretion (SIADH)
- Edematous states: heart failure, cirrhosis, nephrotic syndrome
- Excessive hypotonic IV fluids
- Inadequate sodium intake (NPO status)
- Hyperglycemia
- Age-related risk factors: Older adult clients are at greater risk due to an increased incidence of chronic illnesses, use of diuretic medications, and risk for insufficient sodium intake. Ⓒ

EXPECTED FINDINGS

PHYSICAL ASSESSMENT FINDINGS: Vary with a normal, decreased, or increased ECF volume

VITAL SIGNS: Hypothermia, tachycardia, rapid thready pulse, hypotension, orthostatic hypotension

NEUROMUSCULOSKELETAL: Headache, confusion, lethargy, muscle weakness with possible respiratory compromise, fatigue, decreased deep tendon reflexes (DTRs), seizures, coma

GI: Increased motility, hyperactive bowel sounds, abdominal cramping, anorexia, nausea, vomiting

LABORATORY TESTS

Serum sodium
Decreased: Less than 136 mEq/L

Serum osmolarity
- Decreased: Less than 280 mOsm/kg
- Urine specific gravity: Less than 1.010 (if not due to SIADH)

PATIENT-CENTERED CARE

NURSING CARE

- Report irregular laboratory findings to the provider.
- Monitor I&O, and weigh the client daily at same time of day using the same scale.
- Monitor vital signs and level of consciousness, reporting irregular findings.
- Encourage the client to change positions slowly.
- Follow any prescribed fluid restrictions.
- Monitor respiratory status if muscle weakness is present. Qs

FLUID OVERLOAD: Restrict water intake as prescribed.

RESTORATION OF NORMAL ECF VOLUME: Administer hypertonic IV therapy (3% sodium chloride).

ACUTE HYPONATREMIA
- Administer hypertonic oral and IV fluids as prescribed.
- Encourage foods and fluids high in sodium (cheese, milk, condiments).

Hypernatremia

- Hypernatremia is a serum sodium level greater than 145 mEq/L.
- Hypernatremia is a serious electrolyte imbalance. It can cause significant neurological, endocrine, and cardiac disturbances.
- Increased sodium causes hypertonicity of the serum. This causes a shift of water out of the cells, making the cells dehydrated.

ASSESSMENT/DATA COLLECTION

RISK FACTORS

- Water deprivation (NPO)
- Heat stroke
- Excessive sodium intake: dietary sodium intake, hypertonic IV fluids, hypertonic tube feedings, bicarbonate intake
- Excessive sodium retention: kidney failure, Cushing's syndrome, aldosteronism, some medications (glucocorticosteroids)

- Fluid losses: fever, diaphoresis, burns, respiratory infection, diabetes insipidus, hyperglycemia, watery diarrhea
- Age-related changes, specifically decreased total body water content and inadequate fluid intake related to an altered thirst mechanism ©
- Compensatory mechanisms: increased thirst and increased production of ADH

EXPECTED FINDINGS

VITAL SIGNS: Hyperthermia, tachycardia, orthostatic hypotension

NEUROMUSCULOSKELETAL: Restlessness, disorientation, irritability, muscle twitching, muscle weakness, seizures, decreased level of consciousness, reduced to absent DTRs

GI: Thirst, dry mucous membranes, dry and swollen tongue that is red in color, increased motility, hyperactive bowel sounds, abdominal cramping, nausea

OTHER FINDINGS: Edema, warm flushed skin, oliguria

LABORATORY TESTS

Serum sodium
Increased: Greater than 145 mEq/L

Serum osmolarity
- Increased: Greater than 295 mOsm/kg
- Urine specific gravity: Greater than 1.030

PATIENT-CENTERED CARE

NURSING CARE

- Report laboratory findings outside of the expected reference range to the provider.
- Monitor level of consciousness and ensure safety. Qs
- Provide oral hygiene and other comfort measures to decrease thirst.
- Monitor I&O, and alert the provider if urinary output is inadequate.

FLUID LOSS: Based on serum osmolarity
Administer hypotonic IV fluids (0.225% sodium chloride).

EXCESS SODIUM
- Encourage water intake and discourage sodium intake.
- Administer diuretics (loop diuretics).

Potassium imbalances

- Potassium (K⁺) is the major cation in ICF.
- Potassium plays a vital role in cell metabolism; transmission of nerve impulses; functioning of cardiac, lung, and muscle tissues; and acid-base balance.
- Potassium has reciprocal action with sodium.
- Expected serum potassium levels are 3.5 to 5 mEq/L.

Hypokalemia

- Hypokalemia is a serum potassium level less than 3.5 mEq/L.
- Hypokalemia is the result of an increased loss of potassium from the body, decreased intake and absorption of potassium, or movement of potassium into the cells.

ASSESSMENT/DATA COLLECTION

RISK FACTORS

- Hyperaldosteronism
- Inadequate dietary intake (rare)
- Prolonged administration of non-electrolyte-containing IV solutions such as 5% dextrose in water

EXCESSIVE GI LOSSES: Vomiting, nasogastric suctioning, diarrhea, excessive laxative use

RENAL LOSSES: Excessive use of potassium-excreting diuretics, such as furosemide, corticosteroids

SKIN LOSSES: Diaphoresis, wound losses

ICF: Metabolic alkalosis, after correction of acidosis (treatment of diabetic ketoacidosis), during periods of tissue repair (burns, trauma, starvation), total parenteral nutrition

EXPECTED FINDINGS

VITAL SIGNS: Hyperthermia, weak irregular pulse, hypotension, orthostatic hypotension, respiratory distress

NEUROMUSCULOSKELETAL: Ascending bilateral muscle weakness with respiratory collapse and paralysis, muscle cramping, decreased muscle tone and hypoactive reflexes, paresthesias, mental confusion

ELECTROCARDIOGRAM (ECG): Premature ventricular contractions (PVCs), bradycardia, blocks, ventricular tachycardia, flattening T waves, and ST depression

GI: Decreased motility, hypoactive bowel sounds, abdominal distention, constipation, ileus, nausea, vomiting, anorexia

OTHER CLINICAL FINDINGS: Anxiety, which can progress to lethargy

LABORATORY TESTS

Serum potassium
Decreased: Less than 3.5 mEq/L

Arterial blood gases
Metabolic alkalosis: pH greater than 7.45

DIAGNOSTIC PROCEDURES

Electrocardiogram

NURSING CONSIDERATIONS: Monitor for dysrhythmias, such as PVCs, ventricular tachycardia, flattening T waves, and ST depression.

PATIENT-CENTERED CARE

NURSING CARE

- Report findings outside of the expected reference range to the provider.
- Treat the underlying cause.
- Replace potassium.
  - Provide dietary education and encourage foods high in potassium (avocados, dried fruit, cantaloupe, bananas, potatoes, spinach).
  - Provide oral potassium supplementation.
- Monitor for and maintain an adequate urine output.
- Monitor for shallow, ineffective respirations and diminished breath sounds.
- Monitor cardiac rhythm, and intervene promptly as needed.
- Monitor clients receiving digoxin. Hypokalemia increases the risk for digoxin toxicity.
- Monitor level of consciousness and ensure safety.
- Monitor bowel sounds and abdominal distention and intervene as needed.

IV POTASSIUM SUPPLEMENTATION
- Mixed by a pharmacist and double-checked by two nurses prior to administration.
- Dilute potassium to a concentration of no more than 1 mEq potassium to 10 mL solution and infuse slowly, no faster than 10 mEq/hr. **Qs**
- Monitor for phlebitis (tissue irritant). Discontinue the IV, and notify the provider for infiltration of potassium.

> **!** Never IV bolus (high risk of cardiac arrest) **Qs**

Hyperkalemia

- Hyperkalemia is a serum potassium level greater than 5.0 mEq/L.
- Hyperkalemia is the result of an increased intake of potassium, movement of potassium out of the cells, or inadequate renal excretion.
- Hyperkalemia uncommon in clients who have adequate kidney function.
- Hyperkalemia is potentially life-threatening due to the risk of cardiac arrhythmias and cardiac arrest.

ASSESSMENT/DATA COLLECTION

RISK FACTORS

INCREASED TOTAL BODY POTASSIUM: IV potassium administration, salt substitutes, blood transfusion

ECF SHIFT: Insufficient insulin, acidosis (diabetic ketoacidosis), tissue catabolism (sepsis, trauma, surgery, fever, myocardial infarction)

HYPERTONIC STATES: Uncontrolled diabetes mellitus

DECREASED EXCRETION OF POTASSIUM: Kidney failure, severe dehydration, potassium-sparing diuretics, ACE inhibitors, adrenal insufficiency

AGE: Older adult clients are at greater risk due to decreased kidney function and medical conditions resulting in the use of salt substitutes, angiotensin-converting enzyme inhibitors, and potassium-sparing diuretics. Ⓖ

EXPECTED FINDINGS

VITAL SIGNS: Slow, irregular pulse; hypotension

NEUROMUSCULOSKELETAL: Irritability, confusion, weakness with ascending flaccid paralysis, paresthesias, lack of reflexes

ECG: Ventricular fibrillation, peaked T waves, widened QRS, cardiac arrest Qs

GI: Increased motility, diarrhea, abdominal cramps, hyperactive bowel sounds

LABORATORY TESTS

Serum potassium
Increased: Greater than 5 mEq/L

Arterial blood gases
Metabolic acidosis: pH less than 7.35

DIAGNOSTIC PROCEDURES

ECG will show dysrhythmias (ventricular fibrillation, peaked T waves, widened QRS).

PATIENT-CENTERED CARE

NURSING CARE

- Report findings outside of the expected reference range to the provider.
- Decrease potassium intake.
  - Stop infusion of IV potassium.
  - Withhold oral potassium.
  - Provide a potassium-restricted diet.
  - If potassium levels are extremely high, dialysis might be required.
- Promote the movement of potassium from ECF to ICF. Administer IV fluids with dextrose and regular insulin.
- Monitor cardiac rhythm, and intervene promptly as needed.
- Maintain IV access.
- Prepare the client for dialysis if prescribed.

MEDICATIONS

TO INCREASE POTASSIUM EXCRETION
- Administer loop diuretics, such as furosemide, if kidney function is adequate. Loop diuretics increase the excretion of potassium from the renal system.
- Sodium polystyrene sulfonate is given orally or as an enema. Sodium polystyrene sulfonate increases the excretion of potassium from the gastrointestinal system.

Calcium imbalances

- Calcium is found in the body's cells, bones, and teeth. The expected total calcium level is 9 to 10.5 mg/dL.
- Calcium balance is essential for proper functioning of the cardiovascular, neuromuscular, and endocrine systems, as well as blood clotting and bone and teeth formation.

Hypocalcemia

Hypocalcemia is a total serum calcium level less than 9 mg/dL.

ASSESSMENT/DATA COLLECTION

RISK FACTORS

Increased calcium output
- Chronic diarrhea
- Steatorrhea as with pancreatitis (binding of calcium to undigested fat)

Inadequate calcium intake or absorption
- Malabsorption syndromes, such as Crohn's disease
- Vitamin D deficiency (alcohol use disorder, chronic kidney disease)

Calcium shift from ECF into bone or to an inactive form
- Rapid infusion of blood transfusion
- Post-thyroidectomy
- Hypoparathyroidism

EXPECTED FINDINGS

MUSCLE TWITCHES/TETANY
- Numbness and tingling (fingers and around mouth)
- Frequent, painful muscle spasms at rest that can progress to tetany
- Hyperactive DTRs
- Positive Chvostek's sign (tapping on the facial nerve triggering facial twitching)
- Positive Trousseau's sign (hand/finger spasms with sustained blood pressure cuff inflation)
- Laryngospasms

CARDIOVASCULAR
- Weak, thready pulse, tachycardia or bradycardia
- Cardiac dysrhythmias: prolonged QT interval and ST segments

GI: Hyperactive bowel sounds, diarrhea, abdominal cramping

CENTRAL NERVOUS SYSTEM: Seizures due to overstimulation of the CNS

LABORATORY TESTS

Calcium level less than 9 mg/dL

DIAGNOSTIC PROCEDURES

ECG

PATIENT-CENTERED CARE

NURSING CARE
- Administer oral or IV calcium supplements. (Carefully monitor respiratory and cardiovascular status.)
- Initiate seizure precautions. Qs
- Keep emergency equipment on standby.
- Encourage foods high in calcium, including dairy products and dark green vegetables.

Hypercalcemia

Hypercalcemia is a total serum calcium level greater than 10.5 mg/dL.

ASSESSMENT/DATA COLLECTION

RISK FACTORS

Decreased calcium output: Thiazide diuretics

Increased calcium intake and absorption

Calcium shift from bone to ECF
- Hyperparathyroidism
- Bone cancer
- Paget's disease
- Chronic immobility
- Long-term glucocorticoid use
- Hyperthyroidism

EXPECTED FINDINGS

NEUROMUSCULAR
- Decreased reflexes
- Bone pain
- Flank pain if renal calculi develop

CARDIOVASCULAR
- Dysrhythmias
- Increased risk for blood clot

GI: Anorexia, nausea, vomiting, constipation

CENTRAL NERVOUS SYSTEM
- Weakness, lethargy
- Confusion, decreased level of consciousness

LABORATORY TESTS

Total serum calcium level greater than 10.5 mg/dL

DIAGNOSTIC PROCEDURES

ECG: Shortened QT interval

PATIENT-CENTERED CARE

NURSING CARE
- Increase the client's activity level.
- Limit dietary calcium.
- Encourage fluids to promote urinary excretion.
- Encourage fiber to promote bowel elimination.
- Implement safety precautions if client is confused.
- Monitor for pathologic fractures.
- Encourage fluid intake to decrease the risk for renal calcium stone formation. Qᴇʙᴘ
- Monitor for blood clots; measure calf circumference.

Magnesium imbalances

Most of the body's magnesium is found in the bones. Magnesium in smaller amounts is found within the body cells. A very small amount is found in ECF. The expected magnesium level is 1.3 to 2.1 mEq/L.

Hypomagnesemia

Hypomagnesemia is a serum magnesium level less than 1.3 mEq/L.

ASSESSMENT/DATA COLLECTION

RISK FACTORS

INCREASED MAGNESIUM OUTPUT
- GI losses (diarrhea, nasogastric suction)
- Thiazide or loop diuretics
- Often associated with hypocalcemia

INADEQUATE MAGNESIUM INTAKE OR ABSORPTION
- Malnutrition
- Alcohol use disorder
- Laxative use

EXPECTED FINDINGS

NEUROMUSCULAR: Increased nerve impulse transmission (hyperactive DTRs, paresthesias, muscle tetany), positive Chvostek's and Trousseau's signs, tetany, seizures

GI: Hypoactive bowel sounds, constipation, abdominal distention, paralytic ileus

CARDIOVASCULAR: Dysrhythmias, tachycardia, hypertension

PATIENT-CENTERED CARE

NURSING CARE

- Discontinue magnesium–losing medications.
- Administer oral or IV magnesium sulfate following safety protocols. IV route is used because IM can cause pain and tissue damage. Oral magnesium can cause diarrhea and increase magnesium depletion. QEBP
- Monitor DTRs during infusion to prevent hypermagnesemia.
- Encourage foods high in magnesium, including whole grains and dark green vegetables.
- Implement seizure precautions.

Hypermagnesemia

Hypermagnesemia is a serum magnesium level greater than 2.1 mEq/L.

ASSESSMENT/DATA COLLECTION

RISK FACTORS

Decreased magnesium output
- Chronic kidney disease or acute kidney injury
- Adrenal insufficiency

Increased magnesium intake and absorption:
Laxatives or antacids containing magnesium

EXPECTED FINDINGS

NEUROMUSCULAR
- Diminished DTRs
- Muscle paralysis
- Shallow respirations, decreased respiratory rate

CARDIOVASCULAR
- Bradycardia, hypotension
- Dysrhythmias, cardiac arrest

CENTRAL NERVOUS SYSTEM: Lethargy

LABORATORY TESTS

Serum magnesium level greater than 2.1 mEq/L

DIAGNOSTIC PROCEDURES

ECG: Prolonged PR interval, widened QRS

PATIENT-CENTERED CARE

NURSING CARE

- Perform frequent focused assessments (vital signs, level of consciousness, reflexes). Notify the provider of changes or absent reflexes.
- Monitor respiratory and cardiac status.
- Administer loop diuretics and magnesium free IV fluids if kidney function is adequate.
- Administer calcium for severe cardiac changes.

Application Exercises

1. A nurse is planning care for a client who has hypernatremia. Which of the following actions should the nurse anticipate including in the plan of care?

   A. Infuse hypotonic IV fluids.

   B. Implement a fluid restriction.

   C. Increase sodium intake.

   D. Administer sodium polystyrene sulfonate.

2. A nurse is reviewing the medical record of a client who has hypocalcemia. The nurse should identify which of the following findings as risk factors for the development of this electrolyte imbalance?

   A. Crohn's disease

   B. Postoperative following appendectomy

   C. History of bone cancer

   D. Hyperthyroidism

3. A nurse receives a laboratory report for a client indicating a potassium level of 5.2 mEq/L. When notifying the provider, the nurse should anticipate which of the following actions?

   A. Starting an IV infusion of 0.9% sodium chloride

   B. Consulting with dietitian to increase intake of potassium

   C. Initiating continuous cardiac monitoring

   D. Preparing the client for gastric lavage

4. A nurse is collecting data from a client who has hypercalcemia as a result of long-term use of glucocorticoids. Which of the following findings should the nurse expect? (Select all that apply.)

   A. Hyperreflexia

   B. Confusion

   C. Positive Chvostek's sign

   D. Bone pain

   E. Nausea and vomiting

5. A nurse is providing education for a client who has severe hypomagnesemia due to alcohol use disorder. The client is to receive magnesium sulfate. Which of the following information should the nurse include in the teaching?

   A. "You will receive magnesium in a series of intramuscular injections."

   B. "You should receive a prescription for a thiazide diuretic to take with the magnesium."

   C. "You should eliminate whole grains from your diet until your magnesium level increases."

   D. "You will have your deep-tendon reflexes monitored while you are receiving magnesium."

PRACTICE Active Learning Scenario

A nurse is caring for a client who has hypokalemia as an adverse effect of furosemide. Use the ATI Active Learning Template: System Disorder to complete this item to include the following sections.

ALTERATION IN HEALTH (DIAGNOSIS)

EXPECTED FINDINGS: Identify at least five expected findings.

NURSING CARE: Identify two safety actions for the administration of IV potassium supplementation.

Application Exercises Key

1. A. **CORRECT:** Hypotonic IV fluids, such as 0.225% sodium chloride, are indicated for the treatment of hypernatremia related to fluid loss to expand the ECF volume and rehydrate the cells.

   B. Increased fluid intake is indicated for the treatment of hypernatremia.

   C. Decreased sodium intake is indicated for the treatment of hypernatremia.

   D. Administration of sodium polystyrene sulfonate is indicated for the treatment of hyperkalemia.

   (N) *NCLEX® Connection: Physiological Adaptation, Unexpected Response to Therapies*

2. A. **CORRECT:** Crohn's disease is a risk factor for hypocalcemia. This malabsorption disorder places the client at risk for hypocalcemia due to inadequate calcium absorption.

   B. A thyroidectomy places the client at risk for hypocalcemia due to the possible removal of or injury to the parathyroid glands.

   C. A history of bone cancer increases the client's risk of hypercalcemia due to the shift of calcium from bone to ECF.

   D. Hyperthyroidism places the client at risk for hypercalcemia due to the shift of calcium from bone to ECF.

   (N) *NCLEX® Connection: Physiological Adaptation, Fluid and Electrolyte Imbalances*

3. A. The nurse should initiate an IV infusion of a fluid containing dextrose to promote the movement of potassium from ECF to ICF.

   B. The nurse should withhold oral potassium and provide the client with a potassium-restricted diet.

   C. **CORRECT:** A potassium level of 5.2 mEq/L indicates hyperkalemia. The nurse should anticipate the initiation of continuous cardiac monitoring due to the client's risk for dysrhythmias such as ventricular fibrillation.

   D. Gastric lavage is not indicated for the treatment of hyperkalemia. However, the nurse should prepare the client for dialysis if hyperkalemia becomes severe.

   (N) *NCLEX® Connection: Physiological Adaptation, Illness Management*

4. A. The nurse should expect the client who has hypercalcemia to have decreased reflexes.

   B. **CORRECT:** The nurse should expect the client who has hypercalcemia to have confusion and a possible decreased level of consciousness.

   C. The nurse should expect the client who has hypocalcemia to have a positive Chvostek's sign.

   D. **CORRECT:** The nurse should expect the client who has hypercalcemia to have bone pain.

   E. **CORRECT:** The nurse should expect the client who has hypercalcemia to have nausea and vomiting along with anorexia.

   (N) *NCLEX® Connection: Pharmacological and Parenteral Therapies, Adverse Effects/Contraindications/Side Effects/Interactions*

5. A. Magnesium sulfate is administered either orally or IV. IM administration of magnesium is avoided due to pain and the potential for tissue damage.

   B. Thiazide diuretics increase magnesium output, thereby worsening the client's hypomagnesemia.

   C. The nurse should encourage the client's intake of foods that are high in magnesium, such as whole grains and dark green vegetables.

   D. **CORRECT:** The nurse should instruct the client on the need to monitor deep-tendon reflexes during administration of magnesium. This assessment helps identify hypermagnesemia that can occur during IV administration of magnesium sulfate.

   (N) *NCLEX® Connection: Pharmacological and Parenteral Therapies, Medication Administration*

PRACTICE Answer

Using the ATI Active Learning Template: System Disorder

ALTERATION IN HEALTH (DIAGNOSIS):
Hypokalemia is a serum potassium level less than 3.5 mEq/L that can result from the increased loss of potassium from the body due to the use of potassium-excreting diuretics, such as furosemide.

EXPECTED FINDINGS
- Vital signs: Weak irregular pulse, hypotension, respiratory distress
- Neuromusculoskeletal: Ascending bilateral muscle weakness, muscle cramping, decreased muscle tone, hypoactive reflexes, paresthesias, mental confusion
- GI: Decreased motility, hypoactive bowel sounds, abdominal distention, constipation, nausea, vomiting, anorexia
- Dysrhythmias: PVCs, bradycardia, blocks, ventricular tachycardia, flattening T waves, ST depression

NURSING CARE
- Ensure all infusions containing potassium are mixed by the pharmacist.
- Double-check all infusions containing potassium with another nurse prior to administration.
- Dilute potassium to a concentration of no more than 1 mEq potassium to 10 mL solution and infuse slowly, no faster than 10 mEq/hr.
- Never administer potassium as an IV bolus.
- Monitor vital signs and cardiac and respiratory status closely during administration of IV potassium supplementation.

(N) *NCLEX® Connection: Pharmacological and Parenteral Therapies, Expected Actions/Outcomes*

References

Berman, A., Snyder, S., & Frandsen, G. (2016). *Kozier & Erb's fundamentals of nursing: Concepts, process, and practice* (10th ed.). Upper Saddle River, NJ: Prentice-Hall.

Burchum, J. R., & Rosenthal, L. D. (2016). *Lehne's pharmacology for nursing care* (9th ed.). St. Louis: Elsevier.

Dudek, S. G. (2014). *Nutrition essentials for nursing practice* (7th ed.). Philadelphia: Lippincott Williams & Wilkins.

Eliopoulos, C. (2014). *Gerontological nursing* (8th ed.). Philadelphia: Lippincott Williams & Wilkins.

Grodner, M., Escott-Stump, S., & Dorner, S. (2016). *Nutritional foundations and clinical applications of nutrition: A nursing approach* (6th ed.). St. Louis, MO: Mosby.

Pagana, K. D. & Pagana, T. J. (2014). *Mosby's manual of diagnostic and laboratory tests* (5th ed.). St. Louis, MO: Elsevier.

Potter, P. A., Perry, A. G., Stockert, P., & Hall, A. (2013). *Fundamentals of nursing* (8th ed.). St. Louis, MO: Mosby.

Touhy, T. A., & Jett, K. F. (2012) *Ebersole & Hess' toward healthy aging: Human needs and nursing response* (8th ed.). St. Lois, MO: Mosby.

STUDENT NAME _____

CONCEPT_____ REVIEW MODULE CHAPTER_____

Related Content	Underlying Principles	Nursing Interventions
(E.G., DELEGATION, LEVELS OF PREVENTION, ADVANCE DIRECTIVES)		WHO? WHEN? WHY? HOW?

Diagnostic Procedure

STUDENT NAME _____

PROCEDURE NAME _____ REVIEW MODULE CHAPTER_____

Description of Procedure

Indications

CONSIDERATIONS

Nursing Interventions (pre, intra, post)

Interpretation of Findings

Client Education

Potential Complications

Nursing Interventions

STUDENT NAME _____

DEVELOPMENTAL STAGE _____ REVIEW MODULE CHAPTER_____

EXPECTED GROWTH AND DEVELOPMENT

Physical Development	Cognitive Development	Psychosocial Development	Age-Appropriate Activities

Health Promotion

Immunizations	Health Screening	Nutrition	Injury Prevention

STUDENT NAME _____

MEDICATION _____ REVIEW MODULE CHAPTER_____

CATEGORY CLASS_____

PURPOSE OF MEDICATION

Expected Pharmacological Action

Therapeutic Use

Complications

Medication Administration

Contraindications/Precautions

Nursing Interventions

Interactions

Client Education

Evaluation of Medication Effectiveness

STUDENT NAME _____

SKILL NAME_____ REVIEW MODULE CHAPTER_____

Description of Skill

Indications

CONSIDERATIONS

Nursing Interventions (pre, intra, post)

Outcomes/Evaluation

Client Education

Potential Complications

Nursing Interventions

STUDENT NAME _____

DISORDER/DISEASE PROCESS _____ REVIEW MODULE CHAPTER_____

Alterations in Health (Diagnosis)	Pathophysiology Related to Client Problem	Health Promotion and Disease Prevention

ASSESSMENT

Risk Factors	Expected Findings

Laboratory Tests	Diagnostic Procedures

SAFETY CONSIDERATIONS

PATIENT-CENTERED CARE

Nursing Care	Medications	Client Education

Therapeutic Procedures		Interprofessional Care

Complications

STUDENT NAME _____

PROCEDURE NAME _____ REVIEW MODULE CHAPTER_____

Description of Procedure

Indications

CONSIDERATIONS

Nursing Interventions (pre, intra, post)

Outcomes/Evaluation

Client Education

Potential Complications

Nursing Interventions